INFLAMMATORY CONDITIONS OF THE COLON

INFLAMMATORY CONDITIONS OF THE COLON

JIA-JU ZHENG
EDITOR

Nova Biomedical Books
New York

Copyright © 2008 by Nova Science Publishers, Inc.

All rights reserved. No part of this book may be reproduced, stored in a retrieval system or transmitted in any form or by any means: electronic, electrostatic, magnetic, tape, mechanical photocopying, recording or otherwise without the written permission of the Publisher.

For permission to use material from this book please contact us:
Telephone 631-231-7269; Fax 631-231-8175
Web Site: http://www.novapublishers.com

NOTICE TO THE READER

The Publisher has taken reasonable care in the preparation of this book, but makes no expressed or implied warranty of any kind and assumes no responsibility for any errors or omissions. No liability is assumed for incidental or consequential damages in connection with or arising out of information contained in this book. The Publisher shall not be liable for any special, consequential, or exemplary damages resulting, in whole or in part, from the readers' use of, or reliance upon, this material.

Independent verification should be sought for any data, advice or recommendations contained in this book. In addition, no responsibility is assumed by the publisher for any injury and/or damage to persons or property arising from any methods, products, instructions, ideas or otherwise contained in this publication.

This publication is designed to provide accurate and authoritative information with regard to the subject matter covered herein. It is sold with the clear understanding that the Publisher is not engaged in rendering legal or any other professional services. If legal or any other expert assistance is required, the services of a competent person should be sought. FROM A DECLARATION OF PARTICIPANTS JOINTLY ADOPTED BY A COMMITTEE OF THE AMERICAN BAR ASSOCIATION AND A COMMITTEE OF PUBLISHERS.

Library of Congress Cataloging-in-Publication Data
Zheng, Jia-ju.
 Inflammatory conditions of the colon / Jia-ju Zheng (author).
   p. ; cm.
 Includes bibliographical references and index.
 ISBN 978-1-60692-240-8 (hardcover)
 1. Inflammatory bowel diseases. I. Title.
 [DNLM: 1. Irritable Bowel Syndrome--diagnosis. 2. Irritable Bowel Syndrome--therapy. WI 520 Z63i 2009]
 RC862.I53Z53 2009
 616.3'44--dc22
                              2008037501

Published by Nova Science Publishers, Inc. ✣ New York

Contents

Preface		ix
Section One: Anatomy of the Large Intestine		1
Chapter I	Gross Morphology *Jia-ju Zheng and Yun-di Guo*	3
Chapter II	Histology *Jia-ju Zheng and Yun-di Guo*	5
Section Two: Pathology of Idiopathic Inflammatory Bowel Disease		9
Chapter III	Ulcerative Colitis *Jia-ju Zheng and Yun-di Guo*	11
Chapter IV	Crohn's Disease *Jia-ju Zheng and Yun-di Guo*	17
Chapter V	Site and Extent of Inflammatory Bowel Disease *Jia-ju Zheng and Yun-di Guo*	27
Section Three: Endoscopy in Inflammatory Bowel Disease		33
Chapter VI	Normal Endoscopic Appearance of the Bowel *Jia-ju Zheng*	35
Chapter VII	Colonoscopic Features of Ulcerative Colitis *Ping Xiang*	39
Chapter VIII	Colonoscopic Features of Crohn's Disease *Fu-xing Xu*	43
Chapter IX	Crohn's Disease of the Upper Gastrointestinal Tract: The Value of Esophagogastroduodenoscopic Examination *Wen-jun Zhang and Zhao-shen Li*	49

Chapter X	The Role of EUS in the Diagnosis and Treatment of Inflammatory Bowel Disease and Other Indetermined Colitis *Qi Zhu*	53
Chapter XI	Double Balloon Endoscopy in Diagnosis of Inflammatory Bowel Disease *Jie Zhong*	63
Chapter XII	Capsule Endoscopy in Inflammatory Bowel Disease *Zhi-zheng Ge*	71
Chapter XIII	Narrow Band Imaging: A New Diagnostic Approach in Colorectal Cancer and Inflammatory Bowel Disease *Wei Huang and Yun-lin Wu*	79
Chapter XIV	The Application of Confocal Laser Endomicroscopy for Diagnosis of Inflammation Bowel Diseases *Yan-qing Li*	89
Chapter XV	Magnifying Colonoscopy for Diagnosis of Ulcerative Colitis and Tumor *Si-de Liu*	97
Chapter XVI	Endoscopic Retrograde Cholangiopancreatography in Inflammatory Bowel Disease *Feng Liu and Zhao-shen Li*	109

Section Four: Clinical Aspects of Idiopathic Inflammatory Bowel Disease — 113

Chapter XVII	Management of Inflammatory Bowel Disease in the Asia-Pacific Region *Qin Ouyang*	115
Chapter XVIII	Inflammatory Bowel Disease: Definition and Classification *Jia-ju Zheng*	125
Chapter XIX	Clinical Manifestations and Complications of Ulcerative Colitis *Kai-chun Wu*	129
Chapter XX	Clinical Manifestations, Complications and Diagnosis of Crohn's Disease *Jun Lin and Chang-sheng Deng*	133
Chapter XXI	Severity Assessment of Ulcerative Colitis *Xiao-ping Wu*	139
Chapter XXII	Clinical and Endoscopic Assessments of Activity and Severity of Crohn's Disease *Yi Li and Bing Xia*	147
Chapter XXIII	Perianal Crohn's Disease *Zhi Pang*	155

| Chapter XXIV | Surveillance and Prevention of Colorectal Cancer in Inflammatory Bowel Disease
Zhi-hua Ran | 167 |

Section Five: Medical Treatment in Inflammatory Bowel Disease   175

Chapter XXV	Treatment of Inflammatory Bowel Disease with Aminosalicylates *Zhan-ju Liu*	177
Chapter XXVI	Glucocorticosteroid Therapy in Inflammatory Bowel Disease *Zhi-hua Ran*	185
Chapter XXVII	Chemical Immunomodulator Therapy in Inflammatory Bowel Disease *Jia-ju Zheng*	193
Chapter XXVIII	Topical (Rectal) Therapy in Inflammatory Bowel Disease *Ming Zhang*	201
Chapter XXIX	Nutritional Therapy in Inflammatory Bowel Therapy *Xue-liang Jiang*	207
Chapter XXX	Treatment of Inflammatory Bowel Disease with Traditional Chinese Medicine *Jia-ju Zheng*	215
Chapter XXXI	Conservative Management of Ulcerative Colitis *Fang Gu and Yu-min Lü*	221
Chapter XXXII	Medical Treatment of Crohn's Disease *Zhi-hua Ran*	231
Chapter XXXIII	Biological Therapy for Inflammatory Bowel Disease *Zhan-ju Liu*	239
Chapter XXXIV	Anti-Tumor Necrosis Factor Therapy in Inflammatory Bowel Disease *Zhan-ju Liu*	249

Section Six: Disorders That Simulate Idiopathic Colitis: Non-Infections Colitis   259

Chapter XXXV	Collagenous and Lymphocytic Colitis *Ping Zheng*	261
Chapter XXXVI	Colonic Ischemia *Long-dian Chen*	265
Chapter XXXVII	Eosinophilic Colitis *Ming Zhang*	273
Chapter XXXVIII	Behcet's Disease and Tangier Disease *Fu-xing Xu*	277

Chapter XXXIX	Radiation Colitis *Ping Xiang*	279
Chapter XL	Portal Hypertensive Colopathy *Ping Xiang*	281
Chapter XLI	Solitary Rectal Ulcer Syndrome *Ping Xiang*	283
Chapter XLII	Diverticula-Associated Colitis *Fu-xing Xu*	285
Chapter XLIII	Drug-Induced Proctitis and Colitis *Jia-ju Zheng*	287
Chapter XLIV	Iatrogenic Lesions *Jia-ju Zheng*	289
Chapter XLV	Endoscopic and Pathologic Features and Treatment in Colonic Graft-versus-Host Disease *Wei-chang Chen*	293
Chapter XLVI	Cap Polyposis *Ming Zhang*	299
Chapter XLVII	Watermelon Colon *Ming Zhang*	303

Section Seven: Disorders that Simulate Idiopathic Colitis – Specific Infections — 305

Chapter XLVIII	Intestinal Tuberculosis *Long-dian Chen*	307
Chapter XLIX	Pseudomembranous Colitis *Jia-ju Zheng*	309

Section Eight: Disorders that Simulate Idiopathic Colitis: Other Forms of Acute Infectious Colitis and Acute Self-Limited Colitis — 315

Chapter L	Acute Infectious Colitis and Acute Self-Limited Colitis *Jia-ju Zheng*	317
Chapter LI	Viral Colitis, Bacterial Colitis, Protozoal and Fungal Infections *Jia-ju Zheng*	321

Acknowledgments — 335

Index — 337

Preface

Ulcerative colitis and Crohn's disease, collectively termed infalmmatory bowel disease (IBD), are complex disorders because of their wide variations in clinical manifestations. These two disorders constitute multisystem diseases of idiopathic origin. Both are found worldwide and spare no socioeconomic group in the world.

Recent scientific and technological advances have not only led to greater understanding of the pathogenesis underlying these disorders, but have also enabled us to make a correct diagnosis in the earlier stage and to use better and more efficacious medical therapies for ulcerative colitis and Crohn's disease.

Dr. Zheng from China experienced the research and treatment environment for IBD at the University of Chicago in the United States. He completed his doctoral work in nutrition at Tufts University. He has been an active gastroenterologist in the diagnosis and management of gastrointestinal disease in particular in IBD in China. Thus, he is well suited to the task of bringing together these materials in IBD.

In this handbook, a highly distinguished group of doctors and professors have been invited to present updated knowledge of current status related to the diagnosis and medical therapy of IBD. These articles highlight many advances to date with their clinical experiences. Thus, we are sure that the handbook will greatly increase recognition of the complexity of these conditions in clinical practice, and enhance our experiences of management with IBD patients. We hope the handbook not only reviews the current state of the art, but will also prepare us for the future.

Section One: Anatomy of the Large Intestine

Chapter I

Gross Morphology

Jia-ju Zheng[*] *and Yun-di Guo*[**]

[*]Su-zhou Institute for Digestive Disease and Nutrition, Su-zhou Municipal Hospital,
Nan-jing Medical University, Su-zhou, Jiang-su Province, P.R. China
[**]Su-zhou Municipal Hostipal, Affiliated Soo-chow Hospital,
Nan-jing Medical University,
Su-zhou, Jiang-su Province, P.R. China

Introduction

The large intestine is tubular in its appearance, which runs continuously from the ileocecal valve to the anus (figure 1-1), and is approximately 1.5 m in length and 6.5 cm in diameter in the adult[1]. In comparison with the small intestine, the longitudinal muscle fibers of the muscularis of the large intestine are thickened, forming 3 longitudinal bands located at 120-degree intervals about the colonic circumference, known as teniae coli (figure 1-2), and the intervening colon is gathered into pouches, known as haustra coli (outpouchings of the colon) (figure 1-2) [1,2]. The folds between the haustra are semilunar in appearance if viewed from within the colon, and are called semilunar folds (Plicae Semilunares) (figure 1-2).

Chapter II

Histology

Jia-ju Zheng[*] and Yun-di Guo[**]
[*]Su-zhou Institute for Digestive Disease and Nutrition, Su-zhou Municipal Hospital,
Nan-jing Medical University, Su-zhou, Jiang-su Province, P.R. China
[**]Su-zhou Municipal Hostipal, Affiliated Soo-chow Hospital,
Nan-jing Medical University,
Su-zhou, Jiang-su Province, P.R. China

Layers of the Wall of the Large Intestine

The structure of the wall of the large intestine is fundamentally the same as those in the small intestine, which is made up of four layers: mucosa, submucosa, muscularis and serosa (Figure 2-1) [1,2]. However, the mucosa of the large intestine differs from that in the small intestine, as no circular folds or villi are present [1,2]. Nevertheless, the mucosa does contains many intestinal glands (also call crypts) which penetrate deep into the mucosa, and the mucosal epithelium, which extends into the glands, consists of simple columnar cells and large numbers of mucus-secreting goblet cells. Lymphatic follicles are also present in the mucosa.

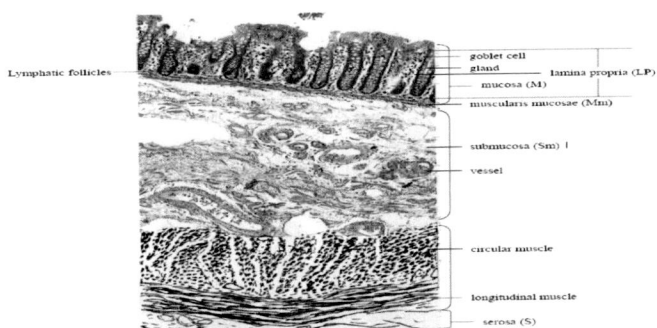

Figure 2-1. Modified light microscopic view of a section of mucosa obtained by endoscopic biopsy specimen from a normal segment of the colon (hematoxylin-eosin stain 6-4×10.bmp).

Cell Types in the Epithelium

In normal colon, plasma cells, eosinophils, and histiocytes are loosely distributed in the upper third of the lamina propria (figure 2-2), and are usually more numerous in the cecum because it is an area of stasis [1,2]. Eosinophil concentrations vary not only by site (cecum greater than rectum) but also by season and geography. Lymphocytes are either intermingled with the crypt and surface epithelium (1 lymphocyte:20 epithelial cells) or aggregated in follicles at intervals along the muscularis mucosae. Neutrophils (inflammatory effector cells) are not normally seen outside the vascular system except in areas of hemorrhage. However, low-grade inflammatory cell infiltration of the colonic mucosa is normal (normal inflammatory cell component) and should not be considered as "colitis" [2].

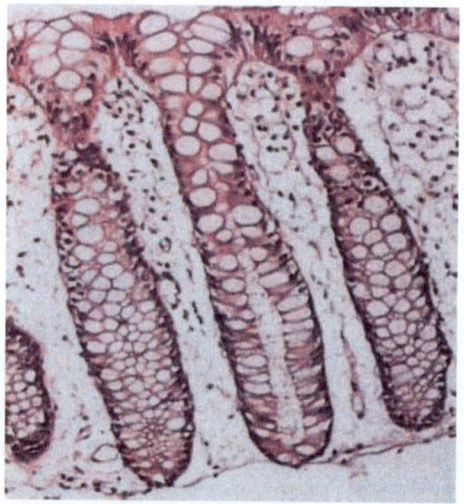

Figure 2-2. Features of the normal colonic mucosa; showing the crypts (they are straight, parallel with each other, and uniformly spaced) and small amount of inflammatory cells, predominantly plasma cells, are most numerous in upper lamina propria (8-10×10 bmp).

Crypt and Its Cells

Crypt is a small cylindric structure that contains the stem cells from which the epithelium is populated, as well as Paneth cells, enteroendocrine cells, goblet cells, and undifferentiated cells (figure 2-1, figure 2-3) [1]. Paneth and stem cells mainly at the base of crypt, whereas the other cells migrate.

Undifferentiated epithelial cells proliferate within the lower half of the crypts and mature as they migrate to the surface, where they undergo apoptosis and slough [2]. Secretion occurs in the crypts and absorption on the surface.

Normal crypts are straight, parallel, uniformly spaced, and uniform in diameter; their base are approximated to the muscularis mucosae (figure 2-2, figure 2-3), and branch is seen only in the region of lymphoglandular complexes (the site of antigen processing) in adults and children ≥9 yr of age [2]. In children ≤ 9 yr, branched crypts may reflect new crypt development in growing, normal colon. Branched crypts otherwise indicate crypt regeneration after crypt destruction.

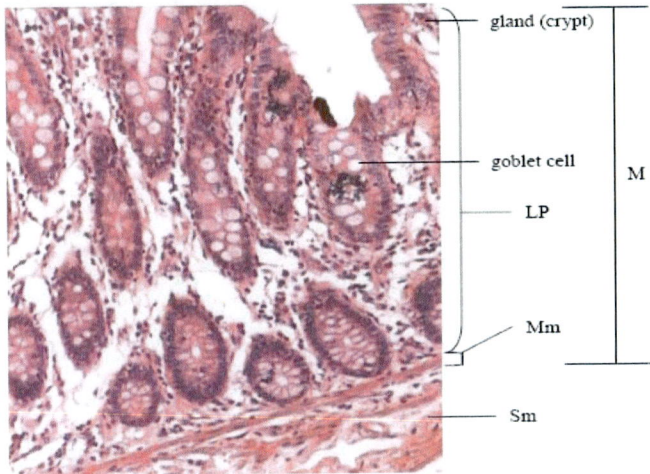

Figure 2-3. Normal colonic mucosa; showing crypts, goblet cells, and the LP, Mm and Sm layers (8-10×10 bmp).

The Normal Inflammatory Cell Component

In evaluating an endoscopic biopsy specimen, it is important to realize that the normal inflammatory cell component (figure 2-2, figure 2-3) may exist in many clinical setting for examples in patients with irritable bowel syndrome, small intestinal disease, self-administered laxatives, or lymphocytic colitis, etc. The normal colonic mucosa with low-grade inflammatory cell infiltration should be distinguished from an inflammatory infiltrate of pathological significance [2].

References

[1] Keljo DJ, Squires, Jr. RH. Anatomy and anomalies of the small and large intestines. In: Feldman M, Scharsehmidt BF, Sleisenger MH. (eds). Sleisenger and Fordtran's Gastrointestinal and liver Disease. 6th ed Printed in China Harcourt Publishers Limited Asia, W. B. Saunders 2001 P. 1419-1436.

[2] Carpenter HA, Talley NJ. The importance of clinicopathological correlation in the diagnosis of inflammatory conditions of the colon: histological patterns with clinical implications. *Am. J. Gastroenterol.* 2000;95(4):878-896.

[3] Zou Z-z. The digestive canal. In: Zou Z-z (ed.) Histology and Embryology: a textbook series of new century. 5th ed. Bei-jing. *People's Medical Publish House.* 2001; P.149-167 (Chinese).

Section Two: Pathology of Idiopathic Inflammatory Bowel Disease

In: Inflammatory Conditions of the Colon
Editor: Jia-ju Zheng

ISBN: 978-1-60692-240-8
© 2008 Nova Science Publishers, Inc.

Chapter III

Ulcerative Colitis

Jia-ju Zheng[*] *and Yun-di Guo*[**]

[*]Su-zhou Institute for Digestive Disease and Nutrition, Su-zhou Municipal Hospital,
Nan-jing Medical University, Su-zhou, Jiang-su Province, P.R. China
[**]Su-zhou Municipal Hostipal, Affiliated Soo-chow Hospital,
Nan-jing Medical University,
Su-zhou, Jiang-su Province, P.R. China

Gross Pathology

The inflammation in ulcerative colitis (UC) affects primarily the mucosa and the most superficial part of the submucosa [1,2]. The gross or endoscopic appearance of the colonic mucosa varies considerably [2]. The changes are usually most significant in the rectum and extend proximally for a variable extent of the colon. In approximately 75% of patients, the disease involves only the left side colon (left-side colitis, figure 3-1), and in the remainder, the entire colon is involved (pancolitis) [3]. However, apparent rectal sparing may be seen as a result of topical treatment and, rarely, in acute severe disease, when the proximal colon tends to be much more severely involved than the rectum [1,4]. In addition, there are two situations in which skip lesions may be seen in UC, i.e., there is evidences of appendiceal inflammation or areas of cecal inflammation associated with left-sided UC [1,2].

In mild cases, the mucosa bleeds easily, and appears granular, friable and hyperemic [3]. Other inflammatory changes include edema, and absence of the mucosal vascular pattern. Endoscopically, fine granularity of the mucosa (like a "wet sandpaper"), pinpoint hemorrhage to mucosa swabbing, and exudation of mucopus have been frequently described [3].

Moderate changes include coarse granularity and ulceration, confluent hemorrhage, confluent mucopus that progresses to gross ulcerations (figure 3-2), spontaneous bleeding, and much more exudation of pus [1,3].

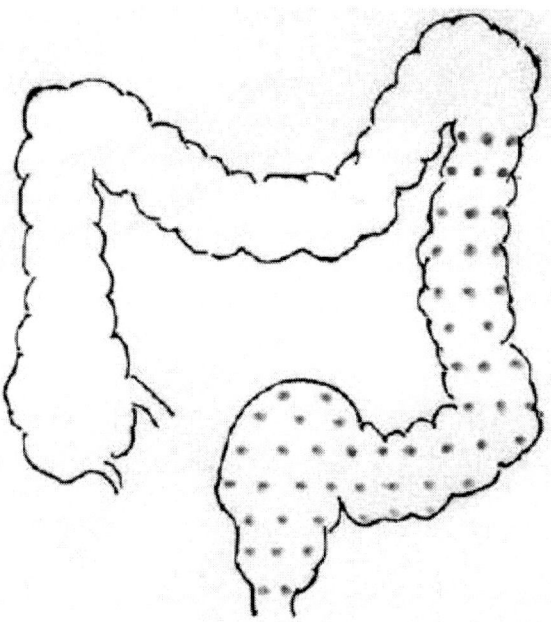

Figure 3-1. Ulcerative colitis (UC). The inflammation involves the left-sided colon in the greater part of the patients.

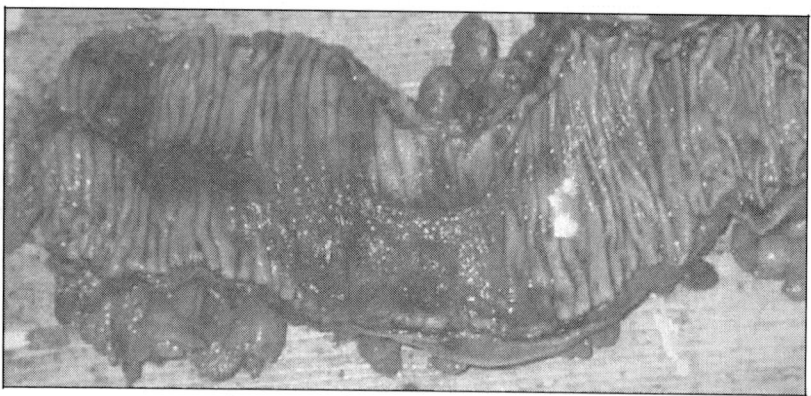

Figure 3-2. Moderately severe UC. Inflammatory changes include coarse granularity, ulcerations and confluent hemorrhage, etc. shown in a resented bowel segment.

In the most severe cases, the inflammation can involve the submucosa and even the serosa and lead to perforation. In toxic dilatation of the colon, a particularly severe and acute form of UC, the diameter of the lumen of the colon is greatly increased ($\geqslant 6.0$ cm in a X-ray plain film) and the bowel wall thinned, with a serious risk of spontaneous perforation[1,3].

With healing the mocosal vascular pattern remains distorted [3]. Alternating processes of superficial ulceration and granulation followed by re-epithelialization can lead to the development of polypoid excrescence [3,6] . These inflammatory polyps (pseudopolyps) may appear as filamentous projections or mucosal bridges, and may be quite friable or indistinguishable from adenomatous polyps [3,7].

Long-standing disease gives rise to hyperplasia of the muscularis mucosae, and this change, accompanied by postinflammatoey fibrosis, causes shortening of the colon. The haustrations are lost, and the large bowel has the appearance of a smooth tube. Strictures may be caused by the localized fibromuscular hyperplasia; a distinction must be made between these and malignant strictures[3].

Histopathology

The histologic changes in UC are nonspecific, but the chronicity and distribution pattern are characteristic [3]. Features that suggest chronicity may help to make the diagnosis of UC with more than 80% probability; these include distorted crypt architecture, crypt atrophy, increased intercrypt spacing to fewer than 6 crypts/mm, an irregular mocosal surface, basal lymphoid aggregate, and a chronic inflammatory infiltrate [2,3].

The inflammation in UC is predominantly confined to the mucosa [1,3]. The lamina propria becomes edematous and the capillaries are congested and dilated, often with extravasation of red cells. The lamina propria contains a mixed inflammatory infiltrate of neutrophils, lymphocytes, plasma cells, and macrophages. Eosinophils and mast cells are also present in increased numbers. The neutrophils invade and accumulate near the tips of the crypt lumen, giving rise to cryptitis and ultimately to crypt abscesses (figure 3-3) [3,7]. The cryptitis is associated with discharge of mucus from goblet cells and increased epithelial cell turnover. Depletion of mucin from goblet cells are apparent (figure 3-4).

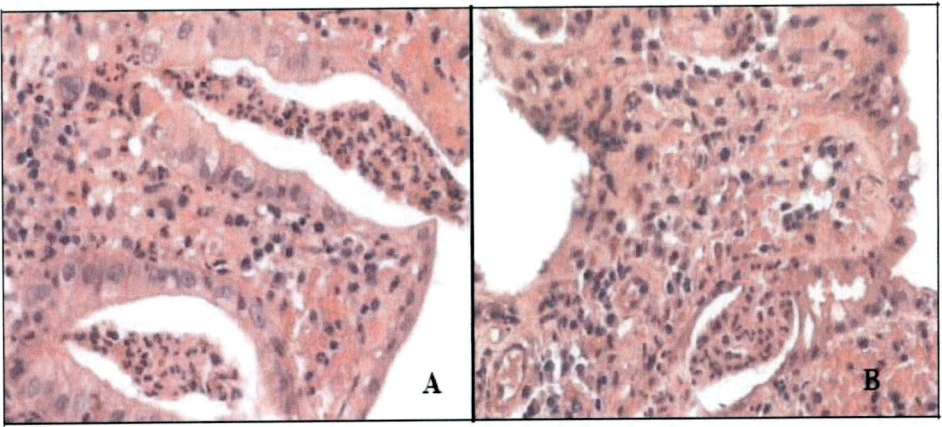

Figure 3-3. Ulcerative colitis - a type of chronic crypt destructive colitis. A. a mixed type of inflammatory cells (primarily plasma cells) uniformly distributed in the depth and superficial lamina propria (H.E.×100); and B. a crypt abscess is indicated in the section (H.E.×100).

With increasing inflammation, the surface epithelial cells become flattened and eventually ulcerate. The ulcers can be deep and undermine the surrounding epithelium. Some inflammation and vascular congestion may be seen in the submucosa. The inflammatory infitrate may extend into the muscularis propria, causing a diffuse pattern of myocytolysis. This is contrast with the transmural inflammation of Crohn's disease, which is in the form of discrete lymphoid aggregate [3,7].

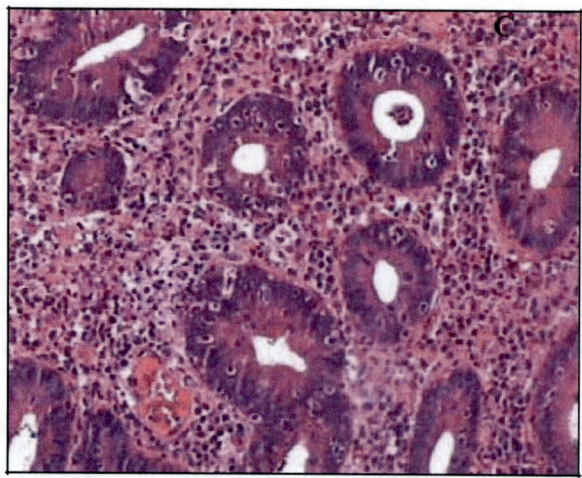

Figure 3-4. Ulcerative colitis, showing a remarkable decreased number of goblet cells (H.E.×400).

Once the disease has gone into remission, the histologic appearances may return to almost normal, especially after mild attacks early in the natural history of the disease. There usually is evidence of altered crypt architecture or actual dropout of glands. Architectural changes include bifid glands and shortened glands that do not extend down to the muscularis mucosae. If there is persistent evidence of acute inflammation despite clinical remission, there is said to be a high risk of relapse. Paneth cell metaplasia is frequently seen.

The histologic features of UC can be summarized as follows [2,3]:

1. Chronicity: prior crypt destruction and subsequent regeneration (most pronounced distally); indicative alterations include crypt architecture with distortion of crypts (called crypt destructive colitis), which may be bifid, irregular, reduced in number, with a gap between the crypt bases and muscularis mucosae;
2. Distribution pattern: basal plasma cells and multiple basal lymphoid aggregate are most apparent, although these also may be seen in other forms of colitis such as Crohn's colitis, microscopic and collagenous colitis;
3. Other features indicative of IBD: Paneth cell metaplasia distal to ascending colon, hyperplasia of argentaffin cells,' mucosal vascular congestion with edema, and focal hemorrage; paneth cell metaplasia in the left colon is not disease-specific but may help to identify inactive chronic colitis when histological changes are subtle [2].
4. Features of disease activity: active disease – neutrophils with crypt abscesses, depletion of goblet cell mucin', shallow superficial mucosal ulcers (erosion); severe colitis – deeper ulcers penetrating the muscularis mucosa into the superficial submucosa.

References

[1] Hanauer SB. Inflammatory bowel disease. In: Bennett JC, Plum F.(eds.) Cecil Textbook of Medicine. 20thed. Philadelphia. W.B. Saunders Company, 1996; 707-715.

[2] Carpenter HA, Talley NJ. The importance of clinicopathological correlation in the diagnosis of inflammatory conditions of the colon: histological patterns with clinical implications. *Am. J. Gastroenterol.* 2000;95(4):878-896.

[3] Riddell RH, Pathology of idiopathic inflammatory bowel disease. In: Kirsner JB (ed). Inflammatory Bowel Disease. Philadelphia. London New York St. Louis Syd. W.B.Saunders. 2000; P.422-488.

[4] Finkelstein SD, Sasatomi E, Regueiro M. Pathologic features of early inflammatory bowel disease. *Gastroeriteril. Clin. N. Am.* 2002;31(1):133-145.

[5] Zheng J-j. Clinical aspects of ulcerative colitis in mainland China. *Chin. J. Dig. Dis.* 2006;7(2):71-75.

[6] Jin R, Xu F-x. Ulcerative colitis. In: Xu F-x (ed.) Endoscopy of the Lower Gastrointestinal Tract (1st ed.). Shang-hai. Shang-hai Science and Technology Press 2003; P.252-269 (Chinese).

[7] Zheng J-j. Endoscopic and histopathologic features in differential diagnosis of inflammatory disease of the colon. *Chin. J. Gastroenterol. Hepatol.* 2006; 15 (4): 339-349 (Chinese).

In: Inflammatory Conditions of the Colon
Editor: Jia-ju Zheng

ISBN: 978-1-60692-240-8
© 2008 Nova Science Publishers, Inc.

Chapter IV

Crohn's Disease

Jia-ju Zheng[*] *and Yun-di Guo*[**]
[*]Su-zhou Institute for Digestive Disease and Nutrition, Su-zhou Municipal Hospital,
Nan-jing Medical University, Su-zhou, Jiang-su Province, P.R. China
[**]Su-zhou Municipal Hostipal, Affiliated Soo-chow Hospital,
Nan-jing Medical University,
Su-zhou, Jiang-su Province, P.R. China

Gross Pathology

As compared with the relatively superficial inflammatory in the mucosa and/or submucosa and solely colonic involvement of ulcerative colitis (UC), the inflammatory process of Crohn's disease (CD) is quite different in many aspects. The disease involves deep into all layers of the bowel wall. In addition, CD may involve any part or combination of segments of the alimentary tract from the month to the anus (figure 4-1) [1,2]. The most commonly affected portions of the bowel are the distal ileum and adjacent right colon.

In the earliest stage, mucosal edma and hyperemia are the macroscopic features and most apparent in affected segments, with other areas of mucosa appearing normal (segmental distribution) [1,2]. In slightly more advanced cases, discrete superficial ulcerations, or aphthae, and erupt are frequently observed.

As the disease progresses, these aphthae enlarge and coalesce. Deep, transverse and longitudinal (linear) or serpiginous ulcers are seen, usually in the long axis of the bowel. These ulcers extend linearly and transversely, and combine with intervening edematous mucosa, isolating normal islands of mucosa, produce the typical cobblestone appearance (nodular swelling of the intervening inflamed edematous islands of the bowel) (figure 4-2) [1,3,4].

Once the disease entrenched, the bowel wall is thickened and hyperemic with some serosal fibrin deposition, and produces adhesions between adjacent loops of bowel (figure 4-3). The bowel wall becomes fibrotic, stiff, and stenotic. The adjacent mesentery is markedly thickened with migration or "creeping" of mesenteric fat onto the serosal surface of the bowel (external fat wrapping, figure 4-4). Mesenteric lymphatics are engorged, and mesenteric lymph nodes are enlarged and matted. Fistulas, presumably formed by the extension of burrowing ulcerations, often develop in the most severely involved areas.

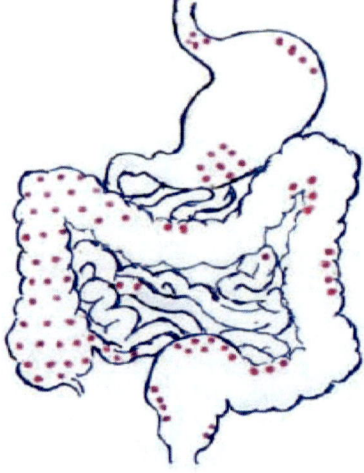

Figure 4-1. Crohn's disease. The inflammatory lesions may involve any part or combination of segments of the alimentary canal.

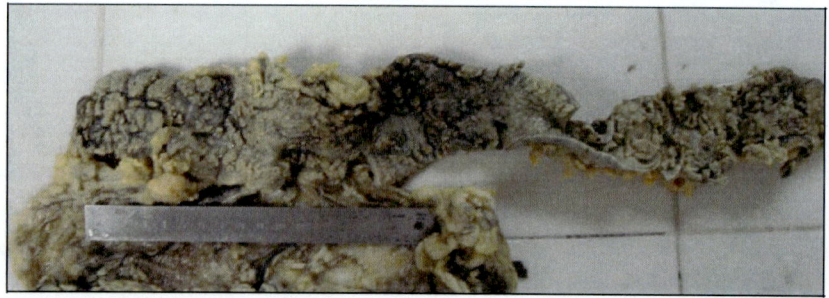

Figure 4-2. A resected bowel specimen showing diverse inflammatory processes including ulcers, cobblestoning (upper-lift site), pseudopolyps and narrowed lumen, etc.

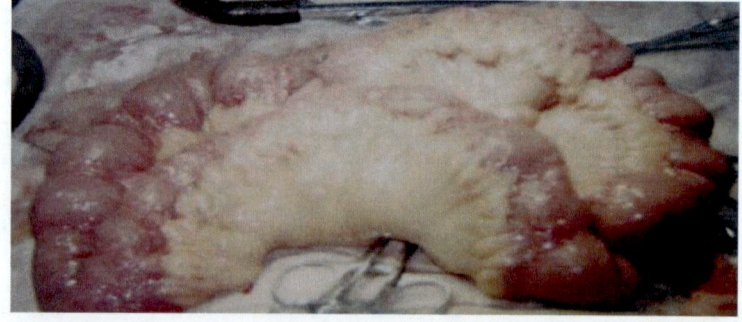

Figure 4-3. Serositis developed on the external surface of the bowel. Adherent loops of the bowel form a large inflammatory mass.

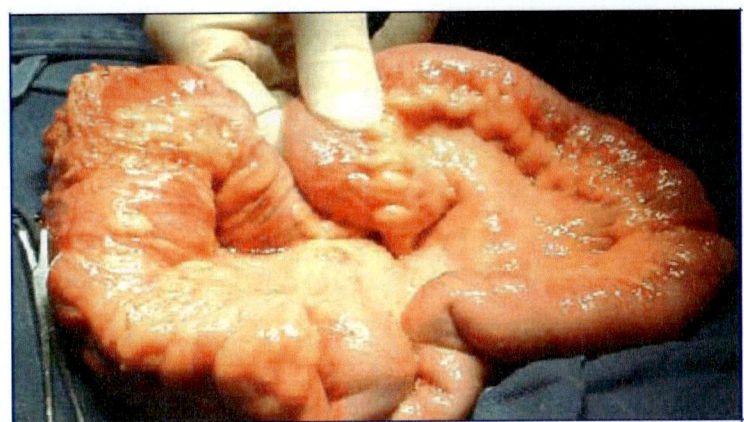

Figure 4-4. External fat-wrapping was found closely correlated with mucosal lesion (transmural inflammation), intestinal fibrosis, muscularization and stricture formation [2].

In summary, the distinct feature of CD is diverse inflammatory processes (multi-staged, both destructive and proliferative or regenerative changes) are simultaneously present in the involved bowel segment (figure 4-2, table 4-1) [5-7].

As described above, a curious and characteristic feature of CD is its segmental nature [2,3,5,7]. The segmental or regional distribution helps distinguish CD of the colon from UC. Involved segments of the bowel are often scattered, separated by apparently uninvolved "skip" areas. These skip areas appear grossly, radiologically, or endoscopically normal, but they may not actually be disease free, because histologic abnormalities are found in widespread segments of the alimentary tract [2,5].

Table 4-1. Pathologic features and frequencies in Crohn's disease [6,7]

Feature	Frequency (%)
Gross morphology	
1. mucosal changes	
destructive lesion	
ulcer	100.0
superficial (or aphthoid)	75.0
serpiginous	75.0
longitudinal	75.0
irregular	50.0
"skip" distributed	62.5
fistula	N
perforation	25.0[1ature, or endoscopically normal])
cobblestoning	75.0
regenerative	
polyps	75.0
mucosal bridge	25.0
2. lumenal changes	
transmural infiltrate	100.0
segmental inflammation	75.0
bowel wall thickened and stiffness	100.0

Table 4-1. (Continued).

Feature	Frequency (%)
stricture	100.0
circumferential lesion	25.0
3. serosal changes	
edema/hyperema	75.0
fibrin exudates	87.5
serosal buble	25.0
adhesion	87.5
4. mesenteric lymphonode	
enlarged	75.0
Histopathology	
lymphocytic infiltration	100.0 (100.0) [2)]
fissuring ulcer	87.5 (23.1)
transmural infiltrate	100.0 (100.0)
granulomas	62.5 (30.8)
submucosal broadening	87.5 (15.4)
fibrosis	87.5 (N)
crypt abscesses	0 (7)

[1.] degree of diagnosis certainty is probable;
[2.] data not within the parenthesis are from resected bowel segments (data within the parenthesis are from biopsy specimens);
N: data not available at publish time or not observable.

Histopathology

In active CD, an early and frequently observed mucosal lesion is crypt injury, which is caused by "crypt seeking" neutrophils[1,2]. This injury takes the form of cryptitis and, subsequently, crypt abscesses consisting of polymorphonuclear cells. These crypt lesions are nearly identical to those occurring in UC, but their distribution is typically more focal in CD [1,8-10].

As abovementioned, the inflammatory changes in CD, unlike UC primarily in the mucosa and submucosa layers, affect the full thickness of the bowel wall. The inflammatory infiltrate extends into the deeper layers, and consists predominantly of macrophages and lymphocytes. [2,8,9]. In addition, the fact that microscopic changes often are identified distant from sites of macroscopic disease indicate again subtle changes exist throught the alimentary tract [11].

The alternating processes of inflammation (ulceration) and repair (granulation) followed by re-epithelialization may lead to formation of polypoid (mucosal tags), or called inflammatory polyps (pseudopolyps) [2]. When they are numerous, they vary considerably in size (most of them are less than 1.5 cm long); they may form a forest of polyps in some cases, and are called "colitis polyposa" (figure 4-5) [2,12]. Inflammatory polyps assume many shapes and sometime form mucosal bridge which can be clearly viewed endoscopically (see Chapter 8 figure 8-6).

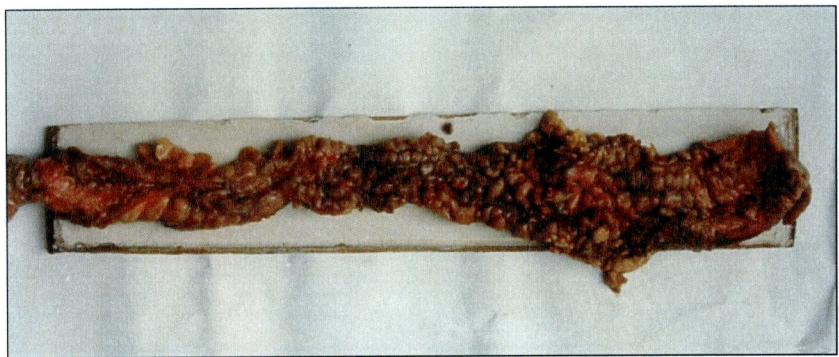

Figure 4-5. Colitis polyposa, which is easily confused with polyposis coli (polyps in different size but usually smaller than 1.0 cm-1.5 cm). [12]

The early crypt injury is followed by microscopic ulceration of the mucosa over a lymphoid follicle. In apparent response to chemotactic signals, macrophages and other inflammatory cells then invade and proliferate in the lamina propria [6,13,14]. Loose aggregations of macrophages ultimately organize into discrete noncaseating granulomas, where consist of epithelioid cells with multinucleated giant cells enmeshed anywhere in the granuloma (figure 4-6).

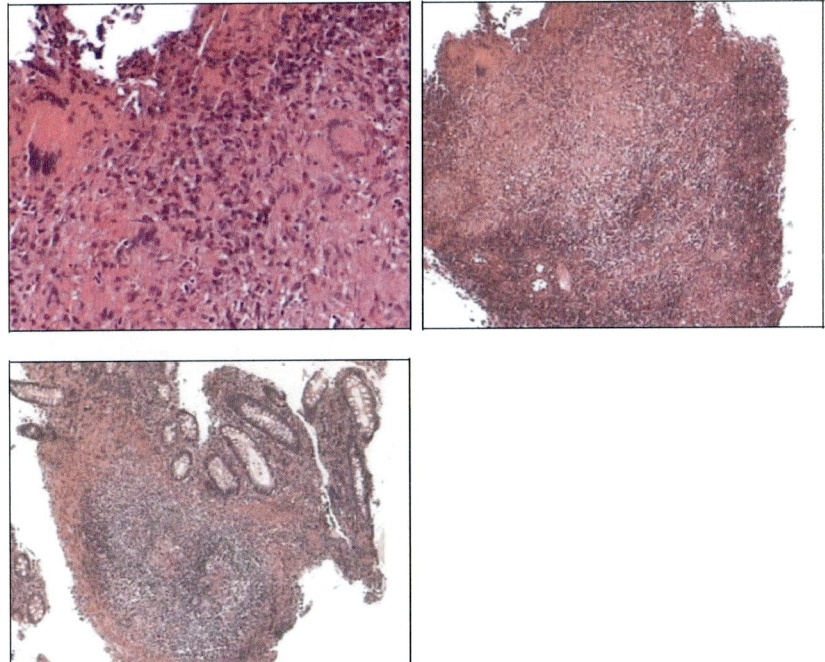

Figure 4-6. Epithelioid granuloma, which is small in size, with eccentrically placed multinucleated giant cell and mixed inflammatory cells clustered at the periphery, and is entirely nonspecific but quiet characteristic in Crohn's disease (H.E.×40).

Lymphoid aggregates were common throughout all layers of the mucosa, submucosa, and serosa, with characteristic aggregations of hiotiocytes and plasma cells forming non easeating granulomas. These granulomas may involve all layers of the bowel wall from the mucosa to serosa; they can occasionally even be seen grossly at laparotomy or lapascopy as military nodules. These lesions are also found in the lymph nodes, mesaentery, peritoneum, and liver as a function of contiguous spread of the disease from the intestine. On occasion they are in the bowel wall without extension to local lymph nodes or mesentery. They are only rarely found in peripheral tissue unless they are also present in the bowel. Although granulomas seem to be a pathognomonic feature of CD, their absence dose not rule out the diagnosis. Only half of CD cases reveal epithelioid granulomas in surgical specimens [2,7,14], and even much lower percentage (<20%)of detection in endoscopic biopsy specimens (table 4-1) [6,11]. Most of the remainder have only nonspecific transmural inflammation or loose aggregations of histiocytes.

A study in a group of Chinese patients with CD reveal that the focal distribution of inflammatory infiltration and lymphoid aggregate were the most frequently observed features in mucosal biopsy specimen, and among others were edematous and widened submucosa (figure 4-7), deep fissuring ulcers (figure 4-8) and hyperplasia and fibrosis respectively. Granulomas were detected in 30% of the group [6].

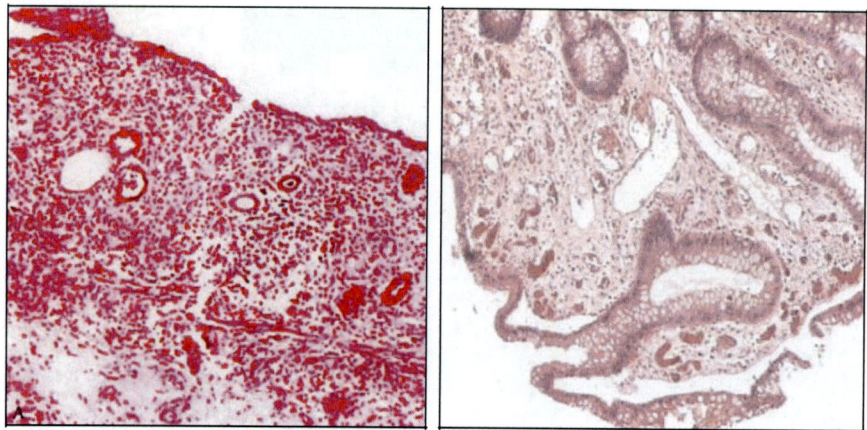

Figure 4-7. Widened submucosa, which is due to edema, lymphagectasis, telangectasis, etc., and may be several times of normal thickness. Lymphocytic aggregation is remarkably seen in the section ((H.E.×100)).

As the invasion by histiocytes and macrophages continnes, other inflammatory cells, including lymphocytes and plasma cells, are recruited to the inflammatory process, which spreads transmurally. Transmural inflammation (figure 4-2, and figure 4-9) is usually present even in the absence of any macrophages or granulomas and may be accompanied by clefts or fissures that penetrate deeply into the wall and sometimes result in frank sinus tract or fistulas [2,10]

Pathologic characteristics with diagnostic significance are summarized in table 4-2.

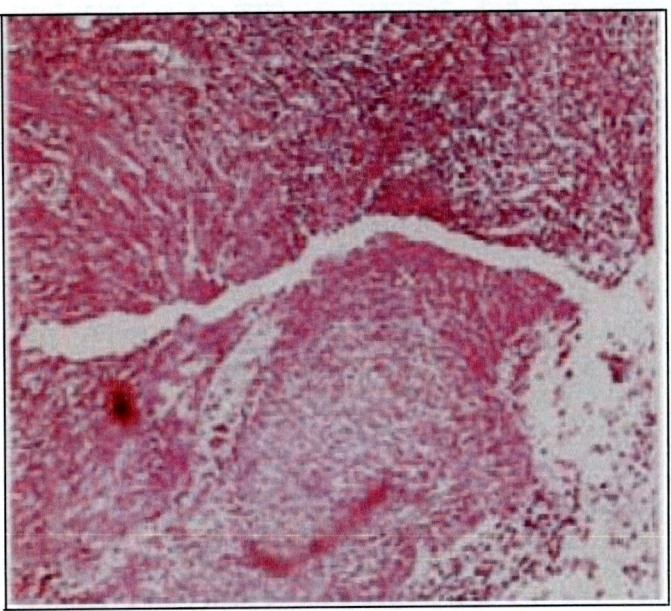

Figure 4-8. Fissuring ulcer, a knife-cutting like ulcer, may be branched, and usually penetrates perpendicularly into the gut wall to different depths, the deepest may reach the serosa or penetrate through the bowel wall resulting in fistula formation (H.E.×40).

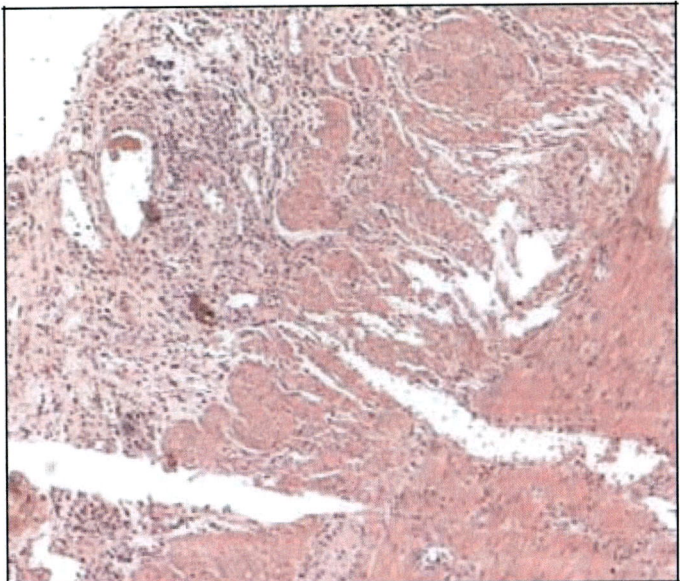

Figure 4-9. Inflammatory process involves all layers of the bowel wall (H.E.×40).

Table 4-2. Pathologic features that support a diagnosis of CD[1,2,14]

Macroscopic	Microscopic (resected bowel specimen)
1. ileum lesion	transmural inflammation
2. rectal sparing	aggregated inflammatory pattern
3. confluent deep linear ulcers	transmural lymphoid hyperplasia
4. aphthoid ulcer	broadened of submucosa layer
5. deep fissures	fibromuscular obliteration
6. fistula	fissures
7. fat wrapping*	sarcoid granuloma (including intralymphonode)
8. skip lesions (segmental lesions)	abnormalities of nervous system of the bowel (proliferation of submucosal nerve fibers, ganglionitis)*
9. cobblestoning	relatively no change of epithelium - mucin retained and most goblet cells are normal
10. thickened intestinal wall*	
11. stricture	

* With more diagnostic values when compared to other macroscopic features.

References

[1] Kornbluth A, Sachar DB, Salomon P. Crohn's disesase In: Feldman M, Scharsschmidt BF, Sleisenger MH. (eds). Sleisenger and Fordtran's Gastrointestinal and Liver disease. 6th ed. Printed in China Harcourt Asia W.B. Saunders Company. 1998, P.1708-1734.

[2] Riddell RH. Pathology of idiopathic inflammatory bowel disease. In: Kirsner JB (ed.) Inflammatory Bowel Disease. 5th ed. Philadelphia: W.B. Saunders Company. 2000; P.453-477.

[3] Pan G-z, Liu T-h, Crohn's disease. In: Pan G-z, Cao S-z (ed.) Modern Gastroenterology. Bei-jing Science Press, 1994 ; P.1152-2265 (Chinese).

[4] ChutKan RK, Waye JD. Endoscopy in inflammatory bowel disease. In: Kirsner JB (ed.) Inflammatory Bowel Disease. 5th ed. Philadelphia: W.B. Saunders Company. 2000; P.453-477.

[5] Lee SD, Cohen RD. Endoscopy in inflammatory bowel disease. *Gastroenterol. Clin. N. Am.* 2002; 31(1):119-132.

[6] Zheng J-j, ChuX-q, Shi X-h, et al. Endoscopic and histologicfeatures of colonic Crohn;s disease in Chinese patients. *J. Dig. Dis.* 2007; 8 (1):35-41.

[7] Zheng J-j, ChuX-q, Shi X-h, et al. Clinical diversity of Crohn's disease. *Chin. J. Dig.* 2002; 22 (4):34-37 (Chinese).

[8] Jin R, Xu F-x. Crohn's disease. In: Xu Fx (ed.) Endoscopy of the lower gastrointestinal tract (1st ed.). Shang-hai Shang-hai Science and Technology Press 2003; P.270-281 (Chinese).

[9] Liu T-h. Esophagus, stomach, intestine and anus. In: Liu T-h (ed) Diagnostic Pathology (1st ed.) Bei-jing People's Health Press 1994; P.78-92, 95-112 (Chinese).

[10] Finkelstein SD, Sasatomi E, Regueiro M. Pathologic features of early inflammatory bowel disease. *Gastroeriteril. Clin. N. Am.* 2002; 31(1):133-145.

[11] Hanauer SB. Imflammatory bowel disease. In: Bennett JC, Plum F (eds.). Cecil Textbook of Medicine. 20thed. Philadelphia. W.B. Saunders Company, 1996; 707-715.

[12] Zheng J-j, ChuX-q, Shi X-h, et al. Colitis Polyposa – uncommon complication of colonic Crohn;s disease. *Chin. J. Dig. Endosc.* 1999; 16 (1):39-40 (Chinese).

[13] Jung B, Carethers JM, Behling C, et al. Aphthous colitis in a young man with diverticulitis. *Gastrointest. Endosc.* 2003; 58(2):301-304.

[14] Stange EF, Travis SPL, Vermeire, et al. European evidence based consensus on the diagnosis and management of Crohn's disease: definition and diagnosis. *Gut.* 2006; 55 (Suppl. 1): i1-i15.

Chapter V

Site and Extent of Inflammatory Bowel Disease

Jia-ju Zheng and *Yun-di Guo*

*Su-zhou Institute for Digestive Disease and Nutrition, Su-zhou Municipal Hospital,
Nan-jing Medical University, Su-zhou, Jiang-su Province, P.R. China
**Su-zhou Municipal Hostipal, Affiliated Soo-chow Hospital,
Nan-jing Medical University,
Su-zhou, Jiang-su Province, P.R. China

Establishing the site and extent of inflammation in inflammatory bowel disease (IBD) is essential and helpful to guide medical therapy, to differentiate Crohn's disease from ulcerative colitis, to establish the risk of colorectal carcinoma, and to decide when to consider surgery [1]. Colonoscopy with multiple biopsies is the standard for defining site and extent of the disease and excluding other forms of inflammation of the colon [1].

Ulcerative Colitis

Although in rare instances the rectum may be spared, ulcerative colitis (UC) usually involves the rectum and extends, in a continuous fashion, down to the anal margin or proximally in the colon for a variable distance [2]. Once the upper demarcation of disease has been identified, it usually remains constant. Up to 40% of patients develop proximal extension of colonic involvement, usually within the first few years after diagnosis [2] . The extent of proximal spread varies but is confined to the colon, with the exception of occasional mild inflammation of the most distal part of the terminal ileum (backwash ileitis or reflux ileitis) in a small group of patients with pancolitis.

As shown in figure 5-1, in approximately one quarter of UC patients, inflammation affects only the rectum (proctitis), and has a clearly delineated upper border [2,3]. In another 25% to 50% of UC patients, the rectum and sigmoid or the descending colon are involved and called proctosigmoiditis or left-sided colitis, respectively; in approximately one third of patients inflammation extends proximal to the splenic flexure (extensive colitis). In pancolitis, the inflammation involves the entire colon. These terms referred to anatomic extent of the disease have been commonly used in practice by most gastroenterologists. However, some patients with proctitis have patches of endoscopic or histologic changes in the cecum or right colon. The prognostic implications of these findings are uncertain [2]. Based on endoscopic and clinical studies, disease distribution of UC has been reported by two Chinese groups (table 5-1) [4,5]. The results are consistent with the data reported by many groups from Western countries.

In a recent world conference of gastroenterology in Montreal in Canada in 2006, the working part on IBD classified the UC based on its anatomic sites as table 5-2 [3].

Table 5-1. Colonoscopic distribution of ulcerative colitis in two cities in China [4,5]

site	Bei-jing		Shang-hai			
	cases (1974-1995)	%	cases (1975-1994)	%	cases (1995-2001)	%
proctitis	35	23.65	140	28.8	182	37.1
proctosigmoiditis	54	36.49	129	26.6	134	27.4
left-sided colitis	25	16.89	84	17.3	68	13.9
sub-total colitis	/	/	57	11.7	26	5.3
right-sided colitis	5	3.38	18	3.7	10	2.0
pancollitis	29	19.59	5	11.9	70	14.3
total	148	100.0	486	100	490	100

Table 5-2. Montreal classification of extent of ulcerative colitis (UC) [3]

Extent	Anatomy
E1 ulcerative proctitis	Involvement limited to the rectum (that is, proximal extent of inflammation is distal to the rectosigmoid junction)
E2 left sided UC (distal UC)	Involvement limited to a proportion of the colorectum distal to the splenic flexure
E3 Extensive UC (pancolitis)	Involvement extends proximal to the splenic flexure

Crohn's Disease

Unlike UC, Crohn's diseases (CD) can affect any segment of the alimentary canal or any combination of segments of the bowel [2]. There are, however, pathologic changes that characterize the inflammatory process in any segment of involved bowel [2]. Table 5-3 provides pathologic features that may help distinguish the two diseases [6]. The most common site of involvement is the terminal ileum, cecum and adjacent right colon [7,8]. Approximately 30-40% of patients have disease confined to the small intestine; 15-25% have colonic disease only, and the remaining 40-55% have involvement of both the small and large intestines [7,8]. A small percentage of patients (<5%) have involvement of the duodenum, stomach or esophagus. Perianal disease is common in CD, affecting up to 50% of patients, while rectal sparing is most common and helps distinguish it from UC [7].

In addition, the inflamed segments are discontinuous with areas of normal bowel separating diseased sections (skip lesions) in CD patients.

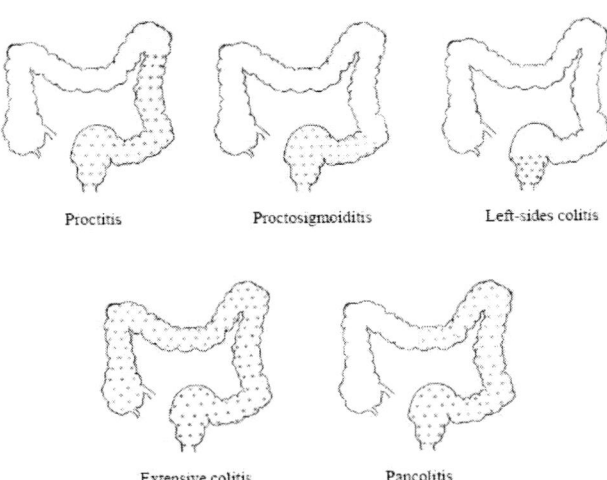

Figure 5-1. Typical patterns of inflammation distribution in Ulcerative colitis.

Table 5-3. Pathologic changes associated with ulcerative colitis and Crohn's disease [6]

Ulcerative colitis	Crohn's disease
Crypt epithelium centered, basally oriented colitis	Irregularly distributed colitis with aphthoid ulceration
Mucin depletion	Mucin retention
Basal plasmacytosis	Histiocytic aggregation
Diffuse distribution in large bowel	Multifocal distribution
Distal-to-proximal progression	Inconsistent and patchy progression, Sharp border between normal and inflamed tissue
Lamina propria infiltration	Transmural infiltration
Diffuse mucosal atrophy	Focal mucosal injury
No sarcois-like granulomatous change	Sarcoid-like granulomatous change
Anal sparing	Anal involvement
Limited to large intestine (except backwash ileitis)	Disease anywhere from mouth to anus (most common site: terminal ileum and proximal colon)

There is an increasing incidence of CD in Asia and in China in particular[9]. It's distribution in gastrointestinal tract has been reported by several Chinese groups [10,11]. Table 5-4 shows the results from a clinical study in Su-zhou in east China [10]. In consistent with reports from most Western countries, the data showed a similar distribution pattern i.e., ileocecal and colonic lesions together account for the major site of the disease. Perianal disease is also common in the study [10]. Among the 75% or more of patients whose Crohn's disease affects the small intestine, the terminal ileum will be involved at lest 90% [12].

Patients with colonic disease alone tend to have more frequent involvement of the distal colon than those with ileocolitis, and have skip lesions in only about one fourth of cases [13].

Table 5-4. Pathologic distribution of CD in a group of Chinese patients [10]

site	frequency	%
esophagus	1	3.3
stomach	1	3.3
small intestine	19	63.3
duodenum	2	6.6
jejunum	8	26.7
ileum	9	30.0
ileocecum	11	36.6
colon	29	96.7
rectum	6	20.0
perianal disease	10	33.3

Multiple sites were involved in many cases. The total number of involvements (frequency) is 76, which is more than the actual number of patients (n =30).
Thus, the sum total of percentage is higher than 100% (%=frequency/cases).

Clinical Importance of Establishing Disease Site and Extent

Proctitis, as for UC, this condition involves only the rectum and may in fact be a variant form of UC, with which it has many features in common. However, proctitis will proceed to left-sided colitis or pancolitis in 25 to 40% of cases. Topical therapy (either suppository or enema) is indicated for distal colitis with promising results [2,7].

The ileocecal region, as for CD, is the most common site for initial presentation, and is observed in approximately 40% of patients [7,12]. The principal symptoms in this region are diarrhea, cramping abdominal pain, and low-grade fever. An inflammatory mass may be palpated in the right lower quadrant of the abdomen. Partial bowel obstruction is common, and severe inflammation of the ileocecal region may lead to localized wall thinning with microperforation, fissuring, and fistula formation to adjacent bowel, skin (figure 5-2), or the urinary bladder or to an abscess cavity in the mesentery [12].

In small bowel disease, as for CD, extensive inflammation is associated with a loss of effective digestive and absorptive surface, resulting in malabsorption and steatorrhea. Hypoalbuminemia, hypocalcemia, anemia, weight loss and growth retardation of children and nutritional deficiencies are all common [12].

In colonic disease (called colonic Crohn's disease or Crohn's colitis), the clinical pattern is inflammatory with symptoms of fever, malaise, diarrhea, and hematochezia [7,12]. The volume of diarrhea and the proportion of patients with hematochezia in CD is less than in UC.

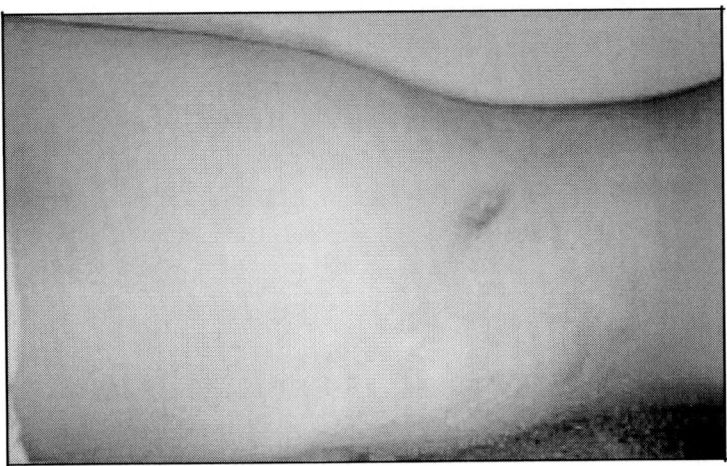

Figure 5-2. A case with ileocecal involvement of Crohn's disease, showing intestinal-skin fistula which is healed after surgical intervention.

Perianal disease (figure 5-3) is common in Crohn's colitis, and is discussed more in detail in chapter 23.

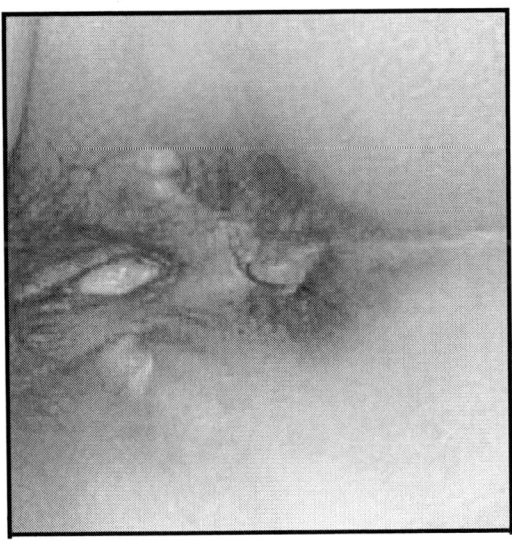

Figure 5-3. A case with ileocecal and colonic involvements of Crohn's disease, showing the orifices of two perianal fistulas, which is recurred with a two-year healing after surgery.

Symptoms of upper gastrointestinal CD can be moderately relieved with antacids. In esophageal CD, ulcerating lesions frequently heal following the initial therapy, and usually do not recur during the course of disease. Duodenal Crohn's disease more often involves the second portion of the duodenum rather than the bulb.

References

[1] Krok KL, Lichtenstein GR. Printed in China. Inflammatory bowel disease. In: Ginsberg GG, Kochman ML, Norton I. Gastout CJ (eds.). Clinical Gastrointestinal Endoscopy. Printed in China, Elsevier Saunders 2005;P.311-332.

[2] Hanauer SB. Inflammatory bowel disease. In: Bennett JC, Plum F (eds.). Cecil textbook of Medicine. 20thed. Philadelpia, W.B. Saunders Company. 1996;P.707-715.

[3] Satsangi J, Silverberg MS, Vermeire S, et al. The Montreal classification of inflammatory bowel disease: controversies, consensus, and implications. *Gut.* 2006;55(6):749-753.

[4] Zhu F, Qian J-m, Pan G-z. Drug therapy in severe ulcerative colitis. *Chin. J. Gastroenterol.* 1996;1(2):78-80 (Chinese).

[5] Xiang P, Bao Z-j, Xu F-x. Endoscopic features and clinical analysis on ulcerative colitis. *Chin. J. Dig.* 2003; 23(4):217-219 (Chinese).

[6] Finkelstein SD, Sasatomi E, Regueiro M. Pathologic features of early inflammatory bowel disease. *Gastroeriteril. Clin. N. Am.* 2002;31(1):133-145.

[7] Zheng J-j. Contemporary drug therapy in ulcerative colitis. In: Zheng J-j (ed.) Inflammatory Bowel Disease – basic and clinical aspects (1st ed.) Bei-jing, Science Press 2001;P.253-269 (Chinese).

[8] Kornbluth A, Sachar DB, Salomon P. Crohn's disease. In: Feldman M, Sacharschmidt BF, Sleisenger MH (eds.). Sleisenger and Fordtran's Gastrointestinal and liver disease. 6th ed. Bei-jing, Science Press, Harcourt Asia, W.B.Saunders 2001; P.1708-1734.

[9] Zheng J-j, Zhu X-s, Huangfu Z, et al. Crohn's disease in mainland China: a systemic analysis of 50 years of research. *Chin. J. Dig. Dis.* 2005; 6(4):175-181.

[10] Zheng J-j, Shi X-h, Chu X-q, et al. Clinical features, diagnosis and treatment of Crohn's disease. In: Zheng J-j (ed.). Inflammatory Bowel Disease-basic and clinical advances. 1st ed. Bei-jing Science Press 2001; P.138-152 (Chinese).

[11] Xiang P, Yin S-m, Xu F-x, et al. Endoscopic and clinical features of Crohn's disease. *Chin. J. Dig. Endosc.* 2006;23(6):426-429 (Chinese).

[12] Zheng J-j, Chu X-q, Shi X-h, et al. Clinical diversity of Crohn's disease. *Chin. J. Dig.* 2002; 22 (4):34-37 (Chinese).

[13] Lashner BA. Clinical features, laboratory findings and course of Crohn's disease. In: Kirsner JB (ed.). Inflammatory bowel disease. 5th ed. Philadelphia, W.B. Saunders Company 2000; P.305-314.

Section Three: Endoscopy in Inflammatory Bowel Disease

In: Inflammatory Conditions of the Colon
Editor: Jia-ju Zheng

ISBN: 978-1-60692-240-8
© 2008 Nova Science Publishers, Inc.

Chapter VI

Normal Endoscopic Appearance of the Bowel

Jia-ju Zheng

Su-zhou Institute for Digestive Disease and Nutrition, Su-zhou Municipal Hospital,
Nan-jing Medical University, Su-zhou, Jiang-su Province, P.R. China

Indications

Endoscopy, including colonoscopy, sigmoidoscopy and esophagogastroduodenoscopy (EGD), is the most sensitive method to evaluate mucosal changes, and is the only method available for providing histologic information of the alimentary tract in inflammatory bowel disease (IBD) [1].

Colonoscopy examination is important in the diagnosis and treatment of suspected colonic disease [2]. It is a diagnostic procedure of choice for patients with diarrhea lasting several weeks to months or for any bloody diarrhea [2]. Colonoscopy has replaced radiology as the initial examination of choice in many clinical situation [2]. Colonoscopy is indicated to evaluate unexplained diarrhea and to aid in the differential diagnosis of IBD [2,3].

It is crucial to determine the extent of disease (also see Chapter 5 in detail), the disease activity, and to evaluate the response to various medical therapies. Colonoscopy is also indicated for all these objectives.

Colonoscopy is indicated in the screening and surveillance for dysplasia and cancer. Screening for colorectal cancer (CRC) can identify premalignant lesions and detect asymptomatic early stage malignancy, and has been shown to decrease mortality. The appropriate choice of screening modalities, age to initiate screening, and frequency of screening is dependent on individual patient factors and risk.

In addition, endoscopy also may offer therapeutic benefits including stricture dilatation, stent placement, and bleeding control [2,3].

Endoscopic retrograde cholangiopancreatography (ERCP) is used often to evaluate for the potential of primary sclerosing cholangitis, and recently a number of newly developed endoscopic techniques, such as video capsule endoscopy, endoscopic ultrasonography, double balloon enteroscopy, narrow band imaging, confocal endomicroscopy and magnifying colonoscopy, etc., has begun to evolve. All those endoscopic techniques will be discussed in detail in following chapters, respectively.

Normal Endoscopic Appeatance

On endoscopy, the normal colonic mucosa is arranged in orderly folds and haustrae. It is uniformly salmon-pink, with a smooth, glistening, transparent surface that reflects the light of the colonoscope. The branching vascular network is visible (figure 6-1) [2,3]. The vessels lie in the submucosa beneath the superficial mucosal layer. Arborization of the vascular pattern is characteristic of normal surface topography [3].

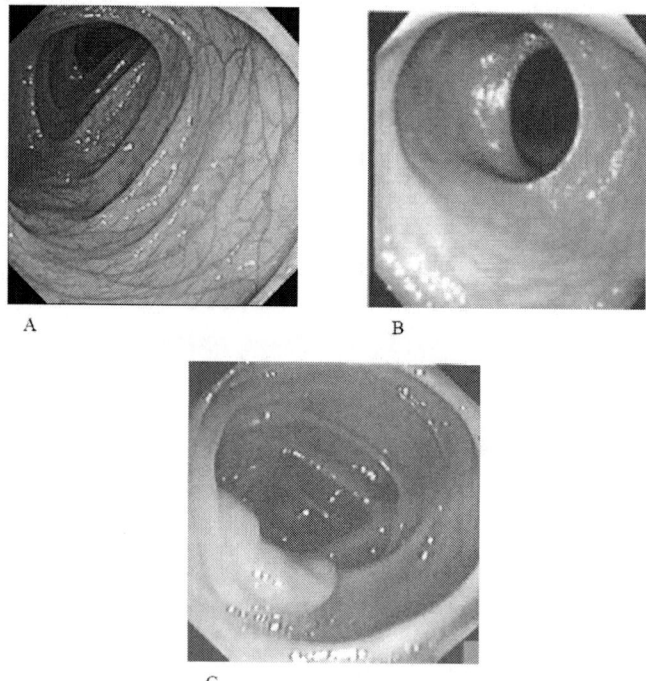

Figure 6-1. The normal colon and rectum. The characteristic features include: "paper-crease" sharp (not indurated) folds and haustral septae, and continually interlacing vascular parttern; exudate is not seen within the lumen. A. the transverse colon. B. the rectum. C. the ileocecal valve.

Mild acute colitis may appear as patchy erythema, granularity, disruption of the light reflex, and edema [2,3]. Edema may interfere with visualization of the submucosal vascular plexus. However, it is important to remember that erythema and edema are not always due to inflammation, which may be caused by congestive colopathy associated with portal hypertension [2]. Branched regenerating crypts are a feature of chronic colitis [2]. In these situations, charateristically the normal vascular pattern, mucosal folds, and haustral markings are lost [4].

The endoscopic features of acute and chronic crypt-destructive colitis overlap; however, a patchy intensely red-to-magenta-colored mucosa suggests acute infection rather than chronic inflammatory bowel disease, as does free pus [2-4]. Contact bleeding (friability) may occur because of minute ulcerations or vascular engorgement. Generally, mucosal folds and haustral markings are preserved [2].

The rectum has a more vascular appearance. Its vessels increase in caliber the further distal they are, producing more prominent vasculature [1-3]. During colonoscopy in rectum, make a reversal procedure to find lesions near the anal zig-line more clearly, such as polyps, inner-hemorrhoids even malignant lesions.

Sigmoidoscopy is best performed in the unprepared bowel so that the earliest signs of ulcerative colitis can be detected without the hyperemia that so frequently follows preparative enemas.

In conclusion, the normal colon, endoscopically, appears to glisten and is salmon-pink in color[1,2]. There is a visible network of branching vessels identified throughout the colon. The smoothness of the mucosal surface and the absence of nodules or irregular polyps are the hallmarks of a healthy colon. There is a classic triangulated or semicircular configuration of the interhaustral markings. Contact bleeding, friability or exudates is not seen in a normal and healthy colon, and should not be explained as a result of the preparation [3].

References

[1] Xu F-x. Structure, principle and type of endoscope. In: Xu F-x (ed.) Endoscopy of the Lower Gastrointestinal Tract (1st ed.). Shang-hai, Shang-hai Science and Technology Press. 2003; P.19-25 (Chinese)

[2] Kruk KL, Lichtenstein GR. Inflammatory bowel disease. In: Ginsberg GG, Kochman ML, Norton I. Gastout CJ (eds.). Clinical Gastrointestinal Endoscopy. Printed in China Elsevier Saunders 2005;P.311-332

[3] ChutKan RK, Waye JD. Endoscopy in inflammatory bowel disease. In: Kirsner JB (ed.) Inflammatory Bowel Disease. 5th ed. Philadelphia: W.B. Saunders Company. 2000;P.453-477

[4] Carpenter HA, Talley NJ. The importance of clinicopathological correlation in the diagnosis of inflammatory conditions of the colon: histological patterns with clinical implications. *Am. J. Gastroenterol.* 2000;95(4):878-896.

Chapter VII

Colonoscopic Features of Ulcerative Colitis

Ping Xiang

Hua-dong Hospital, Fu-dan University, Shang-hai, P.R. China

Active Stage

In active ulcerative colitis (UC), the most typical appearance is that of a diffusely erythematous, edema, erosion and granular friable mucosa, with loss of the normal vascular pattern (table 7-1) [1,2].

In the initial stage, mucosal bleeding point and small erosion appear endoscopically [2-4]. The lesions begin at the anorectal junction and spread upwards in a homogeneous fashion. The upper limit of the diseased mucosa may be anywhere from the rectum. In the rectum, the earliest signs of UC are blurring or actual loss of the vascular pattern, together with hyperemic and edema of the mucosa (figure 7-1). The latter is often detected by thickened and blunted valves of Houston, which are normally sharp, crescentic folds (figure 7-1).

Table 7-1. Endoscopic features of ulcerative colitis [2,6]

features	occurrence
rectum	always involved
colonic lesions	continuous involvement
erythema	diffused distributed[1)
granularity	commonly seen
friability	commonly seen
erosion and/or ulcerations	always in areas of mucosal inflammation
psudopolyps	commonly seen

[1] replaces usual vascular pattern.

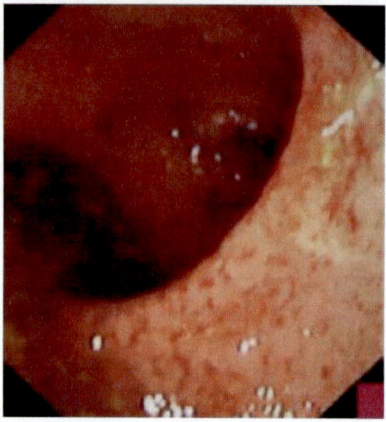 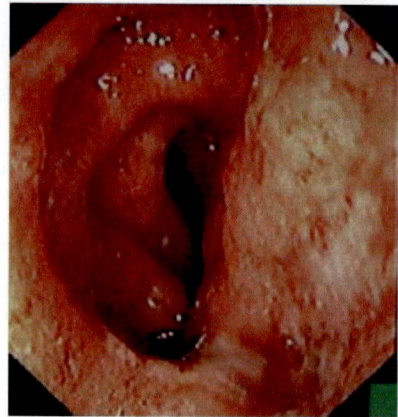

Figure 7-1. Ulcerative proctitis. There is losses of the vascular patient, and congestion, edema, thickened and blunted valves of Houston.

With more severe inflammation, the mucosa becomes granular; friability by the occurrence of small bleeding points when the mucosa is rubbed [5,6].

Finally, severe UC is associated with a mucosa that is spontaneously bleeding and with the presence of ulceration. These changes are diffuse and spread proximally from the rectum. The upper demarcation of disease can be identified endoscopically (figure 7-2). Ulcerations have variable size and depth [4,7]. Colonoscopy is the most accurate means of assessing the depth and extent of colonic ulcerations. They can be superficial, intermediate, or deep. Aphthoid ulcers are never seen in ulcerative colitis. Narrowing of the lumen and loss of haustra occur in long-standing UC. The terminal ileum is usually normal in UC. Nevertheless, UC patients with extensive colitis occasionally can have patchy mild inflammation in the terminal ileum, which is known as "backwash ileitis".

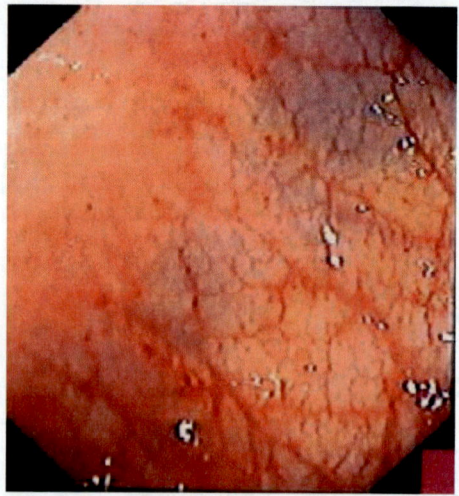

Figure 7-2. Ulcerative colitis. The mucosa with or without normal vascular network can be identified endoscopically.

Chronic Stage

After remission, the mucosa can return to normal, but it may became thin, pale, and atrophic, especially in patients who have had repeated attacks [1,4,6-8]. In chronic phase, there are lumen stenosis and pseudopolyp formation (figure 7-3). Development of colitis-associated colorectal cancer is an important clinical problem in patients with inflammatory bowel disease [4,9]. Endoscopy surveillance may prolongs life expectancy of patients with long-lasting IBD.

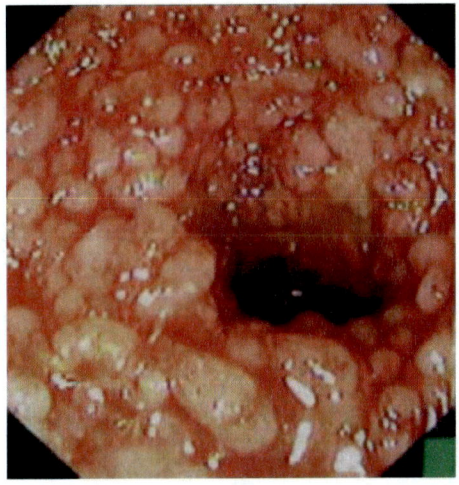

Figure 7-3. Ulcerative colitis involves transverse colon. A large number of pseudopolyps are seen in colonoscopy.

Severe Colitis

Severe attacks of ulcerative colitis are serious, and remain potentially lethal [1,4,6,7]. However, owing to the potential risk of perforation and colonic acute dilation, colonoscopy is often regarded as contraindicated in severe attacks of colitis.

Moreover, as severe lesions are found in more and 90% of patients in the left part of the colon, total colonoscopy is often not mandatory for patients in whom the diagnosis of UC has been previously clearly established.

Interpretation of endoscopic appearances is subject to considerable observer variation, especially in mild changes of hyperemia, edema, and granularity. Thus, any assessment of disease severity is always strengthened by a rectal biopsy specimen.

Colonoscopy is useful for determining the extent of disease [1,4,6-8]. Multiple biopsy specimens throughout the colon should be taken to map the histologic extent of disease as well as to confirm the diagnosis if there is doubt about Crohn's disease. In addition, mucosal hyperemia is frequently produced following preparation enemas.

References

[1] Osterman MT, Lewis JD. The role and importance of endoscopic mucosal healing in ulcerative colitis. *Tech. Gastrointest. Endosc.* 2004;6:144-153.

[2] ChutKan RK, Waye JD. Endoscopy in inflammatory bowel disease. In: Kirsner JB (ed.) Inflammatory Bowel Disease. 5th ed. Philadelphia: W.B. Saunders Company.2000; P.453-477.

[3] Zheng J-j. Clinical aspects of ulcerative colitis in mainland China. *Chin. J. Dig. Dis.* 2006;7(2):71-75.

[4] Xiang P, Bao Z-j, Xu F-x, et al. Endoscopic features and clinical analysis on ulcerative colitis. *Chin. J. Dig.* 2003; 23(4):217-219 (Chinese).

[5] Mamula P, Markowitz J. Special considerations for endoscopy in pediatric and adolescent patients with inflammatory bowel disease. *Tech. Gastrointest. Endosc.* 2004;6:159-164.

[6] Jia L-m, Zhou C-l, Pang Z. Ulcerative colitis. In: Zheng J-j (ed.). Inflammatory Bowel Disease - Clinical aspects, Pathology and Endoscopy. Bei-jing. Science Press 2004; P.51-78 (Chinese).

[7] Jing R, Xu F-x. Ulcerative colitis. In: Xu F-x (ed.). Endoscopy of the Lower Digestive Tract. Shang-hai. Shang-hai Science and Technology Press 2003; P.252-269 (Chinese).

[8] Gao F, Liu X, Ding N, et al. Comparisons of clinical characteristics in patients with ulcerative colitis between Uygur and Han nationality in Xing-jiang. *Chin. J. Dig. Endosc.* 2007; 24(6):423-426 (Chinese).

[9] Vleggaar FP, Lutgens MW, Claessen MM. The relevance of surveillance endoscopy in long-lasting inflammatory bowel disease (Review article). *Aliment Pharmacol. Ther.* 2007; 26:Suppl 2:47-52.

Chapter VIII

Colonoscopic Features of Crohn's Disease

Fu-xing Xu
Hua-dong Hospital, Fu-dan University, Shang-hai, P.R. China

Introduction

Endoscopically, the submucosal branching vascular network decreased or disappeared in the early stage of Crohn's disease (CD) [1,2]. In addition, pale mucosa, with superficial and tiny (pinpoint-like) or small, round ulcers (which are a result of a submucosal lymphoid follicle expansions, and are known as aphthoid ulcers) may be otherwise observed. In a moderate disease, the aphthous ulcers coalesce into larger ulcers. As the disease severity increases in chronicity, submucosal edema and injury result in the cobblestoning appearance of the mucosa, which is seen more often than in ulcerative colitis (UC) (table 8-1). Diverse patterns of mucosal and luminal lesions, representing different stages of the inflammation process can be simultaneously observed during endoscopic examination (table 8-2 and figure 8-1) [3,4]. Segments of normal mucosa are interspersed between and abnormal areas with definite border in springing style.

Table 8-1. Comparison of endoscopic features between ulcerative colitis and Crohn's colitis [1,4,5]

items	CD	UC
rectum	usually spared	involved
disease distribution	segmental, with skip area	continuous, uniform involvement
aphthous ulcer	common	never seen
vascular marking	present	loss
linea or serpiginous	common	not seen
mucosal granularity	may or may not seen	more often fine granular appearance "wet sandpaper-like"
mucosal friability	may or may not seen	more frequently seen than in CD

Table 8-1. (Continued).

items	CD	UC
cobblestoning from submucosa edema	common	not seen
fistulas	commonly seen	not seen
terminal ileum	ulcerations, commonly seen	normal appearance except in "backwash ileitis"
thick interhaustral septam	common	common

Table 8-2. Endoscopic features of Crohn's colitis (colonic Crohn's disease) [1,4,5]

features	occurrence
rectum	usually spared
bowel involvement	discontinuous, segmental
vascular pattern	usually present
aphthous ulcers	common in early stage
linear ulcers	common
mucosal granularity	may or may not seen
cobbestoning	common (often in severe patients)
pseudopolyps	common
mucosal friability	unusual
thick interhaustral septum	yes

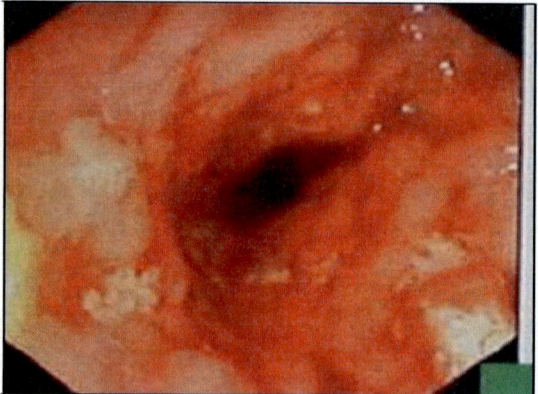

Figure 8-1. The characteristic colonoscopic pattern is a combination of erythema, edema, obscure or loss of the normal vascular pattern, multiple ulcers and/or strictures. Note the fissuring ulcer and stenosis in the margin of the descending colon.

Ulcers

Aphthoid ulcers and indulge-shaped ulcers are features in CD. Ulcers, whether superficial or deep, are frequently surrounded by normal mucosa [1-3]. Aphthoid ulcers usually occur in crops on an otherwise normal mucosa (figure 8-2). They strongly suggest CD, but are not pathognomonic of it. In Crohn's ileocolitis, sampling aphthoid ulcers with biopsy and, to a lesser degree, the edge of other ulcerations gives the best yield for granulomas. Ulcers in CD tend to destroy the initial cluster of epithelioid cells, lowering the incidence of biopsy-demonstrable granulomas. An effective biopsy is also important in helping a diagnosis establishment in CD and UC [1]. The presence of small ulcerations on the ileocecal valve or in the small bowel is virtually pathognomonic of CD [1].

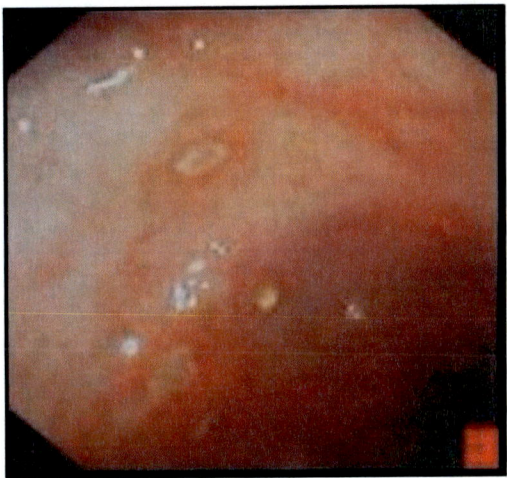

Figure 8-2. Aphthous ulcer in an area of basically normal mucosa (in the sigmoid colon region).

Cobblestoning Lesions

Cobblestoning with a rough irregular nodular mucosal pattern is quite characteristic of CD (figure 8-3) [4,5]. In contrast to pseudopolyps, the base of a cobblestone "island" is wider than its height. Endoscopically, the lesions are projecting, blunt-round at top, semi-spherical from side-view, around with ulcers, in the presence of nodules of every size, looks like cobblestoning street.

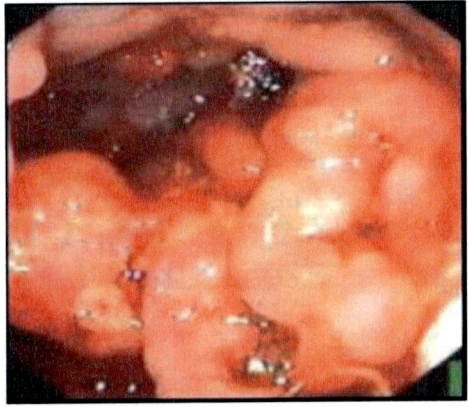

Figure 8-3. Cobblestoned islands of mucosa (that often are histologically normal, surrounded on all sides by fused aphthoid ulcers).

Pseudopolyps

Pseudopolys are, a little different from nodular form of cobblestoning lesion, usually multiple nodules (figure 8-4) [3,4]. They may present as nodular erythema on normal-colored mucosa or myriads of finger-like mucosal projections. Occasionally, pseudopolyps are sufficiently large or numerous to cause narrowing of the lumen. Mucosal bridge can also be frequently observed in patients in chronic stage (figure 8-5) [4,5].

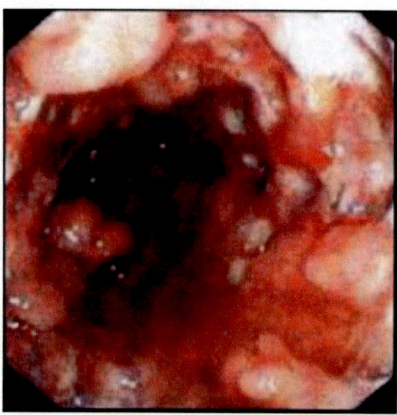

Figure 8-4. Inflammatory pseudopolyps.

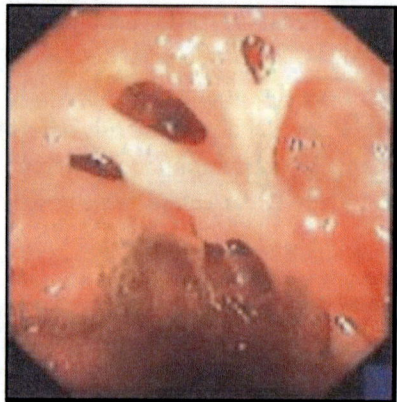

Figure 8-5. A mucosal bridge which is the result of healed inflammation with re-epithelialization of the mucosal tube created by undermining ulcerations.

Stenoses

Fibrotic stenoses in the later term of the disease are induced by extensive fibrosis of colon wall. Stenosed lumina are usually roundly deformed. Any stricture should raise the suspicion of carcinoma. Smooth, inactive-looking strictures in endoscopy are usually benign.

Fistulas

Compared to UC, fistulas are only seen in CD (figure 8-6). Table 8-2.[5]. The fistulous opening may not be readily apparent in endoscopy, and is often surrounded by marked focal edema and erythema.

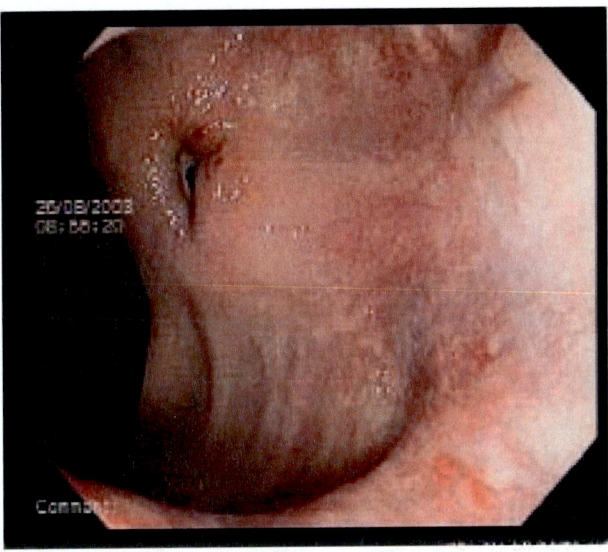

Figure 8-6. Crohn's disease showing fistulous opening, which may not be readily apparent, and is often surrounded by marked focal edema and erythema.

References

[1] Kivsch R, Pentecost M, Hall PM. Role of colonoscopic biopsy in distinguishing between Crohn's disease and intestinal tuberculosis. *J. Clin. Pathol.* 2006 Aug;59(8):840-4

[2] Stange EF, Travis SP, Vermeire S, et al. European evidence based consensus on the diagnosis and management of Crohn's disease: definitions and diagnosis. *Gut.* 2006;55 Suppl 1:i1-15

[3] Jin R, Xu F-x. Crohn's disease. In: Xu Fx (ed.) Endoscopy of the Lower Gastrointestinal Tract (1st ed.). Shang-hai, Shang-hai Science and Technology Press 2003; P.270-281 (Chinese).

[4] Zheng J-j, Cu X-q, Shi X-h, et al. Colonoscopic and histologic features of colonic Crohn's disease in Chinese patients. *J. Dig. Dis.* 2007;8(1):35-41

[5] Lee SD, Cohen RD. Endoscopy in inflammatory bowel disease. *Gastroenterol. Clin. N. Am.* 2002;31(1):119-132.

In: Inflammatory Conditions of the Colon
Editor: Jia-ju Zheng

ISBN: 978-1-60692-240-8
© 2008 Nova Science Publishers, Inc.

Chapter IX

Crohn's Disease of the Upper Gastrointestinal Tract: The Value of Esophagogastroduodenoscopic Examination

Wen-jun Zhang and Zhao-shen Li
Chang-hai Hospital, Second Military Medical University, Shang-hai, P.R.China

Since its first description in the terminal ileum in 1932, Crohn's disease (CD) has been identified in all parts of the gastrointestinal (GI) tract i.e., from mouth to anus [1]. The involvement of the upper GI tract has been considered to be a rare manifestation of CD [2].

Retrospective studies have reported prevalence figures of 0.5% 13% [3]. In adults, reported prevalence figures for each separate localization are: mouth 6–9%, esophagus 1.8%, stomach and or duodenum 1.8 - 4.5%. The diagnosis of CD of the upper GI tract is based on clinical, radiological, endoscopic and histologic features.

Esophagogastroduodenoscopy (EGD or upper endoscopy) - An EGD is a procedure that allows the physician to examine the inside of the esophagus, stomach, and duodenum [2,3]. A thin, flexible, lighted tube, called an endoscope, is guided into the mouth and throat, then into the esophagus, stomach, and duodenum. The endoscope allows the physician to view the inside of this area of the body, as well as to insert instruments through a scope for the removal of a sample of tissue for biopsy.

Esophagus

Patients with advanced esophageal involvement usually present with odynophagia, dysphagia, pyrosis and retrosternal chest pain, and sometimes with severe weight loss [4]. Early lesions, however, can exist without any complaint. Coughing and aspiration pneumonia can be the result of a complicating esophagotrachial fistula. Usually the activity of CD in the esophagus parallels that of the disease of CD elsewhere in the GI tract. The distal part of the esophagus is predominantly involved.

Endoscopic examination may reveal hyperaemia, granularity, slight friability of the mucosa, nodular thickening or cobblestones, mucosal defects such as erosions, aphthoid ulcers, superficial and deep ulcers (figure 9-1), and stenotic parts [2,3]. Huchzermeyer differentiated two stages in the oesophageal inflammatory process [2]: stage I, in which inflammatory changes predominate as a mild or more often erosive-ulcerative esophagitis, and stage II, in which a stenosing form is present. These morphological changes are predominantly limited to the lower part of the esophagus. Upper endoscopic findings have to be differentiated from severe gastroesophageal reflux disease, opportunistic infections in immune compromised patients, and carcinoma. Histological evaluation of biopsies usually demonstrates focal inflammation and infrequently granulomas. With additional sectioning the detection rate of a granuloma can be increased.

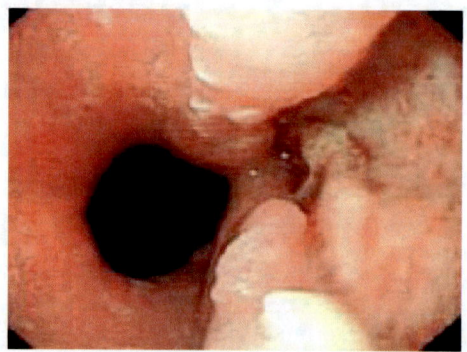

Figure 9-1. Crohn's disease with esophageal involvement showing ulcer in upper GI endoscopy.

The diagnosis is routinely based on radiography and/or endoscopy with histological findings. The use of newer diagnostic tools, like endosonography, can contribute to establishing the diagnosis of esophageal CD. However, the upper endoscopic findings are non-specific and may resemble those of a T2 carcinoma.

Stomach and Duodenum

Symptoms which are frequently encountered in patients with gastroduodenal CD are epigastric pain or dyspepsia, which mimic peptic ulcer or non-ulcer dyspepsia [2,3]. Anorexia is also a common symptom. In more advanced disease, when obstruction has developed, the most predominant symptoms are epigastric distress, early satiety, nausea, vomiting and weight loss. Since patients with gastroduodenal CD nearly always have concomitant lesions in the ileum and/or colon, it is hard to determine whether upper GI symptoms are due to CD of the upper GI tract or not. Wagtmans et al compared the clinical aspects of CD of the upper GI tract with those of distal CD. The main symptoms of the proximal CD group were abdominal pain and/or cramps, diarrhea, weight loss, general malaise, and anorexia and/or nausea. Compared with patients having only distal CD, particularly abdominal pain and/or cramps and general malaise were observed more frequently in the proximal CD group. Complications such as chronic or acute blood loss from the upper GI tract with hematemesis and melaena are rare. Other complications that are seldom seen are: gastric or duodenal fistulae originating from diseased small or large bowel, fistulae between a narrowed bulbus and the common bile duct, and biliary colics or pancreatitis because of CD in the peri-ampullary region. Of the stomach, the antrum is usually involved, and duodenal CD is often associated with antral involvement. Isolated duodenal involvement is more frequent than isolated CD of the stomach. Any part of the duodenum can be involved, but the second part is most commonly affected.

CD of the stomach and duodenum endoscopically resembles distal CD [2,3]. The abnormalities found include patchy erythema, granularity, verrucous changes, aphthoid ulcers, superficial and deep ulcers (figure 9-2), thickened folds and cobblestones. Narrowing may predominantly be seen in the prepyloric region, in the duodenal bulb and the second part of the duodenum (figure 9-3). Mucosal defects were better visualized by endoscopy, whereas features such as diminished expansion and contiguity of lesions were better demonstrated by radiological examination.

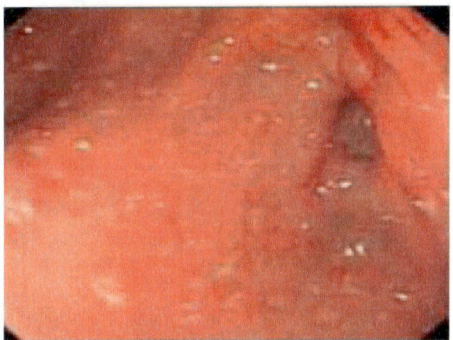

Figure 9-2. Crohn's disease with stomach involvement showing superficial ulcer in gastroduodenoscopy.

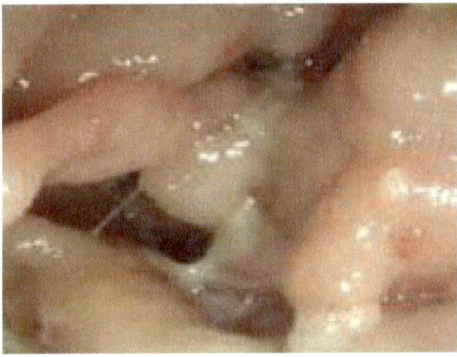

Figure 9-3. Crohn's disease with duodenenal involvement showing proliferative lesions in gastroduodenoscopy.

Microscopical evaluation of biopsies from endoscopically involved mucosa may reveal non-caseating epitheloid granulomas, mucosal inflammation, lymphangiectasy, lymphoid aggregates, fibrosis and 'crypt' abscess [2,3]. It is known that granuloma and mucosal inflammation can also be found in normally appearing mucosa. Studies in which multiple endoscopic biopsies were taken with serial sectioning into a high amount of slices yielded a higher number of granulomas.

References

[1] Crohn BB, Ginzburg L, Oppenheimer GD. Regional ileitis: a pathological and clinical entity. *JAMA*. 1932;99:1323-1328.

[2] Lemberg DA, Clarkson CM, Bohane TD, et al. Role of esophagogastroduodenoscopy in the initial assessment of children with inflammatory bowel disease. *J. Gastroenterol. Hepatol.* 2005; 20(11):1696-1700

[3] Witte AM, Veenendaal RA, Van Hogezand RA, et al. Crohn's disease of the upper gastrointestinal tract:the value of endoscopic examination. *Scand. J. Gastroenterol. Suppl.* 1998; 225:100-105.

[4] Huchzermeyer H, Paul F, Seifert E,et al. Endoscopic results in five patients with Crohn's disease of the esophagus. *Endoscopy.* 1977; 8(2):75-81.

In: Inflammatory Conditions of the Colon
Editor: Jia-ju Zheng

ISBN: 978-1-60692-240-8
© 2008 Nova Science Publishers, Inc.

Chapter X

The Role of EUS in the Diagnosis and Treatment of Inflammatory Bowel Disease and Other Indetermined Colitis

Qi Zhu
Rui-jin Hospital, Shang-hai Jiao-tong University School of Medicine,
Shang-hai, P.R. China

Introduction

The differentiation between ulcerative colitis (UC), Crohn's diease (CD), and other indetermined colitis can be difficult and is currently made through careful interpretation of clinical, endoscopic, barium enema and histologic findings. Furthermore, accurate assessment of the severity of inflammatory bowel disease (IBD) plays an important role in selecting treatment and in evaluating the need for surgery. However, these conventional diagnostic modalities are limited only to evaluate superficial changes in the bowel mucosa. Over the past few years, endoscopic ultrasonography (EUS) has become a useful modality for the diagnosis of gastrointestinal disease, because it allows visualization of the entire bowel wall thickness and changes in tissue density which may be correlated with the histological findings through cross-sectional imaging. These indicated that EUS may be helpful in the evaluation of IBD and other indetermined colitis. Also, EUS can be used in the diagnosis and management of extraintestinal manifestations of IBD, because it has the ability to accurately provide the anatomic details of the perianal and perirectal regions [1].

Equipment and General Principles

A variety of instruments including traditional linear or radial type echocolonoscopy (working frequency varies from 5 to 20 MHz), as well as high frequency miniprobe ultrasonography (MPS, working frequency 15, 20 MHz) can be used in the evaluation of

IBD. Although conventional echocolonoscopy can be more useful in the examination of peri-intestinal lymph node and perianal and perirectal region due to its distant visualization with lower frequency, MPS may be the optimal instrument with the advantage that it can be performed conveniently during colonoscopy and can provide enhanced image resolution, as well as the ability to access the strictures[2]. When evaluating perianorectal diseases, linear probes have an advantage over radial probes because the former potential allows visualization of the entire fistulous tract. On the other hand, radial images can only demonstrate a limited cross-sectional view of the tract [3].

Preparation for EUS and Bowel Evaluation

The preparation of the bowel for EUS was similar to that of conventional colonoscopic examination. Spasmolysant was given before the operation. Sedation was given when necessary. De-aerated water filling, water balloon or both were used to allow acoustic coupling between the transducer and the bowel wall. EUS evaluation was included in the assessment of: 1. the bowel wall thickness including the total wall thickness and the thickness of mucosa, submucosa, muscularis propria, and serosa/adventitia, 2. the structure of the wall including defects in layers, hypoechoic changes, and the boundary of the layer, 3. the presence of pseudopolyp, mucosal bridge as well as its echo pattern, form, boundary and size, 4. the presence of submucosal vessels > 2 mm, 5. the number of peri-intestinal lymph nodes visualized, 6. the presence of perianal and perirectal fistula and abscess as well as its location, echo pattern, boundary and size.

EUS Features of Normal Colonic Layers

Like other parts of the gastrointestinal tract, the normal colonic wall was divided into 5 layers by EUS (figure 10-1). The first hyper echoic and second hypo echoic layer corresponded to the mucosa and lamina propria, the third hyper echoic layer to the submucosa, the fourth hypo echoic layer to the muscularis propria and the fifth hyper echoic layer to the subserosa and serosa or the tunica adventitia. Mean colonic wall thickness was 2.2 mm in normal subject. The total wall (TW), m, sm, and mp were significantly thicker in the rectum than in the colon. There was no significant difference in the thickness between each segment of the colon. The bowel wall thickening was considered when TW was beyond 3.2mm. Tsuga et al [4] classified the boundary of each layer into three patterns (smooth, irregular, and blurred) and then classified the wall into six types (Tsuga types). In type I, both the mucosa-submucosa (m-sm) and submucosa–muscularis propria (sm-mp) boundaries were smooth, and the wall thickness was normal. In type II, both boundaries were smooth but the wall was thickened. In type IIIa, the m-sm boundary was irregular, the sm-mp boundary was smooth, and the wall was thickened. In type IIIb, both boundaries were irregular and the wall was thickened. In type IVa, the m-sm boundary was blurred, the sm-mp boundary was smooth, and the wall was thickened. In type IVb, the m-sm boundary was blurred, the sm-mp boundary was irregular, and the wall was thickened. When the boundary was abnormal but wall thickness was normal, the boundary change took precedence over the wall thickening in determining classification.

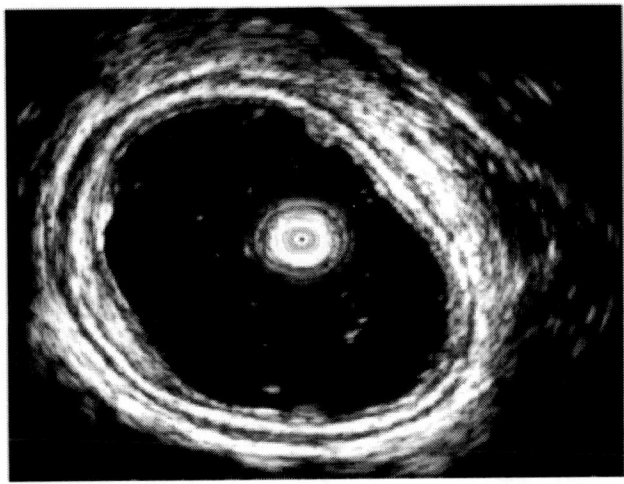

Figure 10-1. The normal colonic wall. The five layers are clearly shown by EUS.

Application of EUS in Inflammatory Bowel Disease

The role of EUS in the evaluation of IBD: The clinical application of EUS includes the assessment of disease severity, differentiation between UC and CD, evaluation for medical or surgical therapy and selection of patients for ileoanal pouch reconstruction. Bowel wall thickness measured by EUS was significantly increased in both UC and CD patients when compared with normal group. Inflammatory changes were observed as hypoechoic changes and defects in the wall layer. The depth of inflammatory change tends to be increased when disease was developed and disappeared when remission. In UC patients, the wall thickness was mainly caused by the thickness of m, mm or sm, or totally. Its structure of layers was blurry but still identifiable (figure 10-2 to figure 10-10). There was a strong correlation between inflammatory depth, colonic wall thickness and severity of colonoscopic changes and a moderate correlation between colonic wall thickness and disease activity score. In the CD group, it was impossible to identify the structure of involved layers with significant thickness of mp layer. Sometimes, the normal structure of the five layers can disappear completely in severe cases (figure 10-7, figure 10-8). There was a strong correlation between identification of wall layers and disease activity score and a moderate correlation between wall thickness and severity of histologic changes in these patients. Furthermore, the EUS imaging of bowel wall structure can be valuable in the prediction of remission and relapse of disease (figure 10-9). Our study showed that although there was no apparent change with total wall in UC patients during remission (3.84+0.64mm/3.62+0.61mm, p=0.15), the thickness of sm decreased significantly when compared with active stage (2.96+0.73mm/2.12+0.35mm, p<0.01), and the boundary of layers were recovered at the same time. In some cases, the presence of submucosal vessels (>2mm) can be detected and it disappeared during remission. But for enlarged lymph node (figure 10-10), there was no obvious change [5]. There was one study also revealed that for those patients who relapsed after remission, the m~sm was significantly thickened compared with those who did not relapse [6]. Most recently, a study shows that although the median thickness of the affected intestinal wall did not differ significantly, inflammation was evaluated to extend to the muscularis propria or deeper on EUS in a significantly greater proportion of patients who underwent surgery than in those who responded to medical treatment (67%vs.19%,p=0.002)[7]. So the conclusion that the structure change of bowel wall detected by EUS can be used to decide the necessity of operations was drawn [8]. Despite of controversy over the selection of surgical treatment for UC patients, when used in combination with the clinical, endoscopic, radiologic and pathologic parameters, EUS may contribute to the differential diagnosis and management of IBD. The different characteristics of EUS imaging between UC and CD see table 10-1.

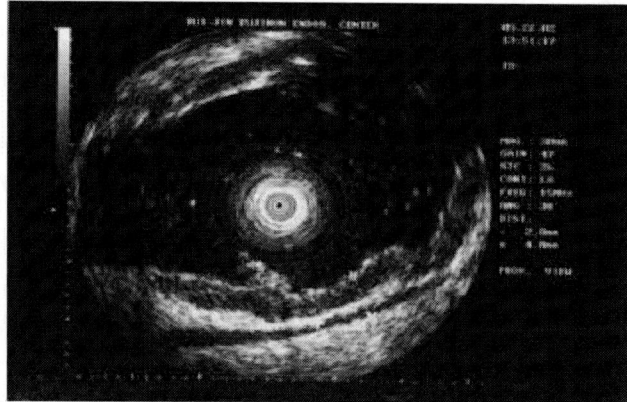

Figure 10-2. The active phase of UC. The increased wall thickness is mainly caused by the thickened m or/and sm.

Table 10-1.

characteristics	UC	CD
depth of inflammation	deeper with severity, mainly m-sm	various but tends transmural disease
bowel wall structure	irregular or blurred but still identifiable	the structure of involved layers disappeared completely
wall thickness	moderately thicken	severely thicken
distribution	continuous lesion	skip lesion
submural vessels > 2mm	Seldom	more frequently
perianorectal complications	Seldom	more frequently
enlarged lymph node	two or more	zero or one

The Role of EUS in the Diagnosis and Treatment... 57

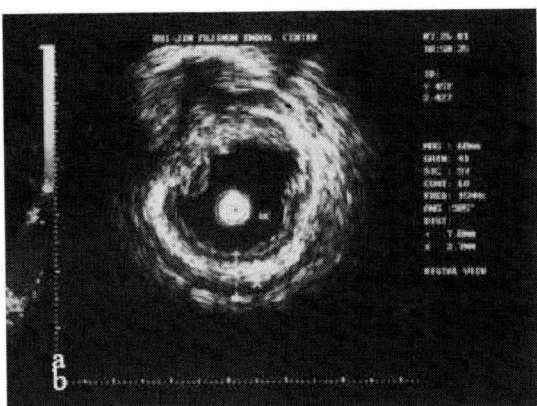

Figure 10-3. The active phase of UC. The increased wall thickness is mainly caused by the thickened sm.

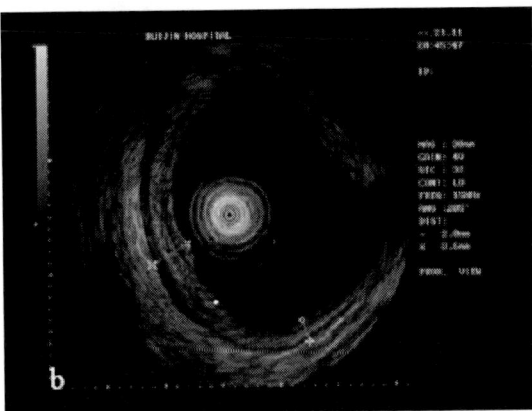

Figure 10-4. The wall thickness is increased in the active phase of UC, with blurred structure.

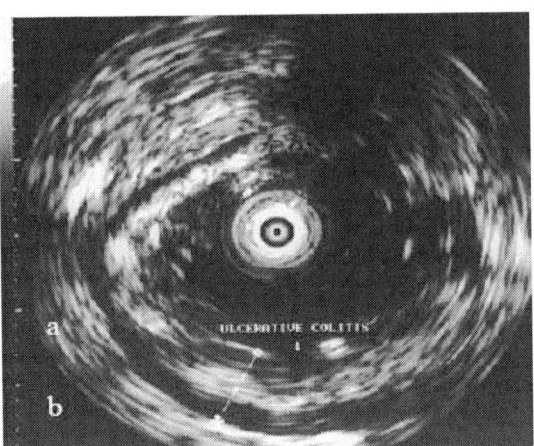

Figure 10-5. The whole bowel wall is thickened in the UC patient, with local ulcerative changes.

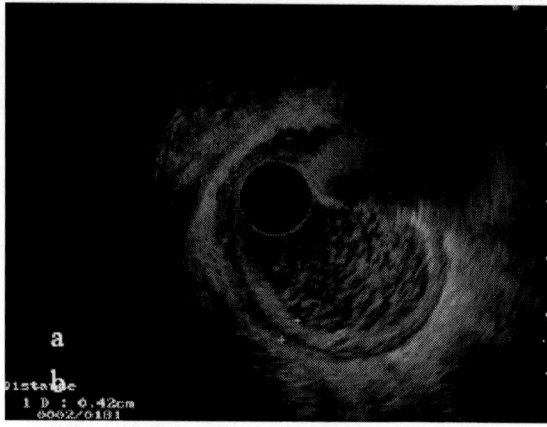
Figure 10-6. The thickened wall is detected by the radial type of EUS in the UC patient, with blurred structures.

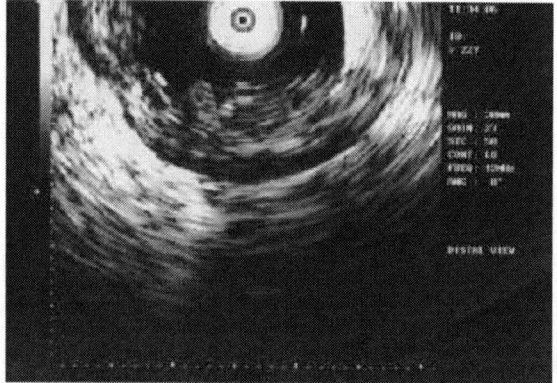
Figure 10-7. The bowel wall in CD is thickened, with destroyed structure.

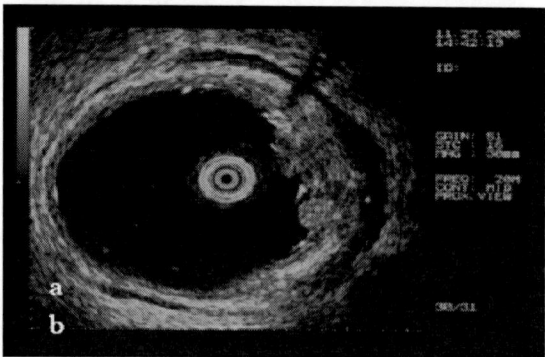
Figure 10-8. The m-sm layers are destroyed in the active phase of CD, with thickened mp.

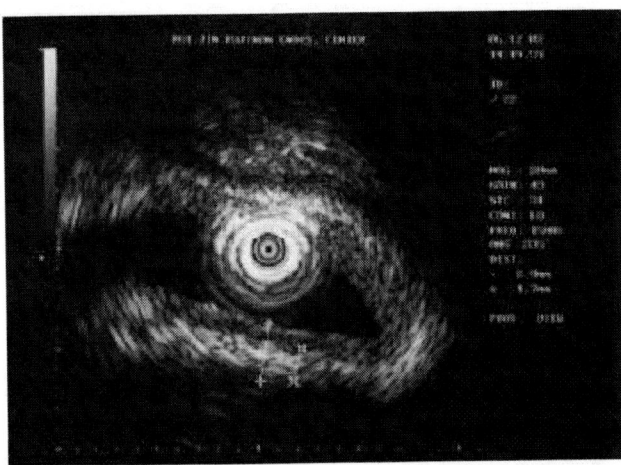

Figure 10-9. The thickness of bowel wall returned to normal in the remission phase.

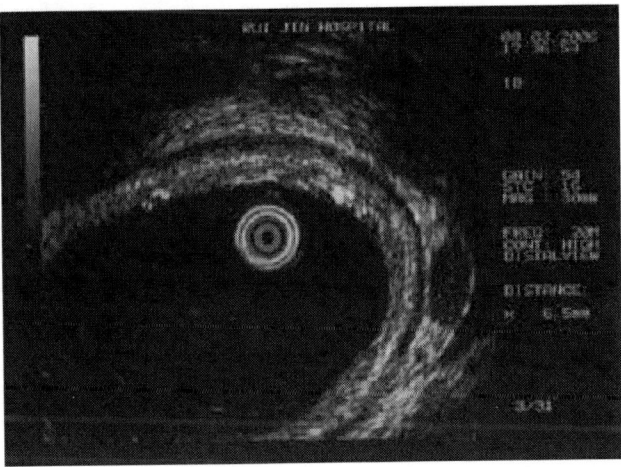

Figure 10-10. The increased peri-intestinal lymph node is shown in the active phase of UC.

EUS in Perianorectal Complications of Inflammatory Bowel Disease

The role of EUS in the management of perianorectal complications: Abscesses and fistulas in perianal and perirectal region were the common complications of IBD. 32 to 50% of Patients with CD will develop perianal complications. EUS can provide excellent information about the local anatomy, thus it has the potential to emerge as a powerful imaging modality in the management of perianorectal complications. The EUS image of the fistula was a hypoechoic or anechoic duct-like structure localized within the perianorectal region with typical hyperechoic focus due to retained air (figure 10-11, figure 10-12). Abscesses were sonographically described as anechoic or hypoechoic cavities localized in the perianorectal structures with or without the presence of fistula. Compared with other imaging methods, EUS has been demonstrated to be superior to conventional ultrasonography, fistulography, CT, and equal with or superior to MRI [9]. Also, EUS can be useful to guide the selection of therapeutic approach. Surgical intervention is only used in cases that are refractory to medical management due to the highly risk of fecal incontinence and thus the accurate anatomic information provided by EUS is required. Recurrence of perianorectal fistulas and abscesses is frequent in IBD. Commonly, this is due to the false healing after medical treatment [10]. Study indicated that EUS can demonstrate the persistence of the internal tract after endoscopic healing and is useful in the guidance of therapy.

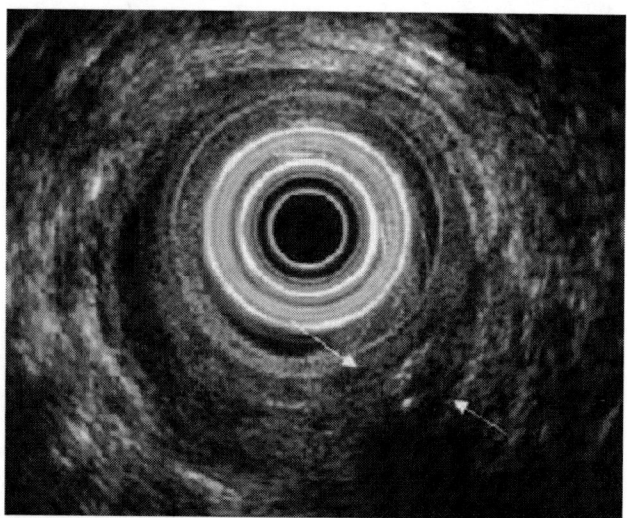

Figure 10-11. Anal fistula in CD which is pointed out by the arrow in the internal and external sphincters as the hypo echoic region with the inflammatory changes around and hyper echoic air shadow inside the fistula. [11]

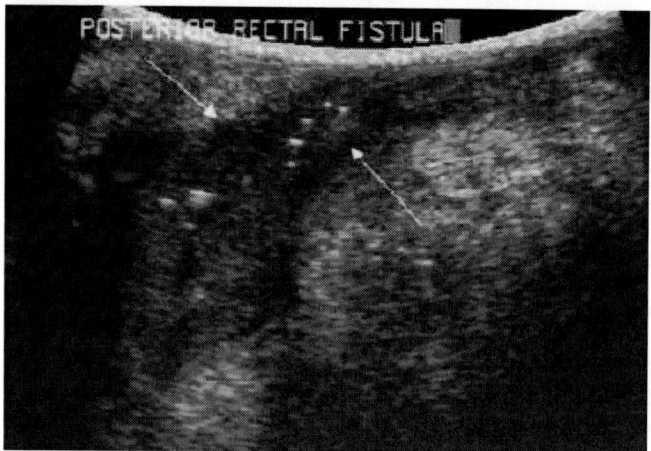

Figure 10-12. Anal fistula in CD. The hyper echoic air shadow inside the fistula is moved with the movement of the tip of the endoscopy when it compressed the wall of the lesion. [11]

The Value of EUS in Colorectal Cancer Associated with Inflammatory Bowel Disease

The value of EUS in the colorectal carcinoma associated with IBD (figure 10-13) [11]: There has been significant increase in the risk of colorectal carcinoma among IBD patients, especially UC. It was estimated that about 5% to 10% of UC patients will suffer from colorectal carcinoma in 20 years. The optimal treatment includes early detection and removal surgically. However, the pseudopolyps and granuloma accompanying IBD patients make the detection of malignancy more difficult, which makes it difficult to accurately launch endoscopic biopsy. For the ability to image the gastrointestinal wall and peri-intestinal structure clearly, EUS has become a useful modality for the diagnosis of malignant disease especially early carcinoma. The EUS imaging of malignancy was the limited disruption of wall structure with irregular hypoechoic changes. Pseudopolyps and mucosal bridge were moderate hyperechoic structures originating from mucosa. EUS can not only accurately detect the bowel malignant lesion, but also conduct precise evaluation of the invasive depth and enlarged lymph node. EUS guided fine-needle aspiration biopsy can also be provided when a metastases lymph node was suspected.

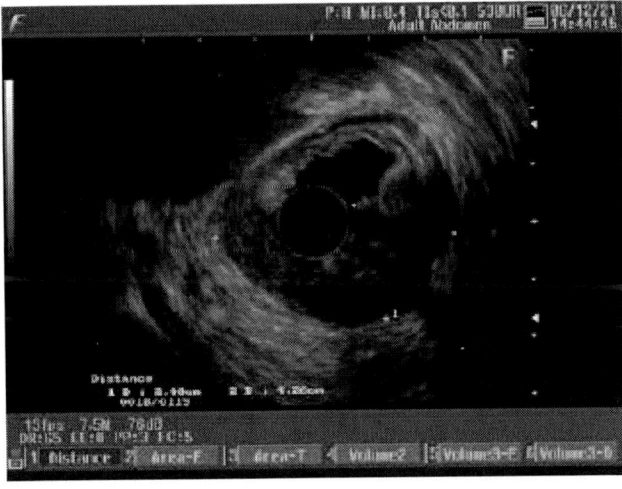

Figure 10-13. UC is complicated with rectal carcinoma.

References

[1] Lew RJ, Ginsberg GG. The role of endoscopic ultrasound in inflammatory bowel disease. *Gastrointest. Endosc. Clin. North Am.* 2002; 12: 561-571.

[2] Parente F, Greco S, Melteni M, et al. Imaging inflammatory bowel disease using bowel ultrasound. *Eur .J. Gastroenterol. Hepatol.* 2005; 17(3):283-91.

[3] Hollerweger A. Colonic diseases: the value of US examination. *Eur. J. Radiol.* 2007; 64(2):239-49.

[4] Tsuga K, Haruma K, Fujimura J, et al. Evaluation of the colorectal wall in normal subjects and patients with ulcerative colitis using an ultrasonic catheter probe. *Gastrointest. Endosc.* 1998; 48: 477-84.

[5] Zhu Q, Xia L, Xu K, et al. The elimentary assessment of high frequency miniprobe ultrasonography (MPS) in estimating the remission of UC. The assembling of the 2nd national IBD conference of China. 2006; P. 4. (Chinese).

[6] Higaki S, Nohara H, Saitoh Y, et al. Increased Rectal Wall Thickness May Predict Relapse in Colitis: A Pilot Follow-Up Study by Ultrasonographic Colonoscopy. *Endoscopy.* 2002; 34:212-219.

[7] Yoshizawa S, Kiyonori K, Katsumata T, et al. Clinical usefulness of EUS for active ulcerative colitis. *Gastrointest. Endosc.* 2007; 65: 253-60.

[8] Rieger N, Tjandra, Slomon M, et al. Endoanal and endorectal ultrasound: applications in colorectal surgery. *ANZ. J. Surg.* 2004; 74(8):671-5.

[9] Orsoni P, Barthet M, Portier F, et al. Prospective comparison of endosonography, magnetic resonance imaging and surgical findings in anorectal fistula and abscess complicating Crohn's disease. *Br. J. Surg.* 1999; 86: 360-364.

[10] Kamm MA, Ng SC. Perianal fistulizing Crohn's disease: a call to action. *Clin. Gastroenterol. Hepatol.* 2008; 6(1):7-10.

[11] Schwartz DA, Harewood GC, Wiersema MJ. EUS for rectal disease. *Gastrointest. Endosc.* 2002 ; 56 :100-109.

Chapter XI

Double Balloon Endoscopy in Diagnosis of Inflammatory Bowel Disease

Jie Zhong
Ru-jin Hospital, Shang-hai Jiao-tong University Medical School,
Shang-hai, P.R.China

Introduction and Indications

Double balloon endoscopy (DBE) is a new diagnostic and therapeutic modality originally described by Yamamoto et al. in 2001 that allows high resolution visualization, diagnosis-making and therapeutic interventions in all segments of the small intestine [1].

At present, the main indications for DBE are as follows: [1,2]

1. the etiologic investigation of obscure gastrointestinal bleeding (OGIB) and intestinal obstruction
2. diagnosis of suspected inflammatory bowel diseases(IBD), small bowel diarrhea, chronic abdominal pain with abnormal radiological studies or capsule endoscopy (CE) findings, and disease severity evaluation.
3. therapeutic interventions such as Argon plasma coagulation(APC), dilation, stenting, polypectomy, endoscopic mucosal resection (EMR) could also be performed under the DBE technique

Contraindications

The contraindications of DBE are as similar as for routine gastroscopy and colonoscopy.

The Instrument

The DBE system consists of four parts:

1. *Endoscopy (EN-450P5, EN-450T5):* Two types of dedicated scope are available. (1) EN-450P5 is a standard scope with better insertability, it has a working length of 2000mm, outer diameter of 8.5 mm, and forceps channel diameter of 2.2mm. (2)EN-450T5 is a treatment scope with more therapeutic capabilities, it has a working length of 2000mm, outer diameter of 9.4mm, and forceps channel diameter of 2.8 mm.

2. *Overtube (TS-12140, TS-13140)*: Two types of overtube are available. One is the TS-12140 (outer diameter 12.2mm, length 1450mm) for use with the EN-450P5, and the other is the TS-13140 (outer diameter 13.2mm, length 1450mm) for use with the EN-450T5.

3. *Scope Balloon (BS-1):* Two latex balloons are attached separately to tip of the enteroscope and the overtube, and are inflated and deflated with a balloon pump controller that supplies and withdraws air.

4. *Balloon Pump Controller (PB-20)*: The pump controller controls inflation and deflation of both balloons.

DBE Procedures

The endoscope could be introduced either by the antegrade (oral) or retrograde (anal) route, the choice of route is mainly determined by the patients' clinical presentation and the results of previous investigations. DBE from oral approach requires no specific preparation other than an 8-12 hour fast before the procedure. When the anal route was indicated, a standard bowel cleaning as for colonoscopy is necessary. Sedation may be achieved with standard conscious sedation, propofol, or general anesthesia.

Before endoscopic insertion, the overtube was slid over the endoscope from the tip with both balloons deflated. When the tip scope and overtube reached to duodenum from the oral approach or the cecum from the anal approach, the overtube balloon was inflated to keep the tube in position, while the endoscope was advanced as much as possible. Then, the balloon of the endoscope was inflated, while the balloon of the overtube was deflated. The overtube was then advanced towards the endoscope tip. When the distal end of the overtube reached the endoscope tip, the overtube balloon was inflated to secure its position within the intestine. Gentle withdrawal of overtube and endoscope (with both balloons inflated) allowed for pleating of the intestine on the overtube in the process shortening the intestine and preventing looping were achieved as well.

In the two-person DBE, the endoscopist controlled and maneuvered the enteroscope while the assistant was responsible for advancement and withdrawal of the instruments, control of the balloons inflation and deflation.

Characteristics of Crohn's Disease (CD) in DBE

1. The lesion could be found in any part of GI tract. The most common involved area was small bowel, especially ileum. In near half patients the colon could be involved. And rectum sparing is frequent.
2. The earlier endoscopic manifestation of CD is the aphthous ulcer, a small discrete ulcer of millimeters in diameter surrounded by a thin red halo of edematous tissue.
3. In active CD, ulcers may be round or long and serpiginous. Large, deep, penetrating ulcers can be surrounded by areas of normal-appearing mucosa. The combination of linear ulceration and transverse fissuring, with submucosal edema and inflammation produces the characteristic "cobblestone" appearance. And the ulcer may merge into a longitude ulcer paralleling with the axis of the bowel. (figure 11-1)
4. Ileocecal involvement often produces a thickened ileocecal valve with deformity of the cecum.
5. Mucosal involvement in CD is not contiguous; patches of involvement are typically interspersed with normal "skip" areas. (figure 11-2)
6. In patients with long-standing disease, persistent inflammatory process and repeated fibrosis may result in intestinal stricture and even obstruction. (figure 11-3)

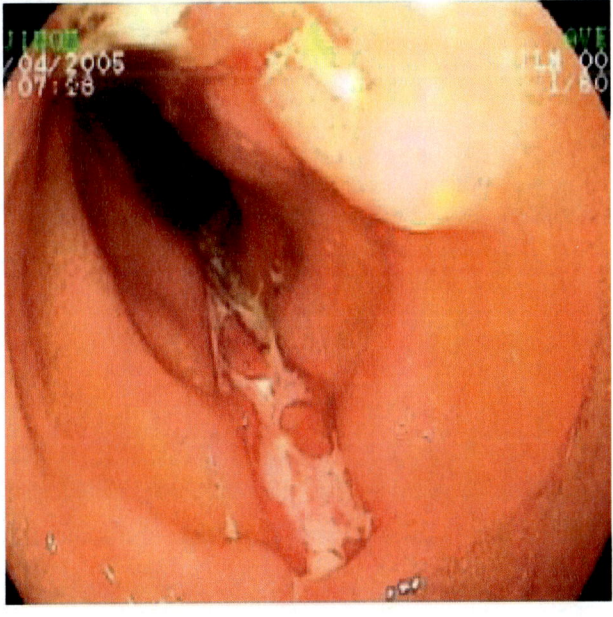

Figure 11-1. Longitudinal ulcer in CD.

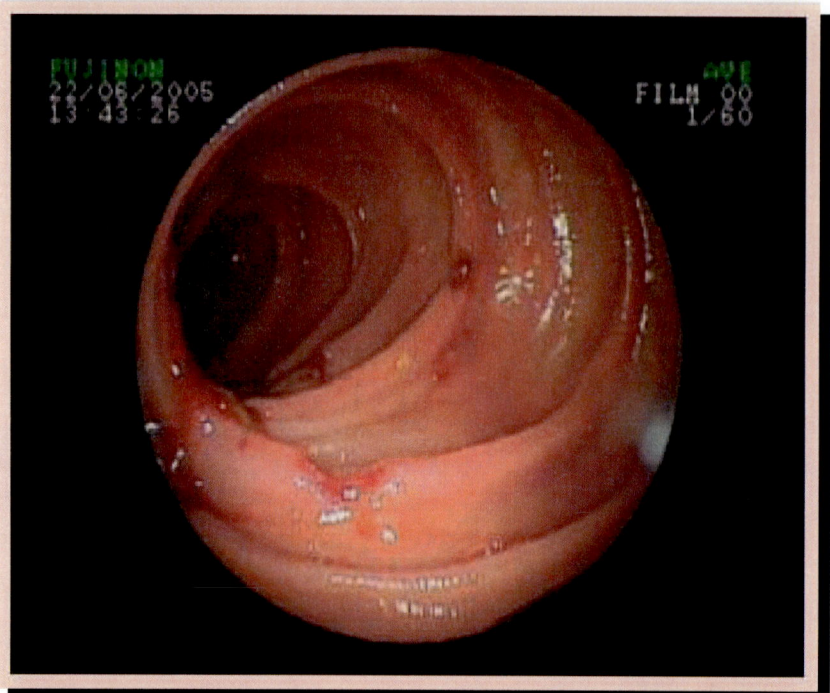

Figure 11-2. Skip lesions in CD.

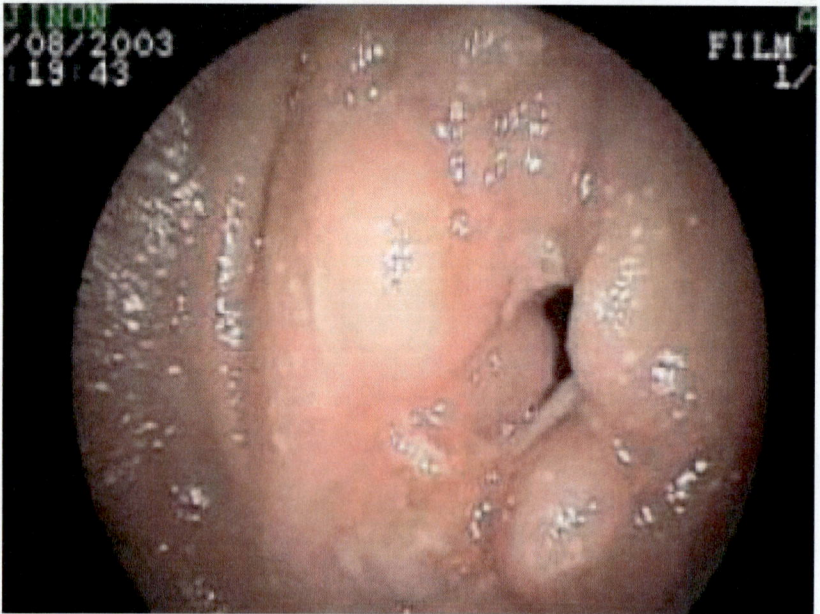

Figure 11-3. Crohn's disease showing intestinal stricture.

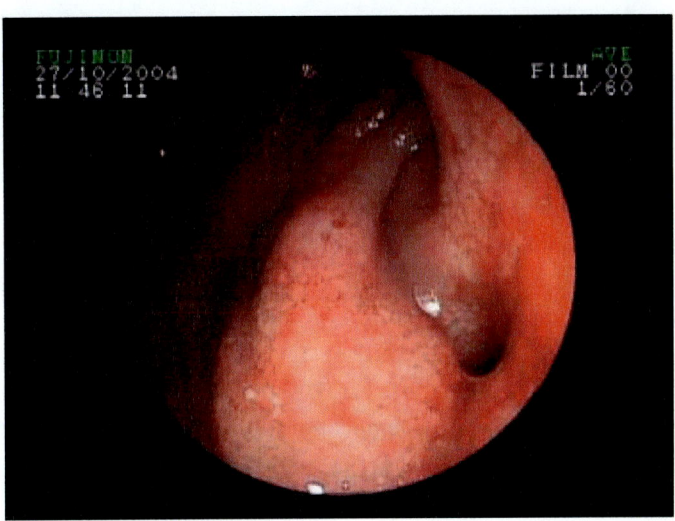

Figure 11-4. Fistula in CD.

Diagnostic Value of DBE in CD

CD is a chronic inflammatory condition which may affect any part of the gastrointestinal tract. It most commonly occurs in small bowel. Evaluation of the entire small bowel could provide precise information for diagnosing and therapeutic decisions in patients with CD.

Up until now, the small bowel was the most difficult part to evaluate by routine endoscopy, because of the length and the convolutions.

Small bowel Enteroclysis (SBE) is a sensitive technique in evaluating both the extensity and the severity of small bowel involvement in CD. The overall diagnosis yield was about 40%[2,3]. It could detect typical skip lesions and stricture, subsequent proximal dilation, and fistula. It fails to evaluate the thickness of the bowel wall and early lesion. But it was an effective screening test.

Computed tomography enteroclysis (CTE) may play an important role in diagnostic and evaluation of small bowel CD. It could clearly demonstrate marked transmural thickening stricture and internal fistula (figure 11-4) [3]. In addition, clinical experience suggests small bowel CTE was an alternative modality for determination of DBE route and a reliable diagnosis work-up while DBE failed to pass the stricture.

CE has reportedly shown to be a useful diagnostic tool for CD, which is capable of demonstrating early or faint or even typical mucosal changes in suspected CD cases [4,5]. However, retention of the capsule caused by small bowel strictures may occur in some percentage of patients (3%).

In intended cases, DBE could have whole small intestine to be scrutinized with combination of oral and anal route procedure, usually which was arranged in different days. Theoretically, DBE was an ideal and gold-standard diagnosis modality for small bowel CD [5,6]. Therapeutic interventions such as biopsy, EUS, or balloon dilation could be available under the therapeutic DBE instruments.

Respecting the advantage of DBE, DBE is a gold-standard modality for diagnosis of small bowel CD, as well as to determine severity, localization, and extensity of the CD.

1. Characteristic endoscopic findings in DBE including aphthous ulceration, pseudo-diverticula, deep fissuring ulceration, skip lesions and asymmetrical wall involvement are all strongly suggestive of CD.
2. Histologically, granulomas may be observed on biopsy specimens in only 25% to 30%. Classic epithelioid granulomas are not necessary for establishing a clinical diagnosis of CD. Detection of epithelioid granulomas is a convincing evidence.
3. DBE is a relatively safe procedure. Low level of serum albumin (<2.6g/dl), medium anaemia, potential existence of various fostala and subsequent adhesion may increase the procedure related complications (abdominal pain, bleeding, perforation). Multiple biopsies may also increase perforation risk.

DBE in Differential Diagnosis of CD from Other Conditions

DBE technique was helpful to make differential diagnostic for CD with following entities

1. (some type of) UC
2. Colonic amebiasis
3. Intestinal tuberculosis(TB)
4. Small bowel lymphoma
5. Epithelial tumors of small intestine

DBE in the CD Following-up

In our recently study, 53 patients of CD were regularly followed up and performed DBE, we found that endoscopic mucosal healing was significantly delayed with the improvements of the clinical symptoms. The first DBE follow-up was at least arranged at 6 months later of regular medication [7].

References

[1] Yamamoto H, Sekine Y, Sato Y, et al. Total enteroscopy with a nonsurgical sterrable double-balloon method. *Gastrointest. Endosc.* 2001, 53:216-20
[2] Zhong J, Zhang C-l, Jin C-r, et al. Double balloon enteroscopy in diagnosis of small bowel Crohn's disease. *Chin. J. Dig. Endosc.* 2006, 23:86-89 (Chinese)

[3] Sailer J, Peloschek P, Schober E, et al. Diagnostic value of CT enteroclysis compared with conventional enteroclysis in patients with Crohn's disease. *Am. J. Roentgenol.* 2005, 185:1575-1581

[4] Papadakis KA, Lo SK, Fireman Z, et al. Wireless capsule endoscopy in the evaluation of patients with suspected or known Crohn's disease. *Endoscopy.* 2005, 37:1018-1022

[5] Nobuhide O, Tomonori Y, Hirokazu Y, et al. Evaluation of deep small bowel involvement by Double-Balloon enteroscopy in Crohn's Disease. *Am. J. Gastroenterol.* 2006, 101:1484-1489

[6] Zhong J, Zhang C-l, MA T-l, et al. Comparative study of double-balloon enteroscopy and capsule endoscopy in etiological diagnosis of small intestine bleeding. *Chin. J. Dig.* 2004, 24:741-744 (Chinese)

[7] Chen M, Zhong J, Tang Y-h, et al. Application of double-balloon endoscopy in diagnosis of small bowel Crohn's disease. *J. Diagn. Concepts Pract.* 2008, 7(1):34-36.(Chinese)

In: Inflammatory Conditions of the Colon
Editor: Jia-ju Zheng

ISBN: 978-1-60692-240-8
© 2008 Nova Science Publishers, Inc.

Chapter XII

Capsule Endoscopy in Inflammatory Bowel Disease

Zhi-zheng Ge

Ren-ji Hospital and Shanghai Institute of Digestive Disease,
Shang-hai Jiaotong University School of Medicine,
Shang-hai, P.R. China

Introduction

Video capsule endoscopy (CE) provides visualization of the GI tract by transmitting images wirelessly from a disposable capsule to a data recorder worn by the patient [1]. The first capsule was approved by the Food and Drug Administration (FDA) in August 2001, mainly to evaluate the small bowel [1,2].The second capsule was approved in October 2004, specifically to evaluate the esophagus. CE plays an important role in the diagnosis of inflammatory bowel diseases. It is useful in the initial diagnosis of CD, for detecting recurrences, for establishing extent of disease, for assessing response to therapy, and for differentiating CD from UC or indeterminate colitis. CE can also play an important diagnostic role in the evaluation of patients with colonic IBD type unclassified (IBDU) [1,2]. Patients who were previously thought to have ulcerative colitis or IBDU underwent CE, the diagnosis may changed to Crohn's disease. PillCam COLON is the third video capsule to be developed to be used as one of the diagnostic tests to visualize abnormalities of the colon [1,3]. The PillCam COLON video capsule visualizing the colon has been cleared for marketing in the European Union and clinical trials are underway in the United States to support submission for marketing clearance from the FDA. Up to date, the first PillCam COLON clinical studies determined it to be a promising new modality for colon polyps and tumors only; there were no correlated evidence on IBD. So in this chapter, we focus on the feature and appearance of IBD(small bowel Crohn's disease) under PillCam SB. It may help us to differentiate CD from UC, indeterminate colitis and IBDU when the diagnosis is ambiguous [1-3].

The Role of CE in Crohn's Disease

Crohn's disease may affect any part of the GI but predominantly involves the SB [1]. Combined colon and distal SB disease is most common (34.6%-58% of patients), followed by Crohn's colitis alone (11%-27.2%) and ileal involvement alone (15%-25.3%). The diagnosis of Crohn's disease (CD) remains a challenge. CE, the noninvasive technology has been shown in several studies to not only have a diagnostic role, but also is related to the management of CD. Firstly, CE has a role in the diagnosis of suspected CD. Secondly, CE may have a role in assessing the extent of disease. We may be able to define those who are more likely to have more aggressive disease when this issue is examined. Third, it may have a role in determining disease activity and, hence, may justify a change of management. This concept has already led to the development of a new disease activity index. Last but not least, because there has been a change in the treatment paradigm for CD from symptomatic control to the induction of tissue healing, the use of CE may be appropriate in any pharmaceutical trial before and after the application of new or previous therapy to look for tissue healing.

Capsule Endoscopic Findings in Crohn's Disease

CD's capsule endoscopic findings consist of absent or blunted villi, mucosal erythema, mucosal edema, mucosal nodularity, mucosal erosion, mucosal fissures, ulcer, and stricture (figure 12-1 to figure 12-6). We performed a study to evaluate the effectiveness of CE in patients with suspected Crohn's disease. Of the 20 patients, 13 (65%) were diagnosed as CD of the small bowel according to the findings of CE. The findings detected by the capsule were mucosal erosions, aphthas, nodularity, large ulcers and ulcerated stenosis. The distribution of the lesions was mainly in the distal part of the small bowel. A plethora of terms have appeared to describe mucosal lesions found by capsule endoscopy as described above. To standardize the terminology a Capsule Endoscopy Working Group has designed a Minimal Standard Terminology (MST) and is in the process of modifying it for use for small bowel capsule endoscopy findings. This is of particular importance in describing these findings because there is limited ability in gauging depth of many mucosal lesions. A partial list of these descriptors has been incorporated into the Lewis scoring system for description of small bowel lesions detected in the evaluation for Crohn's disease (table 12-1). But it has not been universally adopted and has not been validated it's clinical feasibility. Currently, if there are multiple aphthous ulcers; circular, linear or irregular ulcers (≥3); stenosis found in capsule endoscopy in the small bowel, after excluding other small bowel pathological conditions, the final diagnosis of CD can be made [2,5]. Otherwise, it still require further examination to the final diagnosis.

Capsule Endoscopy in Inflammatory Bowel Disease

Table 12-1. Lewis capsule endoscopy scoring table

	duodenum number	jejunum distribution pattern	Regions proximal Ileum lesions longitudinal extent	distal Ileum shape	size (by circumference)
erythema		localized, 1	short segment, 1		
		patchy, 2	long segment, 2		
		diffuse, 3	whole region, 3		
edema		localized. 1	short segment, 1		
		patchy, 2	long segment, 2		
		diffuse, 3	whole region, 3		
nodularity	single, 1	localized, 1	short segment, 1		
	few, 2	patchy, 2	long segment, 2		
	multiple, 3	diffuse, 3	whole region, 3		
ulcer	single, 3	localized, 3	short segment, 3	circular, 3	<1/4, 3
	few, 5	patchy, 5	long segment, 5	linear, 5	1/4-1/2, 5
	multiple, 7	diffuse, 7	whole region, 7	irregular, 7	>1/2, 7
stenosis	none, 0	traversed, 10	nonulcerated, 5		
	single, 10	not traversed, 20	ulcerated, 10		
	multiple, 20				

Score by region by adding points listed.

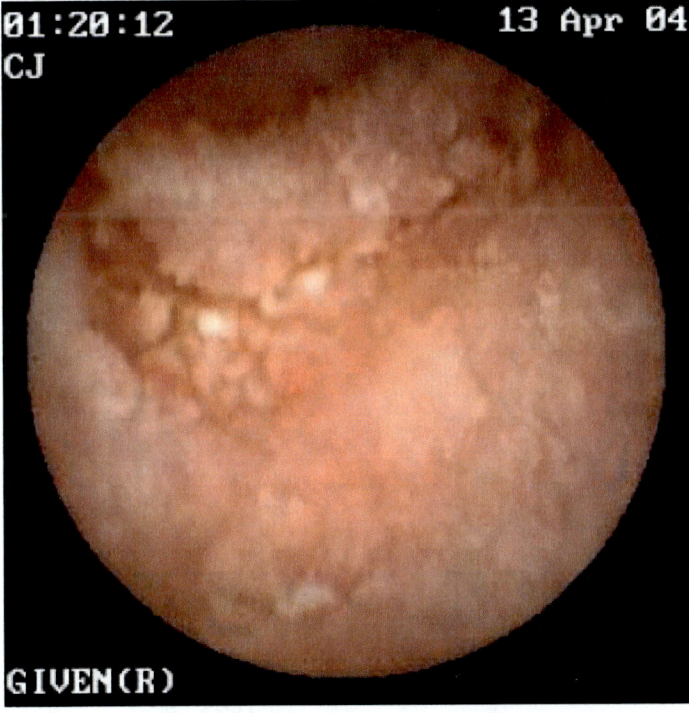

Figure 12-1. Absent mucosal villi.

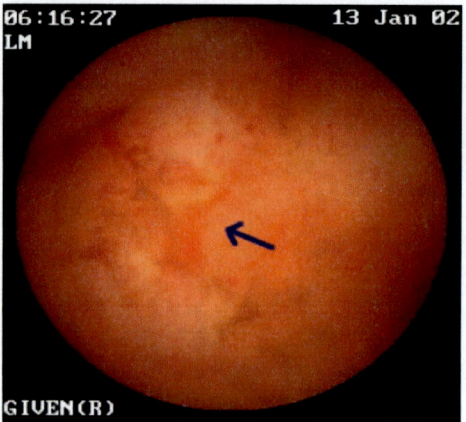

Figure 12-2. Mucosal erosion,

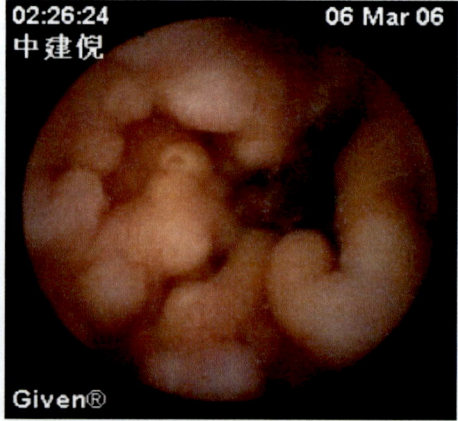

Figure 12-3. Mucosal nodularity.

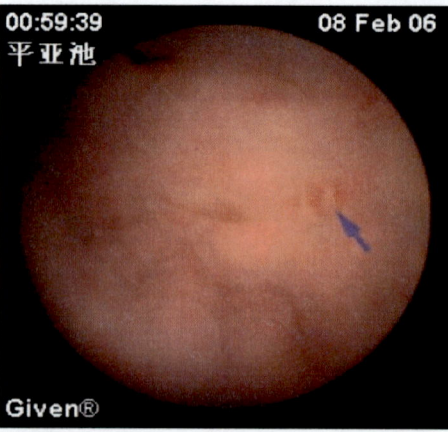

Figure 12-4. Aphthous ulcers.

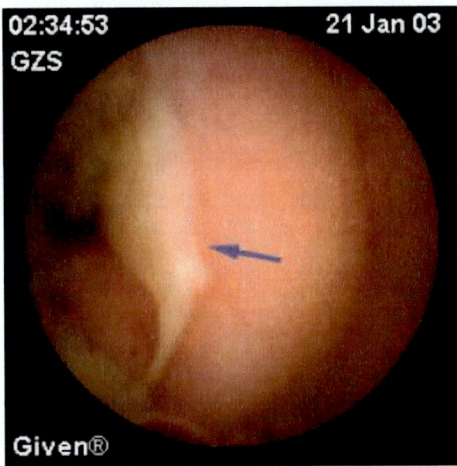

Figure 12-5. A broad, geographic small bowel ulcer.

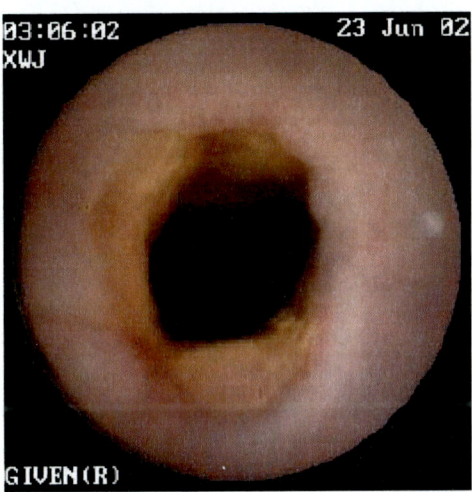

Figure 12-6. Mucosal stricture.

Diagnostic Yield of CE in CD and Compared with Others

The diagnostic yield of CE ranges from 10% to 71%, depending on the clinical setting [1,5]. Data from retrospective studies, case series, and prospective studies have shown that CE is useful for the diagnoses of CD when small bowel follow through (SBFT) and ileoscopy are negative or unsuccessful. CE has been shown to be more sensitive in the detection of small bowel CD than computed tomographic (CT) enterography, SBFT, and enteroclysis. In patients with mild to moderate disease and a normal SBFT, CE may allow for the detection of small bowel changes that are not within reach of push enteroscopy (PE). A recent prospective study of 42 patients compared SBFT, CT enterography, colonoscopy with ileoscopy, and CE in the assessment of small bowel CD. Of these 4 modalities, CE had the highest sensitivity (83%) with the lowest specificity (53%) and colonoscopy with ileoscopy had the highest specificity (100%) with a sensitivity of 74%. A recent study in 39 patients, the majority with known CD, reported CE sensitivity and specificity of 89.6% and 100%, respectively [4,6]. Sample sizes of all included studies were small, and as a result any possible selection bias may have been amplified. Recently, a meta-analysis of the yield of capsule endoscopy compared to other diagnostic modalities in patients with non-stricturing small bowel crohn's disease indicated that CE is superior to small bowel barium radiography, colonoscopy with ileoscopy, CT enterography and push enteroscopy for diagnosing nonstricturing small bowel CD in patients with established non-stricturing CD (table 12-2) [2,4].

Table 12-2. Summary of Incremental Yield (IY) of CE Over Other Modalities

	total yield CE (%)	total yield other modality (%)	% IY for CE (95% CI)
vs. SB radiography	66	24	42 (0.30-0.54)
vs. ileoscopy	61	46	15 (0.02-0.27)
vs. CT enterography	75	37	38 (0.23-0.54)
vs. push enteroscopy	51	7	44 (0.31-0.57)
vs. small bowel MRI	60	40	20 (0.41-0.81)

The Limitations and Risks of CE in the Diagnosis of Crohn's Disease

The main limitation of CE in the assessment of small bowel CD is that it is a visual diagnosis, is the lack of uniform criteria for diagnosis of CD, inability to allow for tissue acquisition or therapeutic intervention [2,5]. Even a biopsy with the new double-balloon push enteroscope may not solve the problem, because biopsy specimens themselves are not always diagnostic. Furthermore, treatment responses may be nonspecific. Some findings, such as scattered mucosal breaks and aphthous ulcers or erosions, may not be sufficient to confirm a diagnosis of Crohn's disease because up to 13.8% of asymptomatic healthy volunteers not taking nonsteroidal anti- inflammatory agents (NSAIDs) may have mucosal breaks and other lesions seen on capsule endoscopy. Altogether, there are 40 pathological conditions such as NSAID intake, lymphoid hyperplasia, lymphoma, radiation enteritis, HIV with opportunistic infection, intestinal tuberculosis, where small bowel permeability is increased and all these conditions may have small intestinal erosions and ulcers. It is, therefore, important to exclude all these pathological conditions before the final diagnosis of CD is made. Misdiagnosis of CD can be harmful because in an unresponsive patient, intensification of therapy can take place and occasionally the patient may even have to undergo an unnecessary operation.

The main risk of CE in CD patients is capsule retention resulting from underlying small bowel strictures, occurring in 1% to 13% of patients with known CD [2,6,7]. Retained capsules may require surgery in patients that may otherwise have not required surgery. A preinitiation radiologic study (CT or SBFT) is recommended because asymptomatic CD strictures occur in as many as 22%. Patients with obstructive symptoms or with endoscopic and radiographic evidence of small bowel narrowing in the setting of CD should not undergo CE. The patency capsule (Given Imaging; Yoqneam, Israel), may have a role to play in this context. This capsule is identical in size and shape to the video capsule, but is composed of dissolvable lactose and barium. The core of the capsule contains a radio-frequency device measuring only 2 mm, which can be detected with a handheld scanning device. In patients in whom a stricture is suspected, the patient ingests the patency capsule and can return for sequential determinations to detect passage prior to ingestion of the M2A video capsule. Capsule retention above a CD stricture may be treated with anti- inflammatory medications, retrieved by double-balloon enteroscopy or by operation.

Finally, capsule endoscopy yields information regarding mucosal lesions only and does not allow assumptions to be made about wall thickness or any extraluminal findings, thus making it an examination complementary to other imaging modalities, rather than a definitive diagnostic tool in its own right.

Pillcam Colon Capsule Endoscopy in IBD

PillCam Colon capsule endoscopy appears to be a promising new modality for colonic evaluation [2,7]. Further studies in the procedure will focus on the populations with various of colonic disease, especially for IBD.

References

[1] Eliakim R. The impact of capsule endoscopy on Crohn's disease. *Dig. Liver Dis.* 2007;39(2): 154-155.

[2] Bar-Meir S. Review article: capsule endoscopy - are all small intestinal lesions Crohn's disease? *Aliment Pharmacol. Ther.* 2006; 24 Suppl 3:19-21.

[3] Voderholzer WA. The role of PillCam endoscopy in Crohn's disease: the European experience. *Gastrointest Endosc Clin. N. Am.* 2006; 16(2):287-297.

[4] Triester SL, Leighton JA, Leontiadis GI, et al. A meta-analysis of the yield of capsule endoscopy compared to other diagnostic modalities in patients with non-stricturing small bowel Crohn's disease. *Am. J. Gastroenterol.* 2006; 101(5):954-64.

[5] Papadakis KA, Lo SK, Fireman Z, Hollerboach S. Wireless capsule endoscopy in the evaluation of patients with suspected or known Crohn's disease. *Endoscopy.* 2005; 37(10): 1018-1022.

[6] Legnani P, Kornbluth A. Video capsule endoscopy in inflammatory bowel disease 2005. *Curr. Opin. Gastroenterol.* 2005; 21(4):438-442.

[7] Ge Z-j, Hu Y-b, Xiao S-d. Capsule endoscopy in diagnosis of small bowel Crohn's disease. *World J. Gastroenterol.* 2004 May 1; 10(9):1349-52.

In: Inflammatory Conditions of the Colon
Editor: Jia-ju Zheng

ISBN: 978-1-60692-240-8
© 2008 Nova Science Publishers, Inc.

Chapter XIII

Narrow Band Imaging: A New Diagnostic Approach in Colorectal Cancer and Inflammatory Bowel Disease

Wei Huang and Yun-lin Wu

Narrow band imaging (NBI) is a new endoscopic technique which uses optical filters to illuminate the mucosa with light from selected or "narrowed" bands of the optical spectrum [1,2]. The filtered light preferentially enhances the mucosal surface and in particular the network of superficial capillaries [1-3]. NBI has been nicknamed "digital chromoendoscopy", and is available to the endoscopist at the push of a button.

Introduction

NBI is an innovative optical technique that can provide clear imaging of the microvascular structure in the mucosal layer [4]. NBI illuminates the tissue surface using special filters that narrow the respective red, green, and blue bands while simultaneously increasing the relative intensity of the blue band. This enhances the tissue microvasculature, mainly as a result of the differential optical absorption of light by hemoglobin in the mucosa associated with the initiation and progression of dysplasia, particularly in the blue range. The resulting images have the appearance of chromoendoscopy without dye staining, focusing on the capillaries. Gono et al. [1,2] found that with narrow-band illumination at 415± 30nm, contrast imaging of the capillary pattern in the superficial layer of the human tongue was markedly improved.

The purpose of introducing optical electronics into video endoscopes is to improve the accuracy of diagnosis through image processing and digital technology [1-4]. NBI technique involves the use of interference filters to illuminate the target in narrowed red, green and blue

(R/G/B) bands of the spectrum. This results in different images at distinct levels of the mucosa, and increases the contrast between the epithelial surface and the subjacent vascular network.

NBI can be combined with magnifying endoscopy with an optical zoom [4,5]. This combined technique can characterize the surface of the distinct types of gastrointestinal epithelia intestinal metaplasia in Barrett's esophagus. The technique may also make the endoscopic possible to demonstrate disorganization of the vascular pattern in inflammatory disorders of the gastrointestinal mucosa, or in superficial neoplastic lesions in the esophagus, stomach, and large bowel.

The morphology of premalignant and malignant precursors of advanced cancer in the gastrointestinal tract mucosa has been categorized in the Paris classification. Endoscopists' cognitive perception of abnormal conditions is changing, as these lesions often have a nonprotruding morphology characterized by slight discoloration and/or variation in relief (elevation or depression), which has been described in various classifications of pit patterns, developed mostly in Japan [5,6].

In addition, superficial vascular structures can change during the process of tumor angiogenesis. Digital reconstruction of the images captured by the video endoscope makes image processing possible. The hemoglobin content in the mucosa (the hemoglobin index) can be assessed by adjusting the color of the reflected light. The new technique of NBI combines the potential of both technological advances of magnifying endoscopy and image processing Technical Background Image Reconstruction in the Electronic Video Endoscope. Video endoscopes use white light from a xenon source for illumination [7-9]. The reflected light is captured by a charge-coupled device (CCD) chip at the tip of the instrument in order to reconstruct the images. The reflectance spectrum differs from the emission spectrum of the light source; during live observation, the spectral composition of the reflected light is influenced by the structure of the tissue and the blood flow.

The depth of penetration into the gastrointestinal tract mucosa depends on the wave length used superficial for the blue band, deep for the red band, and intermediate for the green band (the range of penetration is between 0.15 and 0.30 mm.

Hemoglobin is the major agent responsible for the absorption of visible light, with a principal peak in the blue part of the spectrum (415nm) [4,5]. This explains the red color of the vessels.

The laminar structures of the gastrointestinal mucosa, including those altered by inflammation or neoplasia, act as a scattering element and interfere with the reflectance spectrum. Two different systems are used to reconstruct images from the reflected light. The first is a "color" CCD, in which pixels are selectively assigned to specific wavelength ranges such as red, green, and blue (R/G/B) or cyan, yellow, and magenta (CYMK). The CCD captures the full range of the white light and transfers it in a single step to the processor in order to reconstruct natural color on the video monitor. This system is nonsequential. In a "monochrome" CCD, pixels are not selectively attributed to specific colors and are transferred in a sequential mode in the R/G/B bands to the processor. A rotating R/G/B interference filter is interposed after the white light source, and the mucosa is illuminated alternately in each of the three R/G/B bands. This system is sequential.

NBI is capable of enhancing the clinical value of magnification endoscopy. The improved morphological analysis of epithelial crests on the surface of the mucosa may make the detection of intestinal metaplasia in Barrett's esophagus more reliable.

More precise analysis of the abnormal surface architecture (pit pattern) of neoplastic lesions could be relevant for treatment decisions [10-12]. The most important contribution of the new technique is probably the clear visualization of the vascular network in the mucosa that it provides. This should promote the study of neovascularization in superficial cancers in the gastrointestinal tract and should increase our knowledge of the pathophysiology of inflammatory conditions. It should be noted that chromoscopy is not helpful when the aim of the examination is to study vessels.

Finally, there is considerable potential for further developments by applying NBI technology into non-sequential endoscopic video system and resulting from modifications of the characteristics of the interference filters. This affects the depth of penetration of the light and the morphology of the image, as well as the color rendering. Methodological aspects are critical when correlating magnified images with biopsies from the same area; it has to be ensured that the identical areas are being compared. This may be less of a problem with visible lesions that may have similar characteristics on NBI and histology. However, subtle NBI changes in macroscopically normal mucosa are probably small and focal, so that precise biopsy in the epithelial sampling immediately after NBI imaging is mandatory for reliable assessment of the technique.

NBI is an innovative optical technology that can provide clear imaging of the microvascular structure in the mucosal layer. NBI illuminates the tissue surface using special filters that narrow the respective red, green, and blue bands while simultaneously increasing the relative intensity of the blue band. This enhances the tissue microvasculature, mainly as a result of the differential optical absorption of light by hemoglobin in the mucosa associated with the initiation and progression of dysplasia, particularly in the blue range. The resulting images have the appearance of chromoendoscopy without dye staining, focusing on the capillaries. Gono et al. found that with narrow-band illumination at 415 ± 30 nm, contrast imaging of the capillary pattern in the superficial layer of the human tongue was markedly improved [4-13]. They suggested that this approach could provide an optimal method of visualizing the capillary pattern in vivo and could serve as a complementary technique to conventional magnification assessment.

Detecting Colorectal Lesions

The pit pattern (shape of the opening of a colorectal crypt) classification, proposed by Kudo et al, is reported to be useful for qualitative diagnosis of colorectal tumor [1-4,13]. Assessment of pit patterns is clinically significant in terms of differential diagnosis between neoplasia and nonneoplasia, determining the degree of histologic atypia of a tumor, determining the depth of early carcinoma, detection of minute residual tumors after endoscopic resection, estimating the degree of histologic inflammation in patients with ulcerative colitis (UC), and diagnosis of dysplasia/ colitis-associated carcinoma in patients with UC. In this study of colorectal lesions, pit patterns classified on the basis of NBI magnification without chromoendoscopy were compared with results obtained by standard magnification with chromoendoscopy. Overall concordance in the results between NBI magnification and magnifying chromoendoscopy was 84%, with particularly high concordance for type II, III, IV, and VN pit patterns. Concordance for type VI pit pattern was low [13]. With NBI visualization, the capillaries on the mucosal surface appear an enhanced brown in contrast to the pit itself, which has no capillaries and appears transparent white [13]. These differences in the hues of tissues, which depend on the density of the capillaries, permit indirect assessment of the pit pattern via the capillaries. Low concordance obtained for type VI pit pattern may reflect the difficulty of NBI assessment of type VI pit pattern with mild atypia. It was reported that magnifying endoscopic observation of the microvascular architecture of superficial esophageal carcinoma is useful in determining the depth of invasion. The intrapapillary capillary loops could be seen in the normal esophageal mucosa by magnifying endoscopy. In cancerous lesions, characteristic changes of the intrapapillary capillary loops could be seen in the superficial mucosa according to the depth of tumor invasion [12-14]. Similarly, qualitative diagnosis of colorectal tumor with type V pit pattern was assumed to be possible by using the features of capillaries (including the vessel diameters, irregularity, and capillary network) that are observable with NBI but not by using the pit pattern. The authors frequently encountered patients in whom assessment of the pit pattern by magnifying chromoendoscopy was impossible because of mucus adhesion. Because the NBI method requires neither dye nor stain, the assessment of the pit pattern by this method is possible without the obstruction of mucus. Thus, the NBI method is more powerful than chromoendoscopy for lesions with mucus adhesion. In comparing NBI endoscopic findings between neoplastic and nonneoplastic lesions, the hue of nonneoplastic lesions was very similar to that of normal mucous membranes, whereas the majority of neoplastic lesions appeared brownish. The difference in hue was significant between neoplastic lesions and nonneoplastic lesions, enabling us to differentiate between neoplastic lesions and nonneoplastic lesions by their hue. Previous studies have shown that the diameter and density of capillaries were greater in neoplastic lesions than in nonneoplastic lesions. Similar findings were observed in the current study; that is, NBI magnification depicted no superficial capillaries in nonneoplastic lesions having small capillaries but did depict a brown capillary network in neoplastic lesions having large capillaries, indicating that the difference in hue depicted by NBI depends on the diameter and density of capillaries in the lesions. Nonneoplastic lesion require no specific treatment, and magnified visualization with chromoendoscopy or total biopsy may allow differentiation, but conventional endoscopy may not. NBI permits differentiation between neoplastic and nonneoplastic lesions without chromoendoscopy and thus clarifies whether treatment is necessary [13-15]. In conclusion, NBI magnification is useful for assessment of pit patterns without chromoendoscopy and for differentiation between neoplastic and nonneoplastic lesions. In addition, an advantage of NBI magnification is that it is easy to operate, with the single touch of a button on the scope to alternate between conventional and NBI image. Because there are no complicated devices and no dyes or stains, the procedure time is short, resulting in a reduced burden to the operator and patient. NBI magnification has good potential as an easy-to-use diagnostic tool and will undoubtedly come into wide use in clinical settings

Detection of potentially dysplastic areas and their differentiation from inflammation in colitis is one of the hardest challenges for the endoscopist. Despite this evidence, dye spraying is not routine clinical practice in colitis surveillance in many centers. It takes additional time, equipment, and training to perform and even with specially designed spray catheters mucosal coverage is not guaranteed.

As both adenomas and carcinomas have a richer vascular network than normal mucosa, they are enhanced in wide field view and appear dark brown against a blue green background mucosa. When magnification is combined with NBI, a pit pattern can be distinguished, similar to that described in the Kudo classification, which can be used to estimate whether or not a lesion is dysplastic. To identify the feasibility of the narrow-band imaging (NBI) method compared with that of conventional colonoscopy and chromoendoscopy for distinguishing neoplastic and nonneoplastic colonic polyps. Machida et al. used conventional colonoscope detected lesions, and then the NBI system was used to examine the capillary networks. Thereafter indigo carmine (0.2%) was sprayed directly on the mucosa surface prior to evaluating the crypts using a conventional colonoscope. The pit patterns were characterized using the classification system proposed by Kudo. Finally, a polypectomy or biopsy was performed for histological diagnosis. Of the 110 colorectal polyps, 65 were adenomas, 40 were hyperplastic polyps, and five were adenocarcinomas. The NBI system and pit patterns for all lesions were analyzed. For differential diagnosis of neoplastic (adenoma and adenocarcinoma) and nonneoplastic (hyperplastic) polyps, the sensitivity of the conventional colonoscope for detecting neoplastic polyps was 82.9%, specificity was 80.0% and diagnostic accuracy was 81.8%, significantly lower than those achieved with the NBI system (sensitivity 95.7%, specificity 87.5%, accuracy 92.7%) and chromoendoscopy (sensitivity 95.7%, specificity 87.5%, accuracy 92.7%). Therefore, no significant difference existed between the NBI system and chromoendoscopy during differential diagnosis of neoplastic and nonneoplastic polyps.

Differentiation between neoplastic and nonneoplastic lesions using the NBI system was evaluated in comparison with the results of conventional colonoscopy and chromoendoscopy. NBI and chromoendoscopy had similar levels of sensitivity (each 100%) and specificity (each 75%) in differentiating between neoplastic and nonneoplastic lesions. In addition, both techniques were superior to conventional endoscopy (sensitivity 83%, specificity 44%). NBI provided better visualization of the vascular network, whereas chromoendoscopy was more precise in characterizing the surface pit pattern. Gono et al. reported that NBI clearly enhances the epithelial microvascular pattern. Thus, NBI can be used to differentiate between neoplastic and non-neoplastic gastrointestinal lesions. Yoshida et al. and Muto et al. reported that NBI allows detection of morphological changes in microvascular structure that are useful in the diagnosis of superficial oesophageal carcinomas. Machida et al. demonstrated that NBI is equivalent to magnifying endoscopy for distinguishing colonic neoplasm from non-neoplastic lesions. Our study aimed to prospectively elucidate the diagnostic accuracy of NBI, under both low and high magnification, in distinguishing colorectal lesions and compare this accuracy to the diagnostic accuracies of conventional colonoscopy and of low-magnification and high-magnification chromoendoscopy Machida et al. used a newly developed NBI technique in which modified optical filters are incorporated into the light source of a video endoscope system and can be applied, during colonoscopy in the clinical setting. This pilot study, including 34 colorectal lesions in 34 patients, evaluated the clinical feasibility of the NBI system for colonoscopy.

Machida et al. used a newly developed NBI technique in which modified optical filters are incorporated into the light source of a video endoscope system and can be applied during colonoscopy in the clinical setting [6]. This pilot study, including colorectal lesions in 34 patients, evaluated the clinical feasibility of the NBI system for colonoscopy. Differentiation between neoplastic and nonneoplastic lesions using the NBI system was evaluated in comparison with the results of conventional colonoscopyand chromoendoscopy. NBI and chromoendoscopy had similar levels of sensitivity (each 100%) and specificity (each 75%) in differentiating between neoplastic and nonneoplastic lesions. In addition, both techniques were superior to conventional endoscopy (sensitivity 83%, specificity 44%). NBI provided better visualization of the vascular network, whereas chromoendoscopy was more precise in characterizing the surface pit pattern. In comparison with conventional colonoscopy, NBI and chromoendoscopy with targeted biopsy significantly increased the diagnostic yield for intraepithelial neoplasia and the number of flat neoplastic changes. Chromoendoscopy is a technique in which different dyes are topically applied to the gastrointestinal mucosa during endoscopy in order to better characterize and highlight specific changes in the mucosa. This staining method allows visualization of certain mucosal features that would otherwise not be evident and, thus, improves the accuracy of the endoscopic examination. There are numerous different dyes used in the gastrointestinal tract and they can be classified based on specific characteristics, i.e. absorptive, reactive, and contrast stains. Endoscopists have mainly used indigo carmine and methylene blue and sometimes cresyl violet for enhancing visualization of the mucosa in the colon. The pattern of these pits and other morphological features of the flat and depressed neoplasm have been classified by Kudo et al. The pit pattern classification system identifies 5 types and numerous subtypes. Types I and II are staining patterns that predict nonneoplastic changes, such as hyperplasia, whereas Types III and IV predict neoplastic alterations. Pit pattern analysis has enabled neoplastic prediction, which may determine appropriate treatment, such as endoscopic or surgical therapy based on the results of magnifying chromoendoscopy. A retrospective study using magnifying colonoscopy and dye spraying (indigo carmine) examined the mucosal pit patterns of lesions and compared the results to the histopathological examination. They found that the diagnostic accuracy of magnifying chromoendoscopy for nonneoplastic lesions was 75%, for adenomatous polyps it was 94%, Not only the pit pattern changes during malignant progression but also the superficial microvascular network changes as part of tumor-induced angiogenesis. The term "digital chromoendoscopy" was coined by Sano et al when referring to NBI, which is a novel method to examine the gastrointestinal mucosa by improving imaging of mucosal capillaries. Hemoglobin is the principle agent responsible for the absorption of visible light, with a major peak in the blue part of the spectrum (415 nm) and projecting in red for the endoscopist. NBI is based on reflectance spectral studies of the gastrointestinal mucosa showing that the combination of specific nonoverlapping filters narrowing the blue, green, and red bands creates different images at distinct levels of depth in the mucosa, which increases the contrast between the epithelial surface and subjacent microvascular network. Moreover, the use of these narrow bands enhances the relative intensity of the blue band, which further helps to visualize the superficial capillary network. NBI can easily be incorporated into conventional colonoscopes by introducing a rotation disk with the optical filters interposed after the light source and combined with magnifying endoscopy. Compared with chromoendoscopy, pit pattern alone does not seem to be sufficient for dysplasia differentiation and features specific to NBI such as vascular pattern intensity may need to modify the interpretation of the standard Kudo pattern to maximise differentiation. Pit pattern and vascular pattern intensity both play a role in differentiation of dysplasia with NBI.

Detecting Neoplastic Lesions in IBD

Epidemiological studies have demonstrated an increased risk of colorectal cancer in patients with UC, although this risk has been reported to vary considerably between 7%–30%[1,2].1–3 Nonetheless, this increased risk of cancer in UC is the reason for establishing and improving endoscopic surveillance protocols for patients with UC. Indeed, the development of colon cancer in patients with UC accounts for one-third of UC-related deaths. For a long time the risk of cancer development in Crohn's disease (CD) has been underestimated and most studies on colon cancer surveillance of patients with inflammatory bowel disease (IBD) have therefore focused on UC. Overall, the risk for neoplastic changes in CD is lower than that in UC; however, it has been shown that the risk of cancer in CD involving the colon is similar to that of UC. In fact, study reported a similar incidence of neoplasia in CD patients with extensive colitis compared with that in extensive UC and suggested that the surveillance programs already used in UC should also been considered for use in patients with extensive Crohn's colitis. In general, there is an increased risk for colorectal cancer associated with younger age at onset of IBD, longer duration of colitis, and more extensive disease.

Colonoscopy is considered the gold standard for surveillance of patients with IBD. Colonoscopy may early detect and treat precancerous lesions of colorectal mucosa, and thereby disrupt the classic theoretic sequential change from adenoma to carcinoma, and prevent progression to manifest colorectal cancer. However, standard colonoscopy is far from perfect in detecting adenomas and may miss significant numbers of small lesions. Moreover, it is nowadays generally accepted that flat and depressed adenomas are not limited to Japan but are also a common feature in Western patients. Importantly, flat lesions have malignant potential and their detection poses a great challenge to endoscopists. These circumstances have led to the endorsement of surveillance programs in IBD patients based on multiple nontargeted biopsies. Published guidelines recommend that 2–4 biopsies should be taken every 10 cm in the colorectum, rendering 20–50 biopsies per examination,10 which is not only time-consuming and expensive but may also expose patients to increased risk of complications. Thus, there has been a need for new methods to survey patients with IBD. One such method is chromoendoscopy, which has taken colon cancer surveillance in IBD patients a long step forward by unmasking neoplastic lesions previously missed by standard colonoscopy. Moreover, the introduction of magnifying endoscopy and especially in combination with chromoendoscopy has revolutionized the means to detect malignant transformations in patients with IBD. This review will focus on the role of chromoendoscopy but also mention future alternatives, such as narrow band imaging, to improve colon cancer surveillance in IBD patients.

It has been widely accepted that patients with long-standing UC face an increased lifetime risk of developing colorectal cancer [15]. Factors associated with increased risk include the duration of the colitis (> 8 years), extensive colonic involvement (pancolitis, backwash ileitis), primary sclerosing cholangitis (PSC), and severe chronic active inflammation. NBI with magnification was able to successfully detect and differentiate dysplasia in colitis. The most important features of the NBI system are its speed and ease of use, with rapid push button switching between modes, and no problems with incomplete mucosal coverage associated with dye spray. This has the potential to have a large impact in colitis surveillance as NBI seems to provide many of the benefits of chromoendoscopy without the aforementioned downsides [16], hopefully encouraging greater clinical use of techniques which increase dysplasia detection.

Conclusions

Newly invented technologies can be expected to change and improve colonoscopic diagnosis. Chromoendoscopy is now established as an important diagnostic tool for diagnosing flat adenomas and colitis-associated neoplastic changes in IBD. NBI highlights the surface vasculature and may be able to provide the same diagnostic yield as chromoendoscopy. Further areas of research with NBI in the large bowel include the diagnosis and classification of IBD and, in particular, improved detection of IBD-associated neoplasia. Combining the different technologies and integrating them into a multifunctional endoscope would offer new optical features in gastrointestinal endoscopy.

References

[1] Gono K, Obi T, Yamaguchi M, et al. Appearance of enhanced tissue features in narrow-band endoscopic imaging [J]. *J. Biomed. Opt.* 2004; 9(3): 568-577.

[2] Gono K, Yamazaki K, Doguchi N, et al. Endoscopic observation of tissue by narrow-band illumination [J]. *Opt. Rev.* 2003; 10(1): 1-5

[3] Gono K, Yamaguchi M, Ohyama N. Improvement of image quality of the electroendoscope by narrowing spectral shapes of observation light [J]. *Proc. Int. Congr. Imaging. Sci.* 2002; 5: 399-400

[4] Kuznetsov K, Lambert R, Rey JF, et al. Narrow-band imaging: potential and limitations [J]. *Endoscopy.* 2006; 38(1): 76-81

[5] Fu KI, Sano Y, Kato S, et al. Chromoendoscopy using indigo carmine dye spraying with magnifying observation is the most reliable method for differential diagnosis between non-neoplastic and neoplastic colorectal lesions: a prospective study [J]. *Endoscopy.* 2004; 36(12): 1089-1093

[6] Machida H, Sano Y, Hamamoto Y, et al. Narrow-band imaging in the diagnosis of colorectal mucosal lesions: a pilot study [J]. *Endoscopy.* 2004; 36(12): 1094-1098

[7] Dekker E, Van Deventer S, Hardwick J, et al. The value of narrow band imaging for the detection of dysplasia in longstanding ulcerative colitis [abstract] [J]. *Gastroenterology.* 2004; 126(suppl.): A77

[8] Sano Y, Muto M, Tajiri H, et al. Optical/digital chromoendoscopy during colonoscopy using narrow-band imaging system [J]. *Digestive Endosc.* 2005; 17(suppl.): S43-S48

[9] Hirata M, Tanaka S, Oka S, Kaneko I, Yoshida S, Yoshihara M, Chayama K. Magnifying endoscopy with narrow band imaging for diagnosis of colorectal tumors [J]. *Gastrointest. Endosc.* 2007 Feb 23 [Epub ahead of print]

[10] Thorlacius H, Toth E. Role of chromoendoscopy in colon cancer surveillance in inflammatory bowel disease [J]. *Inflamm. Bowel. Dis.* 2007 Feb 16 [Epub ahead of print]

[11] Su MY, Hsu CM, Ho YP, Chen PC, Lin CJ, Chiu CT. Comparative study of conventional colonoscopy, chromoendoscopy, and narrow-band imaging systems in differential diagnosis of neoplastic and nonneoplastic colonic polyps [J]. *Am. J. Gastroenterol.* 2006; 101(12): 2711-6.

[12] Chiu HM, Chang CY, Chen CC, Lee YC, Wu MS, Lin JT, Shun CT, Wang HP. A prospective comparative study of narrow-band imaging, chromoendoscopy, and conventional colonoscopy in the diagnosis of colorectal neoplasia [J]. *Gut.* 2007; 56(3): 373-9.

[13] East JE, Suzuki N, von Herbay A, et al. Narrow band imaging with magnification for dysplasia detection and pit pattern assessment in ulcerative colitis surveillance: a case with multiple dysplasia associated lesions or masses [J]. *Gut.* 2006; 55(10): 1432-1435

[14] Gheorghe C. Narrow-band imaging endoscopy for diagnosis of malignant and premalignant gastrointestinal lesions [J]. *J. Gastrointestin. Liver Dis.* 2006; 15(1): 77-82

[15] Kiesslich R, Hoffman A, Neurath MF. Colonoscopy, tumors, and inflammatory bowel disease - new diagnostic methods [J]. *Endoscopy.* 2006; 38(1): 5-10.

[16] Dekker E, Fockens P. New imaging techniques at colonoscopy: tissue spectroscopy and narrow band imaging [J]. *Gastrointest. Endosc. Clin. N. Am.* 2005; 15(4): 703-14.

In: Inflammatory Conditions of the Colon
Editor: Jia-ju Zheng

ISBN: 978-1-60692-240-8
© 2008 Nova Science Publishers, Inc.

Chapter XIV

The Application of Confocal Laser Endomicroscopy for Diagnosis of Inflammation Bowel Diseases

Yan-qing Li

Qi-lu Hospital, Shangdong University, Shan-dong Province, P.R. China

Introduction

Ulcerative colitis (UC) is associated with an increased risk for development of colitis-associated colorectal cancer (CRC) [1,2]. Surveillance colonoscopy may detect early neoplastic lesions at a curable stage, and reduce colorectal cancer mortality in UC. However, in contrast to sporadic colorectal cancer, the growing pattern of neoplastic tissue in UC is often flat and multifocal. So the approach of taking 4-quadrant biopsies every 10 cm throughout the colorectum has been currently recommended [3]. Chromoendoscopy has permitted the identification of mucosal lesions and greatly enhanced the endoscopic detection of neoplastic lesions in colitic colon [4-6], however, histological analysis of biopsy specimen still remains the gold standard for the final diagnosis.

Confocal laser endomicroscopy (CLE) is a new endoscopic tool that allows *in vivo* surface and subsurface (*z*-axis) cellular resolution imaging during routine endoscopy, which enables real-time virtual histology at the time of endoscopic examination [7-9].

Recent data suggests that CLE in conjunction with chromoendoscopy can improve the detection of intraepithelial neoplasia in chronic ulcerative colitis (CUC) when compared with chromoendoscopy alone or conventional colonoscopy [10,11]. However, there has not been any report on the application of CLE for the diagnosis of Crohn's disease.

The Confocal Laser Endomicroscope

Confocal endomicroscope is the integration of a miniaturized laser scanning confocal microscope (Optiscan, Notting Hill, Victoria, Australian) into the distal tip of a conventional endoscope (EC-3870K; Pentax, Tokyo, Japan). The distal tip contains an air and water jet nozzle, two light guides, an auxiliary water jet channel (used for topical application of the constrast agent), and a 2.8mm working channel.

Confocal laser endomicroscopy allows conventional white-light endoscopy and confocal microscopy to be done simultaneously. During laser endoscopy, a single-line laser delivers an excitation wavelength of 488 nm and the maximum laser power output is 1 mW or less at the surface of the tissue. Confocal images are collected at a scan rate of 1.6 frames per second (1024 ×512 pixels) or 0.8 frames per second (1024×1024 pixels). The optical slice thickness is 7 μm, and the lateral resolution is 0.7 μm. The range of z-axis is 0-250 μm below the contact surface. The field of view is 475×475 μm[7-9].

Technique of Confocal Laser Endomicroscopy

An exogenous fluorescent contrast agent is needed to achieve high-contrast images using confocal laser endomicroscopy. Potentially suitable contrast agents are fluorescein, acriflavine, tetracycline or cresyl violet. The most common contrast agents are acriflavine hydrochloride (0.05% in saline; topical use only) or fluorescein sodium (5–10 ml of a 10% solution; intravenous application). Fluorescein permits examining the whole spectrum of the Z axis (surface to 250μm depth); cells, vasculature, and connective tissue can be differentiated at high resolution, but the nuclei are not readily visible in the cofocal images with this agent. In contrast, acriflavine can be used topically to stain nuclei and cytoplasm, but it is limited to the surface layers of the mucosa (0-100μm) [7-9].

The confocal endoscope can be handled similar to a standard endoscope. After the systemic application of a contrast dye (e.g. fluorescein), the distal tip of the endoscope is placed in gentle contact with the mucosa and the position of the focal plane within the specimen is adjusted using the buttons on the endoscope control body. In every region of interest, images from the surface to deeper parts of the mucosal layer can be obtained and stored digitally. Targeted biopsies are possible because of the proximity of the working channel and the endomicroscopic window at the distal tip of the endoscope, which allows the position of the confocal scanner on the tissue to be seen via the conventional videoendoscopic view [7,8].

Confocal Imaging Data

In the colon, mucin-containing goblet cells and the columnar epithelial cells can be readily identified by fluorescein-aided CLE. In the confocal images of normal colorectum, superficial and deep "z-axis" crypt architecture appears as regular, oval luminal orifices covered by a homogeneous epithelial layer with evenly distributed goblet cells (figure 14-1a).

The microvascular net architecture is highlighted within the lamina propria in deeper parts of the mucosal layer. The vasculature within the mucosa of the colon shows a typical honeycomb appearance that represents a network of capillaries (figure 14-1b). Red blood cells are not labeled by fluorescein, and appear as moving black dots in the lumen of the vessels.

In regenerative and neoplastic mucosa, the crypt and vascular architecture alter (table 14-1)[7]. The confocal image of neoplastic mucosa is shown in figure 14-2. In the ulcerative colitis, a large number of inflammatory cells infiltrated in the intestinal mucosa stroma can be visible in the confocal endoscopic images. Furthermore, the activity of inflammation in UC can be judged on the basis of the appearance of confocal image (table 14-2) [10].

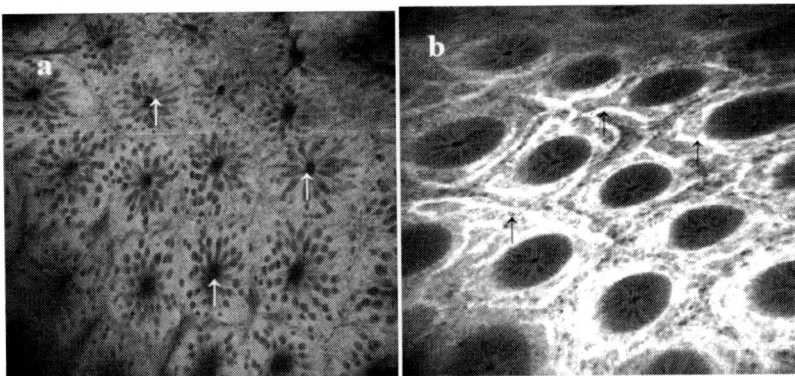

Figure 14-1. Normal colon confocal endoscopic images: a. The luminal openings of the cryptsappear in the horizontal axis as black holes (arrow) projecting onto the surface of the mucosa, and each crypt is covered with a layer of epithelial cells. b. The vasculature within the mucosa of the colon shows a typical honeycomb appearance that represents a network of capillaries (arrow). (The confocal endomicroscopic images were from Qi-lu Hospital).

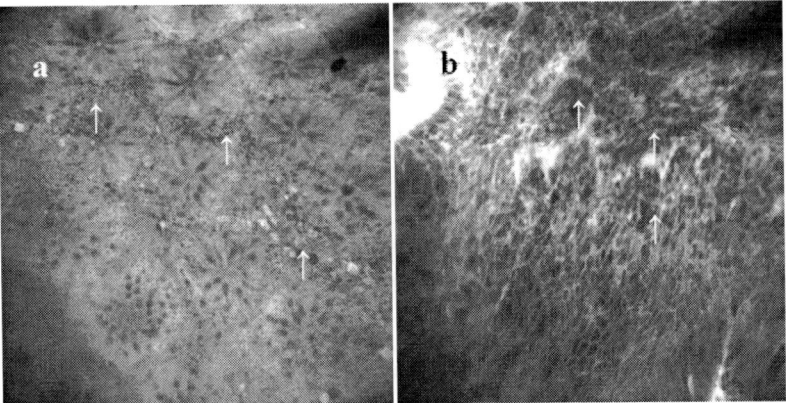

Figure 14-2. Confocal endoscopic images of UC and neoplasia: a. In the ulcerative colitis, a large number of inflammatory cell (arrow) infiltrated in the intestinal mucosa stroma can be visible. b. In the neoplasia, normal crypt and microvascular architecture were destroyed and tumor cells (arrow) with irregular arrangement were visible. (The confocal endomicroscopic images were from Qi-lu Hospital.

Table 14-1. Mainz confocal endomicroscopy criteria for the prediction of colorectal neoplasias

grading	crypt architecture	vessel architecture
normal	regular luminal openings and distribution of the crypts covered by a homogeneous layer of epithelial cells, including goblet cells	hexagonal, honeycomb appearance that presents a network of capillaries outlining the stroma surrounding the luminal openings of the crypts
regeneration	star-shaped luminal crypt openings or focal aggregation of regular-shaped crypts with a regular or reduced amount of goblet cells	hexagonal, honeycomb appearance with no or mild increase in the number of capillaries
neoplasia	ridged-lined irregular epithelial layer with loss of crypts and goblet cells; irregular cell architecture with little or no mucin	dilated and distorted vessels with elevated leakage; irregular architecture with little or no orientation to adjunct tissue

Table 14-2. Mainz confocal endomicroscopy criteria for the prediction of activity of inflammation in UC

grading of inflammation	crypt architecture	Cellularin filtration	vessel architecture
no	regular luminal openings and distribution of crypts covered by a homogeneous layer of epithelial cells, including goblet cells	absent	normal hexagonal, honeycomb appearance that presents a network of capillaries outlining the stroma surrounding the luminal openings of the crypts
mild to moderate	differences in shape, size and distribution of crypts; increased distance between crypts, focal crypt destruction	present;<50% of crypts involved	mild to moderate increase of capillaries, dilated and distorted capillaries
severe	unequivocal crypt destruction	present; >50% of crypts involved	marked increase of dilated and distorted capillaries; leakage of fluorescein

The Diagnostic Accuracy of CLE for Intraepithelial Neoplasias and Colorectal Cancer

To assess the diagnostic accuracy of CLE for intraepithelial neoplasias and colorectal cancer, Kiesslich et al.[7] performed endomicroscopy in 42 patients with indications for screening or surveillance colonoscopy after previous polypectomy. Standardized locations (every 10 cm in the colon and terminal ileum) and 134 circumscript lesions were examined by cnfocal imaging. According to the confocal pattern classification mentioned above, confocal endomicroscopic images were graded as non-neoplastic, regenerative or neoplastic at the time of confocal imaging. Finally, a total of 13020 confocal images from 390 locations were compared with the histological results from 1038 biopsy specimens. The presence of neoplastic changes was predicted with a sensitivity of 97.4 %, a specificity of 99.4% and an accuracy of 99.2%.

Hurlstone et al.[12] performed chromoscopic colonoscopy and subsequent CLE in 40 patients. Chromoscopic colonoscopy revealed 162 lesions in 39 patients. CLE imaging was obtained on all 162 lesions and four segmental "normal" colorectal quadrants in each patients. Similarly, the confocal imaging criteria formulated by Kiesslich et al.[7] were used to predict neoplastic and non-neoplastic CLE images (defined as normal tissue, regenerative and neoplastic; table 14-1). A total of 5422 confocal images were compared with the histological data from 802 targeted biopsy specimens. The study has also showed that the presence of intraepithelial neoplasia was predicted using CLE with high accuracy (sensitivity, 97.4 %; specificity, 99.3%; accuracy, 99.1%).

The Application of CLE for Ulcerative Colitis

According to the above mentioned, CLE can be used to diagnose intraepithelial neoplasias and colorectal cancer with a high level of accuracy *in vivo*. The major application of CLE for IBD is the clinical benefit for the *in vivo* detection of intraepithelial neoplasia in chronic ulcerative colitis surveillance colonoscopy. Because of the long time required by CLE for examination of large surface areas, it is technically impossible to observe the whole colonic mucosa using CLE. Therefore, the role of CLE is to examine the target area where conventional endoscopy has detected some abnormality. Chromoendoscopy can be used to delineate circumscribed lesions and CLE can be subsequently used to determine the qualitative diagnoses of the lesions at cellular level during colonoscopy. And then targeted biopsies of relevant lesions can be performed [13].

Kiesslich *et al.* [10] demonstrated the efficacy of chromoscopic assisted CLE in a trial of 153 patients with long-term ulcerative colitis in clinical remission. Participants were randomized at a 1:1 ratio to either conventional colonoscopy or chromoscopy-guided CLE, to detect intraepithelial neoplasia or colorectal cancer. In the chromoscopic assisted CLE group, circumscribed lesions in the colonic mucosa detected by chromoendoscopy were examined using CLE, and the confocal diagnosis was made according to the confocal pattern classification. Targeted biopsies of the examined areas were subsequently performed and graduated histologically on the basis of the new Vienna classification. In the standard colonoscopy group, randomized biopsies were performed every 10 cm and also targeted biopsy specimens were taken from the areas showing visible mucosal changes. The study has shown that chromoscopic assisted CLE (80 patients) significantly increased the yield of intraepithelial neoplasia detection as compared with standard colonoscopy (73 patients) (19 versus 4; $P = 0.005$). Furthermore, the total number of biopsy specimens required in the chromoscopy with endomicroscopy group was significantly reduced in comparison with those in the standard colonoscopy group (1688 versus 3081; $P=0.008$).

The above study made by Kiesslich et al. has compared the diagnostic yield of chromoscopy-guided endomicroscopy with conventional "white light" endoscopy. Hurlstone et al.[11] performed a prospective randomized controlled study to compare the diagnostic yield of intraepithelial neoplasia and cancer in patients with long-standing ulcerative colitis using chromoendoscopy assisted endomicroscopy versus pan-colonic chromoendoscopy assisted colonoscopy. Patients were randomised at a 1:1 ratio to either chromoendoscopic endomicroscopy (178 patients) or chromoendoscopic colonoscopy alone (175 patients). Circumscribed lesions were characterized using endomicroscopy and chromoendoscopy with pit pattern analysis. There was no significant difference between groups regarding the total number of lesions detected. Targeted biopsies in addition to conventional 10 cm quadrantic biopsies were taken. Compared with pan-chromoendoscopy and biopsy alone, endomicroscopy targeted biopsies significantly increased the yield of intraepithelial neoplasia (79 versus 31; $P<0.001$) and also increased the yield of high-grade dysplastic lesions (21 versus 4; $P<0.001$).

In addition, Kiesslich et al. [10] evaluated the diagnostic accuracy of CLE for grading inflammation in UC. In the chromoendoscopy with endomicroscopy group, randomly selected areas or diffuse changes were graded according to crypt and vessel architecture and cellular infiltration (table 14-2). In the standard colonoscopy group, large areas of inflamed mucosa were graded on the basis of the degree of mucosal destruction. Intact mucosa without visible mucosal changes was classified as normal. A reticular surface pattern with scattered erosions or multiple erosive changes with partially preserved mucosa were classified as mild to moderate inflammatory changes. An ulcerated mucosal surface was classified as a severe inflammartory change. The study has shown that chromoscopy with endomicroscopy significantly increased the agreement of the endoscopic prediction of the extent of inflammatory activity with the histologic results from the corresponding specimens as compared with those in the standard colonoscopy group (95.0% verse 34.2%, $P \leq 0.001$).

In conclusion, CLE in conjunction with chromoendoscopy might lead to significant improvements in the colonoscopic surveillance of patients with CUC. Chromoendoscopy can unmask circumscript lesions, and subsequent targeted CLE permits diagnosing intraepithelial neoplasias with high accuracy *in vivo*. Thus, the reduction of the number biopsy specimens required and improvement of the diagnosis of intraepithelial neoplasias can be achieved [13].

References

[1] Itzkowitz SH, Harpaz N. Diagnosis and management of dysplasia in patients with inflammatory bowel diseases. *Gastroenterology*, 2004, 126: 1634–1648.

[2] Chambers WM, Warren BF, Jewell DP, et al. Cancer surveillance in ulcerative colitis. *Br J Surg*, 2005, 92: 928-936.

[3] Itzkowitz WM, Present DH. Consensus conference: colorectal cancer screening and surveillance in inflammatory bowel disease. *Inflamm Bowel Dis, 2005*, 11: 314-321.

[4] Kiesslich R, Fritsch J, Holtmann M, et al. Methylene blue-aided chromoendoscopy for the detection of intraepithelial neoplasia and colon cancer in ulcerative colitis. *Gastroenterology*, 2003, 124: 880–888.

[5] Rutter MD, Saunders BP, Schofield G, et al. Pancolonic indigo carmine dye spraying for the detection of dysplasia in ulcerative colitis. *Gut*, 2004, 53: 256–260.

[6] Hurlstone DP, Sanders DS, Lobo AJ, et al. Indigo carmine-assisted high-magnification chromoscopic colonoscopy for the detection and characterisation of intraepithelial

neoplasia in ulcerative colitis: a prospective evaluation. *Endoscopy*, 2005, 37: 1186–1192.

[7] Kiesslich R, Bure J, Vieth M, et al. Confocal laser endoscopy for diagnosing intraepithelial neoplasias and colorectal cancer in vivo. *Gastroenterology*, 2004, 127: 706-713.

[8] Kiesslich R, Goetz M, Vieth M, et al. Confocal laser endomicroscopy. *Gastrointest Endoscopy Clin N Am*, 2005, 15: 715-731.

[9] Polglase A, McLaren WJ, Skinner SA, et al. A fluorescence confocal endomicroscope for in vivo microscopy of the upper-and the lower-GI tract. *Gastrointest Endosc*, 2005, 62: 686-695.

[10] Kiesslich R, Goetz M, Lammersdorf K, et al. Chromoscopy-guided endomicroscopy increase the diagnostic yield of intraepithelial neoplasia in ulcerative colitis. *Gastroenterology*, 2007, 132: 874-882.

[11] Hurlstone DP, Kiesslich R, Thomson M, et al. Confocal chromoscopic endomicroscopy is superior to chromoscopy alone for the detection and characterization of intraepithelial neoplasia in chronic ulcerative colitis. *Gut*, 2008, 57: 196-204

[12] Hurlstone DP, Baraza W, Brown S, et al. *In vivo* real-time confocal laser scanning endomicroscopic colonoscopy for the detection and characterization of colorectal neoplasia. *Br J Surg*, 2008, 95: 636-645.

[13] Kiesslich R, Goetz M, Vieth M, et al. Technology Insight: confocal laser endoscopy for in vivo diagnosis of colorectal cancer. *Nat clin pract oncol*, 2007, 4: 480-490.

In: Inflammatory Conditions of the Colon
Editor: Jia-ju Zheng

ISBN: 978-1-60692-240-8
© 2008 Nova Science Publishers, Inc.

Chapter XV

Magnifying Colonoscopy for Diagnosis of Ulcerative Colitis and Tumor

Si-de Liu
Nan-fang Hospital, Nan-fang Medical University,
Guang-dong Province, P.R. China

Equipment for Magnifying Colonoscopy

As early as the electron colonoscope was initially used, Japanese endoscopists had realized that, if the colonic mucosa is observed under the magnifying endoscope, the rate of endoscopic recognition of minute lesions and early cancer may be notably increased, and the earliest equipment for magnifying colonoscope appeared in 1970s. However, it was the Olympus CF-2002 electron magnifying colonoscope system that was actually widely used in clinical practice in 1992, the system used a manual optical zoom system that can magnify the mucosal structure about 100 electron colonoscope. The system was subsequently widely used in Japan because it highly increased the detectable rate of early colorectal cancer, particularly that of flat and depressed lesions. Currently the Olympus 2402 magnifying colonoscope system is the popular type, which belongs to the third generation of electron magnifying colonoscope with a magnifying power of 100 electron colonoscope and an electronic zoom resulting in better quality of images. Recently, Olympus has introduced a new high-quality magnifying colonoscope system, CF-H260AZI, using an HDTV format to output high-definition electronic images, a 70-fold optical zoom that may be advanced to a maximum power of 140 electron colonoscope in combination with an electronic zoom. The system has further incorporated an alternative rigidity control to improve the capability of insertion.

Methods for Magnifying Colonoscopy

Practice of colonoscopy in mainland of China began in 1973, when the initiators in this field were Prof. Pan Qi-Ying and Prof. Zhou Dian-Yuan. In 1977 Prof. Zhou Dian-Yuan concluded basic guidelines as "less inflate, insert and slide the colonoscope through the lumen, straighten out bends and loops, alter the sharp bend to slow bend, alter the acute angle to obtuse angle" and basic skills as "find the lumen, follow the lumen, slide in, position, clasp and pull, twist, prevent loops" for insertion of an endoscope. Following the above principles, the rate of successful ileocecal arrival was increased up to 98.5% even in 1979, and the average duration of each procedure was only 10 minutes, which was at an internationally advanced level [1]. Thereafter, the classical manipulation by two persons was used for insertion of colonoscope all along in China, but disadvantages such as long time of insertion, more pain, inconvenience to observe minute lesions and inconvenience to perform fine diagnostic and therapeutic procedures were associated with this method. Since 1980s, a one man method introduced abroad instead of the two man one appeared to circumvent the shortages above, and numerous new techniques have also been developed and applied based on the one man method. Not until the end of 1990s, the colonoscopy through the one man method was initiated by a few institutions in China [2]. Wang Qiao-Ming et al from Anhui Provincial Hospital reported a rate of successful caecal reaching up to 97.5% using the one man method [2], and in April 2000, started at the "advanced class for one man manipulated colonoscopy" held by the digestive endoscopic center of our hospital as a national project for continuing medical education, the one man manipulated endoscopic insertion was generalized in China, and then the one man colonoscopy has been growing until it is becoming a new tide in China.

The magnifying colonoscopy must use one man endoscopic insertion because when one observe using a zoom magnification, he must know precisely the space between the tip of colonoscope and the mucosa to reach an optimal distance of about 2 mm, and he should also maintain the body of colonoscope stable, and only one man manipulation can precisely control the body and the tip of colonoscope, while two man manipulation is baffled due to the difficult cooperation between the handler and his assistant. Therefore, the one man method is the premise of magnifying colonoscopy.

Diagnosis of Neoplastic Lesions by Magnifying Endoscopy

1. The Value of Pit Pattern in Diagnosing Neoplastic Lesions of Large Bowels

Neoplastic lesions may be diagnosed by the pit pattern of lesion in highly consistent with the pathologic result. Current description regarding the mucosal pit pattern is principally based on the Japanese Kudo's pit pattern classification in 1996 [3], though prior to Kudo, some scholars had preliminarily separately studied and classified the pit pattern derived from each observation, such as, Kosaka et al, through the stero microscopic findings from the mucosal lesions in large intestines of 277 patients, assigned the pits to 4 patterns: i. simple; ii. papillary; iii. tubular; iv. sulcal. Tada modified the above to 6 patterns by addition of mixed and structureless patterns. Furthermore, there were Eto and Nishizawa classifications. None of the classifications above was standardized until 1996, when Shin-ei Kudo presented new criteria of pit pattern classification from his findings by stero microscopy in combination with magnifying endoscopy in 1676 patients. The criteria have been widely accepted in Japanese academia, and have become a current classification of pit pattern. The Kudo's pit pattern is described below with incorporation of magnifying endoscopic findings and pictures.

Kudo concluded 5 types mainly upon the pattern and the size of pits [3], and these types are known as Type I, II, III, IV and V, respectively, among which the Type III consists of two subtypes, IIIs and III_L. The patterns and characteristics of these types are shown in table 15-1.

Table 15-1. Kudo's pit pattern classification (1996)

Type	Pattern	Characteristic	Pit size (mm)
I		Round (normal pit)	0.07±0.02
II		Stella or papillary	0.09±0.02
IIIs		Tubular or discoid, smaller than normal pits	0.03±0.01
III_L		Tubular or discoid, larger than normal pits	0.22±0.09
IV		Sulcal, dendritic or gyrus-like	0.93±0.32
V		Irregular or non-structural (lack of pit structure)	--

When used to diagnose and treat colorectal cancer, zoom colonoscope shows advantages as follows: Firstly: it provides frontal and lateral views of the lesion at short distance, and views at moderate or long distance so that one can find out the visual macroscopic morphology, developmental mode, depression or not, local characters and size of the lesion; secondly, it may change the air volume in large intestines, allow observation on the sclerosis of lesion and the concentration of ruga around it, and alter the shape of lesion by the change of air volume, from which the submucosal invasion of the lesion can be determined; finally, it can approach the lesion and provide vision of its micro-configuration, as well as the specific crypt pattern, which notably increase the accuracy of adjudication for the degree of neoplastic invasion, and make its practicability widely accepted. Type V_I pits incorporates a large proportion of intramucosal cancer (figure 15-1), while type V_N often appears to be submucosal deep cancer (figure 15-2). Use of zoom colonoscope may estimate presence of a tumor where a mucosal biopsy is absent, and give information of the histological type of the lesion. When an excision of colorectal tumor is indicated, the magnifying view for the area around the resected lesion is also advisable to confirm the complete removal of the lesion.

This is quite significant in the treatment for colorectal cancer. Furthermore, when practice the piecemeal mucosal resection to resect major tumors similar to laterally spreading tumors (LST), it is also very important to perform a one-off resection of parts with higher malignancy using zoom colonoscope prior to the resection of other parts.

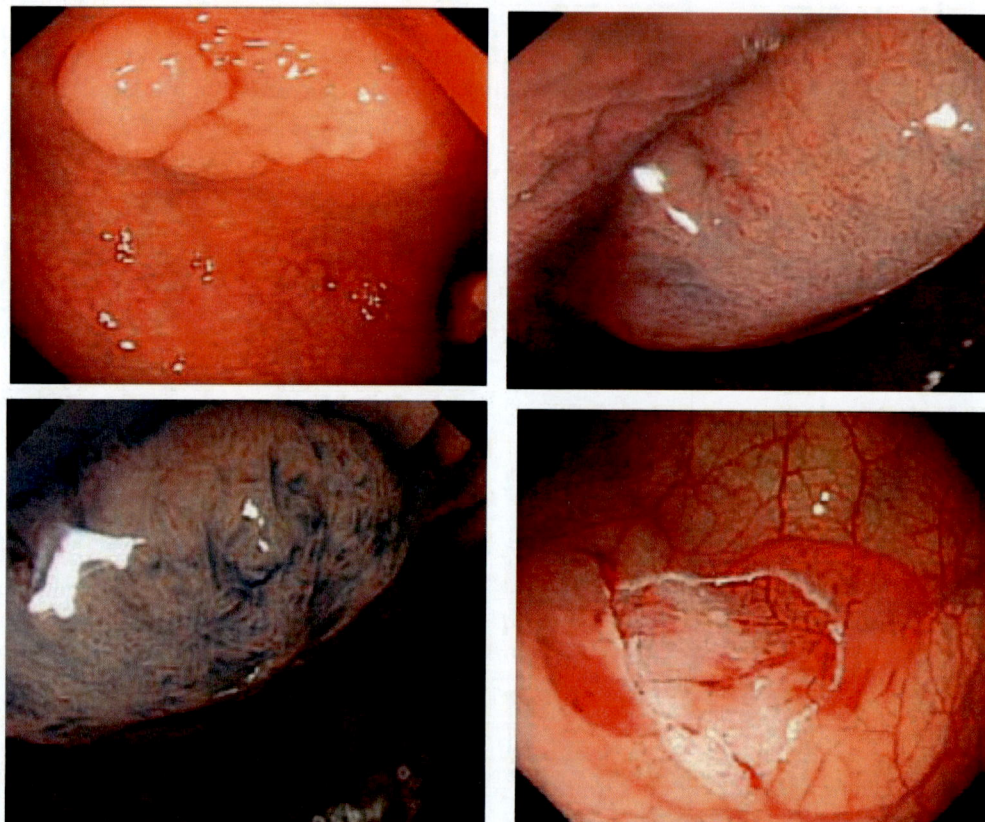

Figure 15-1. Magnifying endoscopic view of early colorectal cancer: irregular arrangement of pits on the surface of tumor, disappearance of pits in some regions, presence of type V_1 pits. EMR resection was done for this case, and a intramucosal cancer was indicated by pathological analysis.

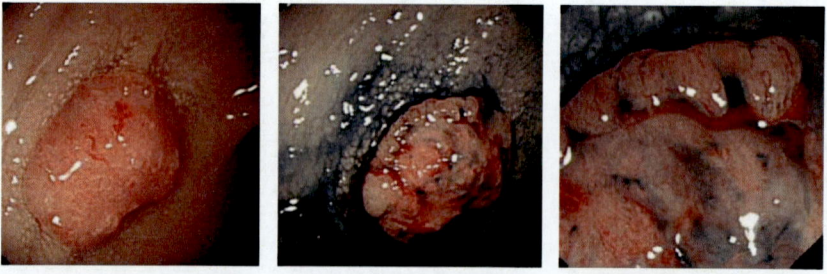

Figure 15-2. Minute progressive cancer in the upper segment of rectum with diameter about 0.9cm, the left is a typical endoscopic image, the middle is the image after mucosal staining, and the right is the 70-fold magnified image by magnifying endoscopy, where normal pits are completely disappeared, and non-structural type V pits are presented.

Magnifying colonoscopy was introduced later to China, where the earliest one was a second generation electron colonoscope, Olympus CF-Q200Z coloscope with manual zoom at a magnification of 100 times, was imported by our hospital in mid-1990s. Since then, large hospitals in Shanghai and Beijing have subsequently purchased newest electron magnifying colonoscope. In 2000, our hospital began to use the third generation magnifying colonoscope, Olympus CF-Q240Z, instead of the general electron colonoscope. It uses magnifying colonoscope in combination with mucosal staining and has detected a number of intramucosal cancers and large intestinal tumors with special morphologies [4-15], among which 46 cases of laterally spreading tumor of colon, 4 cases of type IIc colorectal cancer, 7 cases of serrated adenoma of large intestine and 8 cases of flat early colorectal cancer were reported.

Magnifying Endoscopy Together with Mucosal Staining for Diagnosis of Ulcerative Colitis

Diagnosis for ulcerative colitis is principally based on the colonoscopic findings. Due to the complexity and multiplicity of the mucosal lesions and the ulcers in ulcerative colitis, the inflammatory lesions are lacking of specific exhibition by mucosal biopsy, and some cases are hardly distinguished from Crohn disease, intestinal tuberculosis, lymphoma and other intestinal ulcerative lesions by endoscopy. Magnifying endoscopy can magnify the mucosal structure by 30~100 folds, and is able to effectively detect mucosal tiny lesions and the morphological characteristics of lesions; for protrusive lesions it may produce diagnoses highly consistent with pathological conclusions based on the pit pattern on the mucosal surface, and for inflammatory lesions and depressed lesions it also allows finding the characteristics of the micro structures of mucosal surface for differentiation. Endoscopic mucosal staining enhance significantly the ability of endoscopists to identify mucosal microstructures and lesions, and in combination with magnifying endoscopy the accuracy of diagnosis for ulcerative colitis can also be highly increased [21].

Under the magnifying endoscope, ulcerative colitis mainly shows the following 6 characteristics:

1. Normal Pits (Normal Crypts)

Mostly seen in the normal intestinal mucosa of ulcerative colitis, where since the mucosa is not involved in the lesion, the mucosal morphosis is normal both by standard endoscopy and by magnifying endoscopy, and a typical type I pits are shown under the magnifying endoscope (figure 15-3).

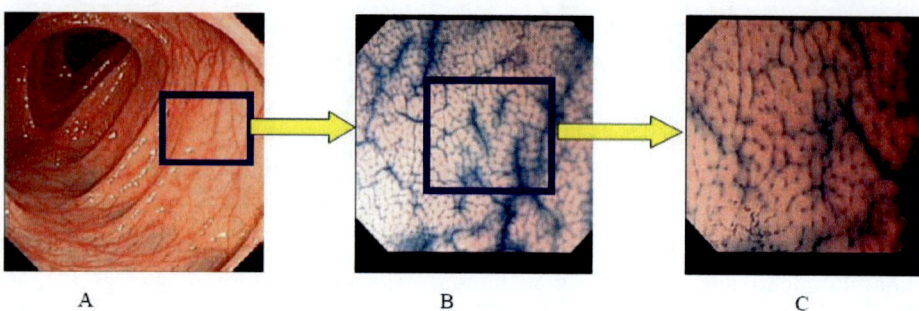

Figure 15-3. A: View of mucosa in a normal transverse colon by standard endoscopy; B: Normal type I pits observed by local 40-fold magnification after mucosal staining; C: Normal type I pits observed by 100-fold magnification after mucosal staining.

2. Reduced Normal Crypts, Deformed Crypts

Mostly seen in the early stage of inflammatory activities of ulcerative colitis, mucosal congestive edema is visible by standard endoscopy, the vascular net disappears, but the mucosal integrity is not destroyed. The histological shape in this stage appears as large amounts of inflammatory infiltration in the lamina protria of the mucosa, but integral crypt structures still, indicating crypt abscesses were not formed. Deformed crypts can be seen by magnifying endoscopy, and reduced crypts are seen in some regions (figure 15-4).

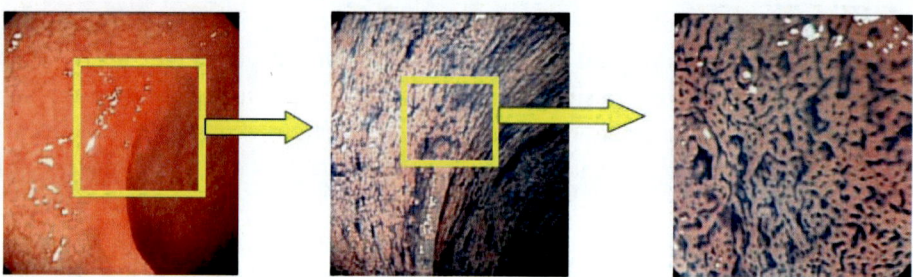

Figure 15-4. Reduced normal crypts, deformed crypts.

3. Enlarged Crypts and Granular Structure

This is a typical figure of mucosal lesion in the progression of ulcerative colitis in the active stage, with rough and fine granular structures, fine abrasive paper-like surface seen by standard endoscopy. After staining, by magnifying endoscopy a typical fine granular structure is observed (figure 15-5), and this histopathological alteration is caused by the inflammatory cell infiltration in the underlayer of the crypt mucosa that resulting in the swelling of crypts. The granular structure by magnifying endoscopy is a typical figure of ulcerative colitis in its active stage, and is highly valued for diagnosis.

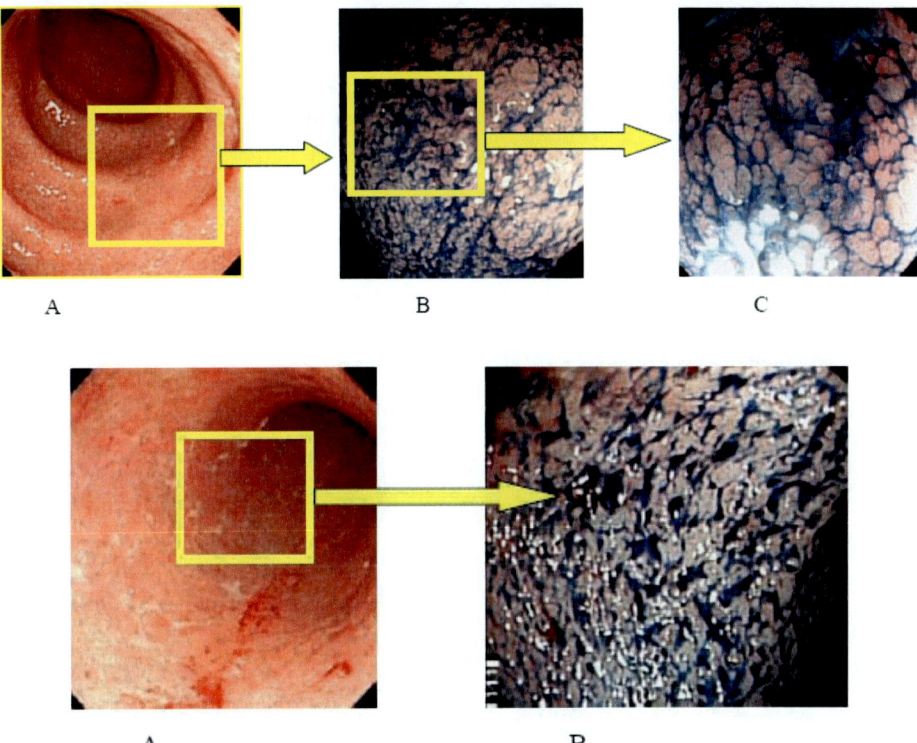

Figure 15-5. Image A show the general coloscope view of ulcerative colits, image B and C show the staining and magnifying view of the marked area, it appear the enlarged crypts and granular structure.

4. Crypt Damage, Coarse Villiform Structure

This is one of the typical figures of mucosal lesion in ulcerative colitis, with crypt swelling showing short villiform seen by magnifying endoscopy, distributed in normal density, and partial crypt damages among the short villiform crypts present as irregular depressions and superficial ulcers (figure 15-6.), and usually more inflammatory exudates appear on the mucosal surface, which incorporates characteristic significance for diagnosis.

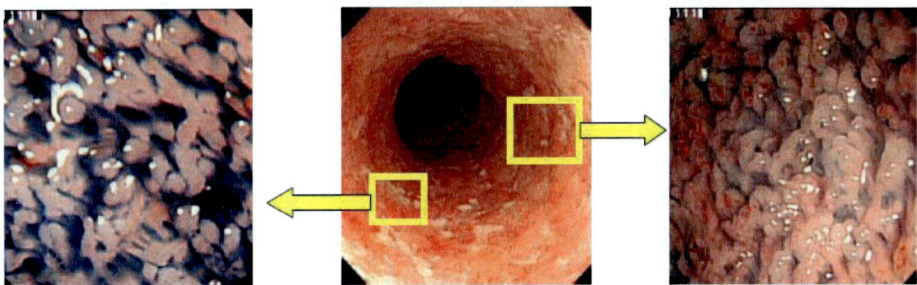

Figure 15-6. Crypt damage, coarse villiform structure.

5. Crypt Fusion and Formation of a Cribriform Structure

The sieve texture formed by destroyed crypts that mutually merge is the inflammatory activity of ulcerative colitis. The characteristic alterations indicating apparent mucosal damage are seen in highly affected intestinal segments in patients with active ulcerative colitis, and usually evident surface inflammatory exudation as well, and if the crypts fuse extensively, superficial ulcers will be formed (figure 15-7). A typical cribriform structure is the major characteristic of the magnifying endoscopic findings for mucosal lesions of ulcerative colitis, since it seldom occurs in lesioned mucosa of other colitises including infective colitis, Crohn disease and intestinal tuberculosis, et al. Consequently, a sieve structure of the lesioned mucosa seen by magnifying endoscopy will conclude a endoscopic diagnosis of ulcerative colitis.

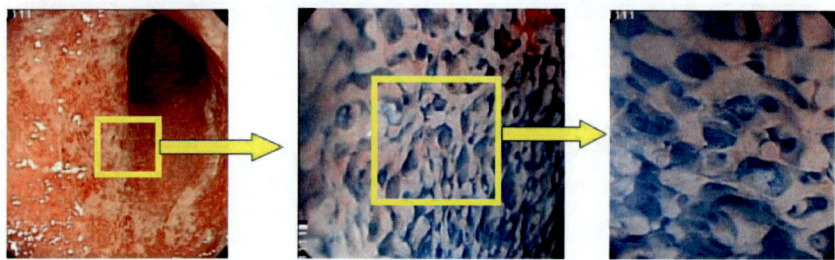

Figure 15-7. A: Diffuse damage, extensive erosion and large amount of effusion of the mucosa observed by standard endoscopy; B: After staining, complete disappearance of normal surface structure seen by magnifying endoscopy, and extensive damage of crypts that fuse to a vertically and horizontally interlaced sieve texture; C: Further magnifying shows destroyed crypts with necrotic tissues and fibroid exudates insides.

6. Ulcers

Irregular superficial ulcers may be formed after the crypts are extensively destroyed and merged. The ulcers form a very irregular figure with high multiformity, and it is hardly found that two ulcers in an entirely same shape. They are usually polygons or asterisms, densely distributed with a large amount of inflammatory exudation on the surface, and without normal mucosal distribution among the ulcers (figure 15-8.).

The pathological manifestation of ulcerative colitis under the magnifying endoscope is typical crypt lesions characterized in the enlargement, damage and fusion of crypts, and may appear as granular, cribriform structures and ulceration, while the remaining normal crypts may proliferate to form coarse villiform structure. Table 15-2 shows the magnifying endoscopic morphological characteristics in 116 patients with ulcerative colitis diagnosed in the Southern Hospital. Magnifying endoscopy together with mucosal staining can notably increase the rate of identification for tiny lesions of crypts, and thus help the endoscopic diagnosis and differentiation for ulcerative colitis.

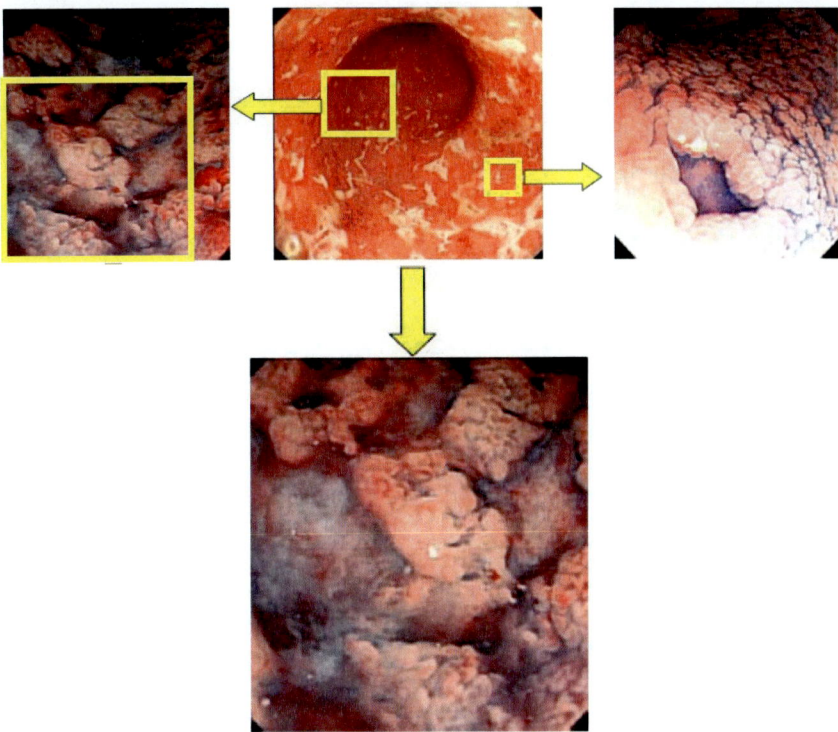

Figure 15-8-1. A great variety of ulcers and a large amount of inflammatory exudation on the surface, and without normal mucosal distribution among the ulcers.

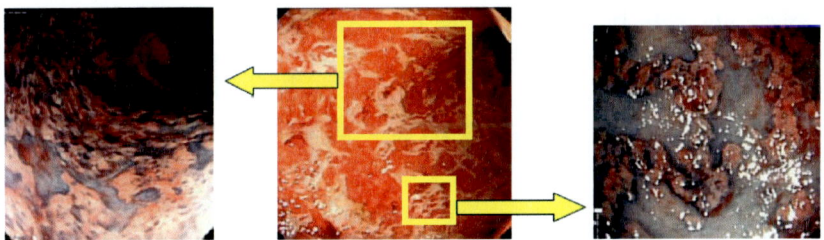

Figure 15-8-2. The ulcer's shape is irregular under magnifying coloscope and appears like map.

Table15-2. The magnifying endoscopic morphological characteristics in 116 patients with ulcerative colitis diagnosed in the Southern Hospital

Magnifying endoscopic characteristics	Cases (n)	Percent (%)
Reduced normal crypts, deformed crypts	41	35.3
Enlarged crypts and granular structure	91	78.4
Crypt damage, coarse villiform structure	16	13.8
Crypt fusion and formation of a cribriform structure	108	93.1
Ulcers	82	70.7

References

[1] Zhou Dian-Yuan. Experience of enhancing the rate of success to insert a fiber-colonoscope. *Chinese Journal of Internal Medicine.* 1979;18:180-183.

[2] Wang Qiao-Min, Zheng Bang-Hai, Jia Yong, et al. The clinical prctice and evaluation of the one-man colonoscopy. *Chinese Journal of Digestive Endoscopy.* 2003;20:405-406.

[3] Shin-ei Kudo (工藤淮英). Early colorectal cancer-detection of depressed types of colorectal carcinoma. P50-51. Igaku-Shoin Medical Publisher, Inc. Tokyo, 1996.

[4] Jiang Bo, Zhi Fa-Zhao, Liu Si-De, et al. Pit pattern and endoscopic mucosal resection in diagnosis and treatment of colorectal tumors. *National Medical Journal of China.* 2003;83:294-297.

[5] Liu Si-De, Jiang Bo, Zhi Fa-Zhao, et al. Serrated adenoma of large intestine: report of 7 cases. *Journal of First Military Medical University.* 2002;22:283.

[6] Jiang Bo, Liu Si-De, Zhi Fa-Zhao, et al. The diagnosis and treatment of 25 cases of laterally spreading tumor of large intestine. *Journal of First Military Medical University.* 2002;22:189-191.

[7] Jiang Bo, Liu Si-De, Zhi Fa-Zhao, et al. Diagnosis and management of laterally spreading tumor of colon by dyeing and Magnifying colonoscopy. *Chinese Journal of Digestive Endoscopy.* 2003;20:9-12.

[8] Liu Si-De, Li Ming-Song, Chen Xue-Qing, et al. Diagnosis and treatment of laterally spreading tumor (LST) through endoscopy. *Medical Journal of Chinese People's Liberation Army.* 2004;29:928-931.

[9] Liu Si-De, Yue Hui, Li Ming-Song, et al. Report of unusual flat lesions and serrated adenoma of large intestine in 2 cases. *Medical Journal of Chinese People's Liberation Army.* 2004;29:941-942.

[10] Liu Si-De, Li Ming-Song, Chen Xue-Qing, et al. Report of endoscopic resction for the macro flat early cancer of rectum in one case. *Medical Journal of Chinese People's Liberation Army.* 2004;29:943.

[11] Liu Si-De, Yue Hui, Bai Lan, et al. Endoscopic mucosal resections and follow-up study for 8 patients with colonic laterally spreading tumors with early carcinomatous change. *Medical Journal of Chinese People's Liberation Army.* 2004;29:932-933.

[12] Zhi Fa-Zhao, Jiang Bo, Liu Si-De, et al. Comparison of curative effect for colon flat lesion between mucosa resection and fulguration with high frequency current after mucosa staining under magnifying endoscope. *National Medical Journal of China.* 2002;82:180-182.

[13] Bai Lan, Liu Si-De, Zhi Fa-Zhao, et al. The diagnostic value with analysis of pit pattern classification on early cancer of large intestine detection. *Chinese Journal of Digestion.* 2004;24:78-82.

[14] Jiang Bo, Liu Si-De. Pay emphasis to the diagnosis and treatment of flat tumors of colon. *Medical Journal of Chinese People's Liberation Army.* 2004;29:925-927.

[15] Shen Shou-Rong, Jiang Xi-Wang, Xu Can-Xia, et al. Application of midazolam combined with propofol or fentanyl to colonoscopy. *China Journal of Clinical Medicine.* 2003;9:7-9.

[16] Luo Jun, Zhao Ying, Wang Xiao, et al. The Comparison of Clinical Application between Gatroscopy and Conoloscopy in General Anesthesia Painlessly. *West China Medical Journal*. 2004;19:273-274.

[17] 工藤進英. 側方發育型腫瘍 (Laterally spreading tumor; LST) について. *Early Colorectal Cancer*. 1998;2:477-481.

[18] 寺井毅, 今井靖, 二瓶英人, 他. LSTの臨床的意義 (3) 臨床病理學的檢討かうみたその特殊性. *Early Colorectal Cancer*. 1998;2:505-516.

[19] Takashi Hirooka, Hiroaki Ohchi, Shinichi Kataoka, et al. 大腸結節集簇樣病變がBorrmann 2型病變に進展した1症例. *Early Colorectal Cancer*., 1998;2:517-519.

[20] Jiang Bo, Liu Si-De. Laterally spreading tumors (LST) of large intestine and options of endoscopic treatment for it. Compilation of papers from the 3rd annual session of Guangdong Society of Endoscopy. 2005:53-60.

[21] Liu Si-De, Jiang Bo, Zhou Dian-Yuan, et al. Diagnosis of ulcerative colitis by magnifying endoscopy and colonic mucosal staining. Compilation of papers from the 3rd annual session of Guangdong Society of Endoscopy. 2005:174-176.

Chapter XVI

Endoscopic Retrograde Cholangiopancreatography in Inflammatory Bowel Disease

Feng Liu and Zhao-shen Li
Chang-hai Hospital, Second Military Medical University, Shang-hai, P.R. China

Introduction

Inflammatory bowel disease (IBD) includes ulcerative colitis and Crohn disease, which is of unknown origin and chronic inflammatory disorder involving any parts of the gastrointestinal (GI) tract. Endoscopy plays an important role in the diagnosis, follow-up and malignancy surveillance of IBD. As a special autoimmune disease, IBD usually involves in arthrosis, skin, eyes, biliary and liver system in addition to the GI tract. Some extraintestinal manifestitions in IBD patients may develop earlier than GI symptoma of IBD. The pathogenesis of extraintestinal manifestitions in IBD remains unknown Some autoantibodies occurred in IBD patients may reflect an immune deregulation triggered by bowel mucosal ulcerations, or a cross-reaction as has been shown important in other autoantibodies. Primary sclerosing cholangitis (PSC) and IBD[1] related pancreatitis are two extraintestinal manifestitions of IBD. Cholangiography or pancreatography, preferably endoscopic retrograde cholangiopancreatography (ERCP) is the current standard method for imaging the biliary and pancreatic tract in patients with PSC and chronic pancreatitis.

The Role of ERCP in PSC

Primary sclerosing cholangitis is a chronic cholestatic liver disorder that is characterized by multiple fibrotic strictures of the intrahepatic and extrahepatic biliary ducts. During the course of PSC many patients experience worsening of symptoms such as pruritus, abdominal pain, fever with chills, and jaundice due to impeded biliary drainage[1]. Liver failure and cholangiocarcinoma are cause of death of patients with PSC. About 2% -10% of patients with IBD suffer from PSC. Approximately 50-70% of patients with PSC have IBD,and the others will develop IBD in few years. ERCP is golden standard for diagnosis of PSC.

According to ERCP imaging of PSC, There are three types in PSC. 1.extrahepatic type: patients with PSC typically have multifocal areas of stricture of extrahepatic bile ducts on ERCP, with intervening segments of normal or dilated ducts, like "a string of beads" (figure 16-1). 2. intrahepatic type: the intrahepatic bile ducts become spare and stiff, like "stick" (figure 16-2). The shape of intrahepatic bile ducts is irregular. 3. diffused type: On ERCP, patients with PSC have abnormity of both extrahepatic and intrahepatic bile ducts.

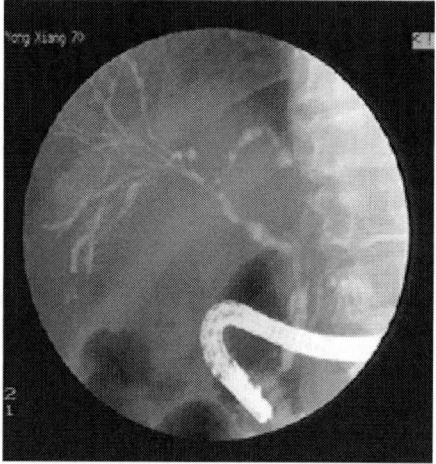

Figure 16-1. Both intra-and extrahepatic bile ducts have mulifocal areas of strictures, with intervening segments of dilated ducts imaging like "a string of beads" on ERCP.

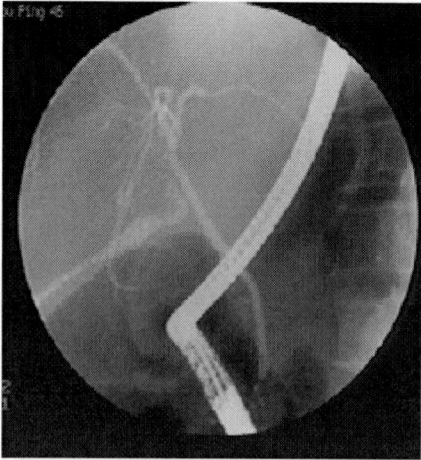

Figure 16-2. ERCP showed spare and stiff intrahepatic bile ducks, like "stick".

Over time, 10–20% of patients with PSC are known to develop cholangiocarcinoma with a very dismal prognosis. It is very important to diagnosis the cholangiocarcinoma early to improve the prognosis of PSC, but few methods can be used. Brush cytology from bile duct strictures in PSC patients can detect cholangiocarcinoma. ERCP can be performed using standard technique. After radiographic documentation of biliary stricture and placement of a Glidewire, a Geenen brush system was used to obtain cytologic samples under fluoroscopic control[2,4]. Cluster of malignant cells in a bile duct brushing exhibits marked crowding of enlarged cells and coarse granularity of nuclear chromatin. Boberg et al reported the sensitivity, specificity, positive- and negative predictive values, and accuracy of brush cytology in diagnosis of biliary malignancy were 100%, 84%, 68%, 100%, and 88%, respectively[2,4].

Approximately 20% of patients with PSC have dominant strictures. In patients with such strictures, it is generally agreed that biliary tract patency should be restored promptly if technically feasible. The endoscopic modalities that have been used to restore biliary patency include catheter or balloon dilation with or without biliary stent placement[4,5]. The endoscopic attempts to maintain biliary patency may improve the five years survival of patients with PSC.

The Role of ERCP in Pancreatitis Related to IBD

Episodes of pancreatitis occur in many patients during the course of IBD. Gallstones and alcohol intake were found in some of the cases, whereas drug-induced pancreatitis was found in IBD. The cause of the other cases with pancreatitis was unknown. We recognize this pancreatitis as idiopathic pancreatitis. The final rate of idiopathic pancreatitis was 8% in this series[6]. Autopsy studies in UC have revealed the presence of macroscopic or icroscopic pancreatic lesions in 14–53% of cases. The pathogenesis of IBD-related pancreatitis remains unknown. The pancreatic autoantibodies may reflect an immune deregulation triggered by bowel mucosal ulcerations. The main manifestation of pancreatitis related IBD is pancreatic duct abnormalities and exocrine pancreatic insufficiency. The main pancreatic ductal changes could be due to severe periductal inflammation, periductal lymphocytic inflammatory infiltrates, perilobular fibrosis. On ERCP, patients with IBD-assotiated to pancreatitis have these anomalies included irregularities , short stenosis or upstream dilation of the main pancreatic duct.

References

[1] Huang C, Lichtenstein DR. Pancreatic and biliary tract disorders in inflammatory bowel disease. *Gastrointest. Endosc. Clin. N. Am.* 2002; 2(3):535-59.

[2] Boberg KM, Jebsen P, Clausen OP,et al. Diagnostic benefit of biliary brush cytology in cholangiocarcinoma in primary sclerosing cholangitis. *J. Hepatol.* 2006; 45(4):568-74.

[3] Barthet M, Lesavre N, Desplats S,et al. Frequency and characteristics of pancreatitis in patients with inflammatory bowel disease. *Pancreatol.* 2006; 6(5):464-71.

[4] Baluyut AR, Sherman S, Lehman GA,et al. Impact of endoscopic therapy on the survival of patients with primary sclerosing cholangitis. *Gastrointest. Endosc.* 2001; 53(3):308-12.

[5] Moff SL, Kamel IR, Eustace J, et al. Diagnosis of primary sclerosing cholangitis: a blinded comparative study using magnetic resonance cholangiography and endoscopic retrograde cholangiography. *Gastrointest. Endosc.* 2006; 64(2):219-223.

[6] Jiang X-y, Rong L, Son D-y. Extraintestinal manifestations of inflammatory bowel disease. *J. Gastroenterol. Hepatol.* 2006; 15(4):350-352

Section Four: Clinical Aspects of Idiopathic Inflammatory Bowel Disease

In: Inflammatory Conditions of the Colon
Editor: Jia-ju Zheng

ISBN: 978-1-60692-240-8
© 2008 Nova Science Publishers, Inc.

Chapter XVII

Management of Inflammatory Bowel Disease in the Asia-Pacific Region

Qin Ouyang
West China Hospital of Si-chuan Unversity, Si-chuang Province, P.R. China

Introduction

In recent years a significant increase in the incidence and prevalence of inflammatory bowel disease (IBD) observed in Asia–Pacific countries has prompted the gastroenterologists in this region to work out an optimal diagnostic and management strategy for patients with IBD. The clinical epidemiology, diagnosis and treatment of IBD in this region are somewhat different from those in Western countries. For example, infectious diseases, especially intestinal tuberculosis and other intestinal infections, are common in this region; they have added to the complexity in the diagnosis and treatment of patients with IBD. Asia-Pacific Working Party-IBD has been presented a management guideline of IBD, and was ratified at the Asia-Pacific Digest Week (APDW) in 2004. We now revised as follows.

Epidemiology of Inflammatory Bowel Disease in Asia

The incidence of UC ranged from 1.0 to 2.0 per 100 000 person years[1–4]. The incidence of CD ranges from 0.5 to 1.0 per 100 000 person years[4,5]. The prevalence of UC has ranged from 4.0 to 44.3 per 100 000 and that of CD from 3.6 to 7.7 per 100 000[6,7]. Ulcerative colitis appears to be more common than CD in Asia. In China the speculated prevalence varies between 11.6/100 000 and 1.4/100 000, respectively. Several recent Asian studies confirm that the incidence and prevalence of both UC and CD are lower than those in North America and Europe. Compared to time trends in the West, there appears to be a time lag phenomenon involving incidence and prevalence of IBD with regard to the Asian experience.

Diagnosis of Inflammatory Bowel Disease

Various diagnostic classifications of IBD are available, including Mendeloff's criteria,[8], the Lennard-Jones criteria[9], the international multicentre scoring system of the Organization Mondiale de Gastroenterology (OMGE), [10] and the diagnostic criteria of Japanese Research Society on IBD.[11]

Modified Mendeloff Criteria

UC: Definite (i) History of diarrhea or rectal bleeding for 6 weeks or more with: (ii) at least one sigmoidoscopy or colonoscopy revealing one or more of the following: mucosal friability, petechial hemorrhage, diffuse inflammatory ulceration; radiological evidence of ulceration or narrowing/shortening of the colon; characteristic macroscopic and microscopic changes in a specimen obtained by surgical resection or biopsy. Probable (i) A compatible sigmoidoscopy, colonoscopy, or barium enema with inadequate history; (ii) a compatible history with dubious sigmoidoscopic or colonoscopic appearance and no barium enema; (iii) an adequate history but dubious radiological findings and no sigmoidoscopy or colonoscopy report; and (iv) a characteristic macroscopic appearance of the operative specimen with an uncertain histology.

After exclusion of infectious colitis, ischemic colitis, radiation colitis, solitary rectal ulcer, findings compatible with CD, if compatible histology is found, such as continuous mucosal inflammation without granulomas and rectal involvement with continuity of the colon, the diagnosis is regarded as 'definite'; in the absence of histological confirmation, the diagnosis is regarded as 'probable'.

CD: Definite Characteristic pathological and histological findings in an operative specimen showing segmental, transmural lesions, fissuring ulcers, and non-caseating granulomas and lymphoid aggregates in the lamina propria and submucosa. Probable (i) A laparotomy report of characteristic naked-eye appearance of the bowel but no specimen for histology; (ii) an equivocal histological report from an operative specimen with characteristic macroscopic features; (iii) a colonoscopic report compatible with CD, and biopsy histologic features strongly suggestive of CD; and (iv) a radiologic examination showing chronic inflammation with obstruction or fistulae.

After exclusion of infections (particularly intestinal tuberculosis [TB]), ischemia, radiation, lymphoma or carcinoma, if granulomas are present with at least another criteria or, in the absence of granulomas, with three of the characteristic lesions, such as skip lesions, discrete ulcers, fissuring ulcers, fistulae, strictures or aphthoid ulcers etc., a diagnosis of CD is regarded as 'definite'; if two criteria without granuloma are present, the diagnosis is regarded as 'probable'.

The term 'indeterminate colitis' should be used when only the colon is involved, and the diagnosis of UC or CD is impossible based on the aforementioned criteria.

The Criteria Used by the Japanese Research Society on IBD

Ulcerative colitis:(A) Symptoms: continuous or repeated bloody diarrhea; (B) endoscopy: diffuse inflammation, loss of vascular pattern, friability (bleeding at contact), abundant mucus and (i) granular appearance; (ii) multiple erosions, ulcers; and (iii) pseudopolyps, loss of haustration (lead-pipe pattern), lumen narrowing, and colonic shortening.(C) Histology: active: inflammatory cells infiltration, crypt abscess, goblet cell depletion. Remission: crypt architectural abnormalities (distortion branching), atrophic crypts. These changes usually begin in the rectum and extend proximally in continuity.

Definite Diagnosis: A+ One Item of B and C

Crohn's disease: Major findings: (A) Longitudinal ulcer, (B) cobblestone appearance, (C) non-caseating granuloma. Minor findings: (D) Irregular-shaped ulcer or aphthoid ulcers, (E) irregular-shaped ulcer or aphthoid in upper and lower gastrointestinal tract.

Definite diagnosis: (i) C along with either A or B; (ii) C and D or E. Suspect: (i) A or B, but cannot exclude ischemic colitis or ulcerative colitis; (ii) C; (iii) D or E. The criteria are quite simple and easy to apply, but the exclusion criteria should be applied first; in particular the epidemic infectious disease should be excluded first in this region.

A suggested guideline from China paid more attention to the scrutinizing and evaluation of the patients, and the exclusion criteria applied first.

Differential Diagnosis of Inflammatory Bowel Disease

Differentiating IBD from acute self-limiting colitis and amoebic colitis: ASLC by definition resolves generally in <4 weeks. An infectious etiology is often suspected, such as Salmonella, Shigella, Clostridium difficile, Escherichia coli,E. histolytica. Acute onset of illness with fever and more than 10 bowel movements/24 h is seen in more than three-fourths of the patients. Stool cultures are positive in less than half of cases, but they may help the diagnosis. Fecal leukocytes are insensitive markers of infection because they are seen in both ASLC and IBD, but increased platelet is not commonly seen in ASLC[12]. The colonic mucosa crypts are generally normal, which is characterized by a predominantly polymorphonuclear infiltrate in the lamina propria; giant cells and rarely granulomas may be seen in the upper part of the mucosa (e.g. in lymphogranuloma venereum, syphilis). The diagnosis of amoebiasis is made by identifying trophozoites in fresh stools, mucosal exudates or mucosal biopsies. Serology may be useful.

Differentiating Crohn's disease from TB: Because of the similarity of clinical, endoscopic, radiologic and pathological findings of CD and TB, there may be a 50–70% misdiagnosis rate between the two conditions. Diagnosis of CD should always be made with caution in this region and TB must be excluded first. Distinguishing clinical features include perianal involvement and intestinal fistulae for CD, and past or present history for TB. Endoscopic features may help distinguish these two conditions. Helpful endoscopic features include longitudinal ulcers for CD and transverse ulcers for TB [13,14]. Histopathological features are most useful in distinguishing between the two conditions [15]. The presence of small, discrete and loose granulomas without caseation both in the bowel and in mesenteric lymph nodes are characteristic of CD. But large, dense, confluent granulomas with caseation and acid-fast bacilli (AFB) positive are characteristic of TB. In cases where TB cannot not excluded, a therapeutic trial of antituberculosis therapy for a period of 4–8 weeks is justified. A TB DNA analysis on the tissues with TB-specific primer could be helpful.

Differentiating Crohn's disease from Behcet's disease: The following diagnostic criteria for Behcet's disease are recommended by the International Study group for Behcet's disease[16]: (i) recurrent oral ulcers: occurring at least three times in the past 12 months; (ii) recurrent genital ulceration; (iii) ocular lesions: anterior uveitis, posterior uveitis, retinal vasculitis; (iv) skin lesions: erythema nodosum, pseudofolliculitis, papulopustular lesions, aceniform nodules; (v) positive pathergy test: pricking a sterile needle into the patient's forearm; an aseptic erythematous nodule or pustule >2 mm in diameter at 24–48 h are judged as positive. For a definitive diagnosis the patient must have recurrent oral ulceration plus two other features in the absence of clinical explanations.

Other differential diagnoses: included ischemic colitis, microscopic colitis, radiation colitis, diversion colitis, and non-steroidal anti-inflammatory drug enteropathy, Henoch-Schonlein purpura, malignant lymphoma, colon cancer et al.

For some cases difficult to differentiate, 3-6 months of follow up is recommended to make a definite diagnosis of IBD.

Essentials for Diagnosis of Inflammatory Bowel Disease

A complete diagnosis of IBD should include clinical type, distribution and extent of disease, severity and activity of disease for better therapeutic strategy and prognostic evaluation. Extraintestinal manifestations and complications should also be included. The most important aspects of diagnosis are the distribution, activity and severity of the disease.

Management of IBD from an Asia–Pacific Standpoint

Guidelines for IBD management in the USA, UK and other Western countries should serve as a major reference for our management consensus.

The Goals of IBD Treatment

The goals of IBD treatment are to induce and maintain remission of both clinical symptoms and mucosal inflammation, and to re-establish the intestinal barrier, so as to reduce relapse and complication, and to improve quality of life[17]. A simplified DAI can be helpful for a quantitative estimate of disease activity and response to therapy. The Sutherland index (also called Mayo indices) for UC and the Harvey–Bradshaw index for CD are recommended in practice, as described in tables 1 and 2. (Sutherland index: <2, remission; 3–5, mildly active; 6–10, moderately active; 11–12, severe active. Harvey-Bradshaw CDAI <4: remission; 5–8:moderate; >9:severe.)

Treatment Recommendations for Induction and Maintenance of Remission in UC

Induction of Remission

For mild active distal UC with disease <25 cm, topical 5-aminosalicylic acid (5-ASA) is the first line therapy. For colitis from >25 cm up to the splenic flexure, oral 5-ASA + topical 5-ASA is indicated. Combined therapy is better than single treatment.

For moderate active UC extending beyond the splenic flexure and up to the cecum (extensive), optimal oral 5-ASA combines with topical 5-ASA/steroid should be given depending on rectal symptoms. After 2–4 weeks of 5-ASA, if the patient fails to respond with the treatment, then oral glucocorticoids (GCS) should be started. Optimal dose: sulfasalazine at 3–6 g/day; mesalamine at 2–4.8 g/day; balsalazide at 4–6.75 g/day; olsalazine at 2 g/day.

For severe extensive colitis if an oral GCS approach fails or disease is refractory to oral treatment, the patients should be hospitalized for i.v. GCS. If GCS have been used for 7–10 days and failed, cyclosporine can be considered, although approximately 50% of patients will eventually need colectomy at 1-year follow up. Antibiotics should be considered for infectious complications, or if the patient appears clinically toxic, until the blood culture reports come back negative. Patients with fulminant colitis are treated similarly but observed closely and a decision regarding surgery should be made within 7–14 days of.

Maintenance of Remission

Maintenance therapy is recommended for all patients, except those with a mild first attack or limited lesions who went into complete remission with initial treatment; it is also recommended if the relapses occur within 6 months of remission induction. Regardless of how remission was induced, oral 5-ASA is recommended at the same dose that induced remission, and dose reduction is not recommended, except for sulfasalazine (SASP) because of intolerance of side-effects. The 5-ASA maintenance is always recommended for long-term utility. The patient should be informed to take 5-ASA for the 'foreseeable future', which can be defined as a 3–5-year period or even lifelong. Glucocorticoids are not recommended for maintenance. if failure of maintenance, you should check treatment adherence and medication of patients carefully. Add immunosuppressives with doses of 6-mercaptopurine (6-MP) at 0.75–1.5 mg/kg per day; or azathioprine (AZA) at 1.5–2.5 mg/kg per day. If relapse is severe, use the same regimen that achieved the initial induction of remission and follow closely until the remission is achieved. Probiotics could be tried.

Chronic Active Recurrent Disease

An optimal dose of oral 5-ASA and immunosuppressives is recommended. The patient should be advised to take 5-ASA for lifelong maintenance therapy or for the foreseeable future, which can be defined as a 3–5-year period or remission for 2 years. If 5-ASA and immunosuppressives fail, colectomy or biologicals should be considered, such as infliximab, or probiotics. But GCS are not recommended. Colectomy is indicated for severe dysplasia and cancer.

The Treatment Recommendations for Induction and Maintenance of Remission in CD

Induction of Remission

For all CD patients it is mandatory to stop smoking. For mild disease of the small bowel, high-dose 5-ASA as initial therapy or antibiotics (metronidazole or ciprofloxacin) are recommended, but usually not as first-line therapy because of side-effects. For colonic CD, 5-ASA and/or antibiotics, SASP is effective, but beware of side-effects.

For moderate disease in small bowel, budesonide/prednisone and/or antibiotics are recommended, but 5-ASA is not recommended. For colonic moderate CD, GCS, 5-ASA or antibiotics are recommended. Topical 5-ASA may be effective in left-sided colonic CD.

For severe disease of the small bowel and colon, i.v. GCS and antibiotics are appropriate, but 5-ASA is not recommended. Consider immunosuppressives as adjunctive therapy, AZA and 6-MP act slowly, which precludes their use as a sole therapy. Biologicals, such as infliximab, are effective, but are better to be avoided for obstructive CD cases. For all severe cases, nutritional therapy should be considered, either elemental or polymeric diets are adjunctive. Total parenteral nutrition should be used in cases of significant nutritional deficiency.

Maintenance of Remission

Cessation of Smoking Is of Critical Importance

Start maintenance therapy during the induction phase regardless of disease severity. The 5-ASA has limited benefit for CD maintenance. Salfasalazine is not recommended because of the high incidence of side-effects. The patient should be advised to take 5-ASA for the foreseeable future, which can be defined as a 3–5-year period or even longer. Azathioprine and 6-MP are effective for maintenance of remission, but are reserved as second-line therapy because of the potential toxicity. Methotrexate could be used i.m. or s.c. in cases of failure or intolerance to AZA or 6-MP. The GCS are not effective for maintenance, although budesonide has been used for long periods, in chronic active CD. Infliximab is effective in patients who responded to initial therapy, if used at regular intervals, but it is better to combine it with other options. In cases of failure of remission or maintenance, new biologicals or surgery should be considered. For gastroduodenal involvement The same therapy as for small bowel is recommended, plus acid suppression (proton pump inhibitors).

Perianal disease: Antibiotics are first-line therapy. Drainage of abscesses and placement of setons should be used if appropriate. Infliximab is effective for active disease. For maintenance also consider antibiotics, drainage of abscesses, infliximab, and immunosuppressives.

Complications: For obstruction/strictures, consider surgery. For inflammatory complications, the same therapy as for induction of remission, is recommended. For fistulas, apply the same therapy as for induction of remission, also consider infliximab and/or surgery. For entero-enteric, -vesical, -vaginal fistulas, apply the same therapy as for the induction of remission, and consider surgery on a case by-case basis.

New Biological Agents for the Treatment of IBD in the Asia–Pacific Region

Advances in the understanding of the mechanisms of gut inflammation have led to the development of a whole series of new agents that specifically block molecules with pro-inflammatory activity or supply an excess of molecules with natural anti-inflammatory activity. Such agents, called 'biological agents,' or simply 'biologicals', are revolutionizing the treatment of IBD in Western countries. Although not readily accessible, these agents will eventually become available in the Asia–Pacific region. Based on their biological properties, they can be classified as agents that neutralize the cytokine tumor necrosis factor-a (TNF-a), agents that block cell adhesion molecules, natural anti-inflammatory agents, and miscellaneous agents. Anti-tumor necrosis factor-a agents is a potent pro-inflammatory molecule and its blockade has proven to be beneficial in IBD. The infliximab, that neutralizes the biological activity of TNF-a and induces apoptosis of TNF-a-bearing immune cells, is now recognized as the most effective biological for the treatment of CD[18], not only for active disease, but also for maintaince and treatment of fistulas[19, 20]. The apparent beneficial effects of infliximab in UC have been recently reported [21].

References

[1] Morita N, Toki S, Hirohashi T et al. Incidence and prevalence of inflammatory bowel disease in Japan: nationwide epidemiological survey during the year 1991. *J. Gastroenterol.* 1995; 30 (Suppl. 8): 1–4.

[2] Radhakrishnan S, Zubaidi G, Daniel M, Sachdev GK, Mohan AN. Ulcerative colitis in Oman. A prospective study of the incidence and disease pattern from 1987 to 1994. *Digestion.* 1997; 58: 266–70.

[3] Yang SK, Hong WS, Min YI et al. Incidence and prevalence of ulcerative colitis in the Songpa-Kangdong District, Seoul, Korea, 1986–1997. *J. Gastroenterol. Hepatol.* 2000; 15: 1037–42.

[4] Leong RW, Lau JY, Sung JJ. The epidemiology and phenotype of Crohn's disease in the Chinese population. *Inflamm. Bowel Dis.* 2004; 10: 646–51.

[5] Al-Ghamdi AS, Al-Mofleh IA, Al-Rashed RS et al. Epidemiology and outcome of Crohn's disease in a teaching hospital in Riyadh. *World J. Gastroenterol.* 2004; 10: 1341–4.

[6] Sood A, Midha V, Sood N, Bhatia AS, Avasthi G. Incidence and prevalence of ulcerative colitis in Punjab, North India. *Gut.* 2003; 52: 1587–90.

[7] Lee YM, Fock K, See SJ, Ng TM, Khor C, Teo EK. Racial differences in the prevalence of ulcerative colitis and Crohn's disease in Singapore. *J. Gastroenterol. Hepatol.* 2000; 15: 622–5.

[8] Calkins BM, Lilienfeld AM, Garland CF, Mendeloff AI. Trends in incidence rates of ulcerative colitis and Crohn's disease. *Dig. Dis. Sci.* 1984; 29: 913–20.

[9] Lennard-Jones JE. Classification of inflammatory bowel disease. *Scand. J. Gastroenterol. Suppl.* 1989; 170: 2–6;discussion 16–19.

[10] Myren J, Bouchier IA, Watkinson G, Softley A, Clamp SE, de Dombal FT. The OMGE multinational inflammatory bowel disease survey 1976–1986. A further report on 3175 cases. *Scand. J.Gastroenterol. Suppl.* 1988; 144: 11–19.

[11] Shivananda S, Hordijk ML, Ten Kate FJ, Probert CS, Mayberry JF. Differential diagnosis of inflammatory bowel disease. A comparison of various diagnostic classifications. *Scand. J. Gastroenterol.* 1991; 26: 167–73.

[12] Anand BS, Malhotra V, Bhattacharya SK et al. Rectal histology in acute bacillary dysentery. *Gastroenterology.* 1986; 90: 654–60.

[13] Liu TH, Pan GZ, Chen MZ. Crohn's disease. Clinicopathologic manifestations and differential diagnosis from enterocolonic tuberculosis. *Chin. Med. J. (Engl.)* 1981; 94: 431–40.

[14] Bhargava DK, Tandon HD, Chawla TC, Shriniwa S, Tandon BN, Kapur BML. Diagnosis of ileocecal and colonic tuberculosis by colonoscopy. *Gastrointest. Endosc.* 1985; 31: 68–70.

[15] Tandon HD, Prakash A. Pathology of intestinal tuberculosis and its distinction from Crohn's disease. *Gut.* 1972; 13: 260–9.

[16] Lee RG. The colitis of Behcet's syndrome. *Am. J. Surg. Pathol.* 1986; 10: 888–93.

[17] Fiocchi C. Inflammatory bowel disease pathogenesis: therapeutic implications. *Chin. J. Dig. Dis.* 2005; 6: 6–9.

[18] Targan SR, Hanauer SB, van Deventer SJH et al. A short-term study of chimeric monoclonal antibody cA2 to tumor necrosis factor a for Crohn's disease. *N. Engl. J. Med.* 1997; 337: 1029–35.

[19] Hanauer SB, Feagan BG, Lichtenstein GR et al. Maintenance infliximab for Crohn's disease: the ACCENT I randomised trial. *Lancet.* 2002; 359: 1541–9.

[20] Present DH, Rutgeerts P, Targan S et al. Infliximab for the treatment of fistulas in patients with Crohn's disease. *N. Engl. J. Med.* 1999; 340: 1398–405.
[21] Rutgeerts P, Sandborn WJ, Feagan BG et al. Infliximab for induction and maintenance therapy for ulcerative colitis. *N. Engl. J. Med.* 2005; 353: 2462–76.

In: Inflammatory Conditions of the Colon
Editor: Jia-ju Zheng

ISBN: 978-1-60692-240-8
© 2008 Nova Science Publishers, Inc.

Chapter XVIII

Inflammatory Bowel Disease: Definition and Classification

Jia-ju Zheng

Su-zhou Institute for Digestive Disease and Nutrition, Su-zhou Municipal Hospital,
Nan-jing Medical University, Su-zhou, Jiang-su Province, P.R. China

The term "inflammatory bowel disease" (IBD) is broadly used to refer to idiopathic chronic inflammatory disease of the intestine, principally ulcerative colitis (UC) and Crohn's disease (CD), which together affect as many as 1/1000 individuals in Western societies [1,2], and an increasing frequency of IBD has been reported in Asia, and China in particular [3,4].

Etiologic Classification

In the strict sense, the generic term "IBD" encompasses all the various inflammatory conditions affecting the bowel [1,2]. From clinician's perspective, a classification shown in table 18-1 was proposed as an attempt to group all the inflammatory conditions into categories based on etiology (if known) or other associations [1].

In the table, the term "idiopathic IBD" applies in the restrictive sense to refer only to UC, CD and cases believed to be UC or CD but in which the diagnosis is uncertain because they show the characteristics of both disease - (colitis of indeterminate type, which accounts for approximates 10-15 % of idiopathic IBD (figure 18-1) [1,5,6]. However, the term "indeterminate colitis" should be reserved only for those patients where colectomy has been performed and pathologists are unable to make a definitive diagnosis of either UC or CD after full examination [6,7].

The diagnosis of idiopathic IBD can be established only after all the other inflammatory disorders listed in table 18-1 have been excluded. For many of the entities listed in the table, the final diagnosis dependent on the clinical presentation and the findings on imaging studies, or sometime requires microbiological confirmation or a response to specific therapy. Thus, all the available information concerning the patient must be considered before a final diagnosis is established.

Table 18-1. Classification of inflammatory diseases of the intestine [1]

Idiopathic inflammatory bowel disease (idiopathic IBD)
Ulcerative colitis
Crohn's disease
Colitis of indeterminate type
Inflammation caused by infectious agents
Viruses
Chlamydiae
Bacteria
Fungi
Parasites
Inflammation associated with motor disorders
Diverticulitis
Solitary rectal ulcer syndrome
Inflammation secondary to vascular hypoperfusion
Ischemic colitis
Colitis complicating colonic obstruction
Inflammation Induced by therapeutic intervention
Effects of *enema* and *laxative*
Drug-induce colitis
Colitis due to therapeutic *radiation colitis*
Colitis in graft versus host disease (GVHD)
Colitis *following small intestinal bypass* and *Diversion of the fecal stream*
Miscellaneous causes of intestinal inflammation
Collagenous and lymphocytic colitis
Nonspecific (idiopathic) ulcer of the colon
Necrotizing enterocolitis in cancer patients
Eosinophilic colitis and allergic proctitis

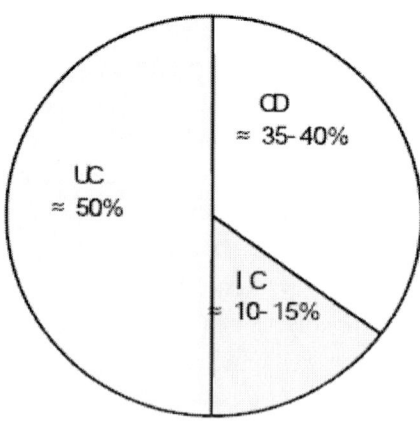

Figure 18-1. The frequency of indeterminate colitis (IC) was reported approximate 10-15% of all idiopathic IBD patients.

International Classification

After the first proposed IBD classification (based on anatomical distribution, operative history, and clinical behavior including inflammatory, fistulizing, or stenotic disease) reported in Rome in 1991, and the second Vienna Classification in 1998 (based on the predominant phenotypic elements such as age of onset, disease location and behavior), a third classification of IBD was reported by a Working Party(formed by investigators from with an interest in disease subclassification in 2003) at the 2005 Montreal World Congress of Gastroenterology (see the chapter of " site of inflammation" in details) [6]. In the conference , the term " inflammatory bowel disease, type unclassified" (IBDU) was suggested for patients in whom there is evidence on clinical and endoscopic grounds for chronic inflammatory bowel disease affecting the colon, without small bowel involvement, and no definitive histological or other evidence to favor either CD or UC [6]. However, clearly infection would have been excluded for these patients before IBDU was considered.

References

[1] Haggitt RC. Pathology of Bowel Inflammatory. In: AGA Postgraduate Course: Idiopathic Inflammatory Bowel Disease. New Orleans, Louisiana, 1984;P.53-63

[2] Carpenter HA, Talley NJ. The importance of clinicopathological correlation in the diagnosis of inflammatory conditions of the colon: histological patterns with implications. *Am. J. Gastroenterol.* 2000;95(5):878-896

[3] Zheng J-j. Pathophysiological researches of ulcrative colitis in China. *Chin. J. Dig.* 2005; 25(10): 637- 638 (Chinese)

[4] Jia Ju ZHENG, Xia Shuang ZHU, Zao HUANG-FU et al. Crohn's disease in mainland China: a systematic analysis of 50 years of research. *Chin. J. Dig. Dis.* 2005; 6(4):175-181

[5] Tremaine WJ. The other colitides. In: Kirsner JB (ed.) 5th ed. *Inflammatory Bowel Disease.* Philadelphia: W. B. Saunders Company 2000;P.410-423

[6] Satsangi J, Silverberg MS, Vermeire S, et al. The Montreal classification of inflammatory bowel disease: controversies, consensus, and implications. *Gut.* 2006;55(6):749-753

[7] Yokoyama H, Takagi S, Utsunomiya K, et al. A case of indeterminate colitis undergoing subtotal colectomy. *Dig. Endosc.* 2004;16(4):347-352

In: Inflammatory Conditions of the Colon
Editor: Jia-ju Zheng

ISBN: 978-1-60692-240-8
© 2008 Nova Science Publishers, Inc.

Chapter XIX

Clinical Manifestations and Complications of Ulcerative Colitis

Kai-chun Wu
Xi-jing Hospital, Fourth Military Medical University,
Shan-xi Province, P.R. China

Intestinal Symptoms

The major intestinal symptoms of ulcerative colitis (UC) in approximate order of frequency are rectal bleeding, diarrhea, the passage of mucus and abdominal pain [1]. In general, the severity of the symptoms correlates with the extent of bowel involvement and the intensity of inflammation in the affected colon. Usually the symptoms start gradually with a chronic and relapsing nature.

For patients with inflammation confined to the rectum (proctitis), rectal bleeding is the most common presentation, with loss of fresh blood on the outside of a normal stool or as a blood-stained mucus. With more extensive disease, the blood is mixed with the stool or with pus and mucus presented as bloody diarrhea.

Bloody diarrhea is the classical presenting symptom of UC, although a small number of patients with proctitis may have constipation and never experience diarrhea. When inflammation affects mainly the rectum and sigmoid colon, patients may complain of urgency, tenesmus, and fecal incontinence [1,2]. Patients with severe disease pass frequent stools as many as six or more daily. Mucus and pus are often appeared in the stool of patients with active ulcerative colitis.

Abdominal pain may also be present in patients with UC although it is usually mild and relieved by defecation. Severe pain may occur in patients with severe disease.

There are few abnormal physical signs in patients with mild disease of UC. However for patients with moderate or severe disease, abdominal examination reveals marked tenderness along the affected colon and reduced bowel sound. Rebound tenderness may be present.

Extra-Intestinal Manifestations

Approximately 20% of patients with ulcerative colitis have extra-intestinal manifestations in their chronic course of the disease, and in some cases patients may present with symptoms of arthritis, or eye and skin disorders [1]. Sometimes extra-intestinal manifestations are the presenting feature and precede intestinal symptoms. The extra-intestinal symptoms may improve with effective medical treatment or surgical resection.

Arthritis can present in UC with three types: axial arthritis affecting the spine and sacroiliac joints; rheumatoid-like arthritis; or peripheral large joint arthritis. The severity of the latter type of arthritis tends to reflect the severity of colitis, while the other two forms are independent of underlying bowel disease. Sacroileitis and ankylosing spondylitis are slowly progressive. Effective treatment of the colitis does not alter the clinical course of the arthritis.

There are about 4% of patients with UC develop eye diseases. The most common eye disorder in patients with UC is uveitis and the next being episcleritis. Conjunctivitis and iritis may also present with pain, photophobia and blurring of vision.

Erythema nodosum is usually present symmetrically in lower limbs of patients with ulcerative colitis, while a smaller number of patients develop pyoderma gangraenosum mainly in the trunk with ulceration and necrosis of the skin (figure 19-1) [3].

Sclerosing cholangitis, aphthous ulceration of the mouth and thromboembolic disorders occur less frequently but may be associated with ulcerative colitis [4,5].

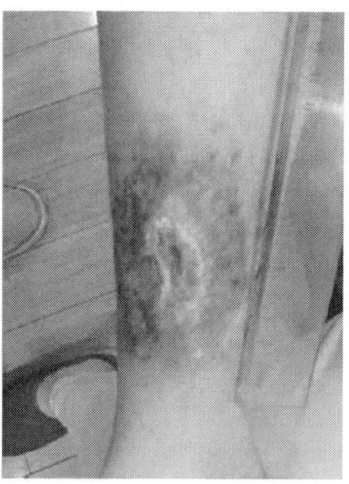 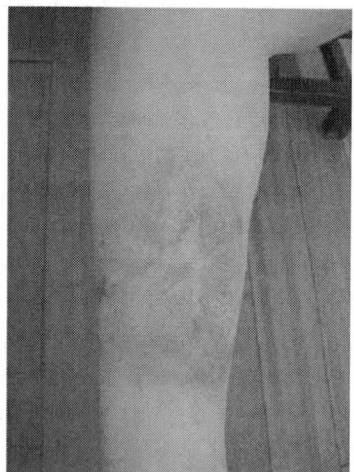

Figure 19-1. A patient with ulcerative colitis complicated with pyoderma gangraenosum before (a) and after treatment [3].

Complications

A major complication of ulcerative colitis is toxic megacolon which occurs in 3 to 5% of adults and 5% of children, and is characterized by progressive dilatation of the colon, with stretching of the bowel wall, and ultimately perforation. This is a life-threatening condition, presenting with tachycardia, pyrexia, abdominal tenderness and distension, and requiring emergency colectomy.

Patients with longstanding disease of over a 10-year duration have an increased risk of developing colorectal carcinoma, and this risk is further increased in patients with extensive colonic involvement. The incidence of colorectal carcinoma in patients with ulcerative colitis appears to peak at approximately 50 years of age, compared with 60 years in the normal population. Risk is significantly greater in younger patients relative to an age-matched general population. So patients with history of ulcerative colitis greater than 8-10 years need to be closely followed-up by colonoscopy every 1-2 years and have the bowel removed if there is dysplasia occurred.

References

[1] Kornbluth A, Sachar DB; Practice Parameters Committee of the American College of Gastroenterology. Ulcerative colitis practice guideline in adults (update): American College of Gastroenterology, Practice Parameters Committee. *Am. J. Gastroenterol.* 2004; 99(7):1371-85.

[2] Satsangi J, Silverberg MS, Vermeire S, et al. The Montreal classification of inflammatory disease: controversies, consensus, and implications. *Gut.* 2006; 55(6): 749-753.

[3] Zheng J-j. Treatment of Pyoderma gangrenosum complicated with ulcerative colitis with Sanguis Draconis and steroids. *Chin. J. Dig. Endosc.* 2008; 25(5):273-274 (Chinese).

[4] Bo W-l, Yin S-h, Jiang A-m, et al. High blood agglutination and thrombosis of intracranial vein in ulcerative colitis. *Chin. J. Dig.* 2007; 27(3):184 (Chinese).

[5] Zheng J-j. Treatment of thrombosis of left calf vein with Lovenox (Enoxaparin sodium) in ulcerative colitis: one case study. *Moder. Dig. Intervent.* 2007; 12(12):260-261 (Chinese).

In: Inflammatory Conditions of the Colon
Editor: Jia-ju Zheng

ISBN: 978-1-60692-240-8
© 2008 Nova Science Publishers, Inc.

Chapter XX

Clinical Manifestations, Complications and Diagnosis of Crohn's Disease

Jun Lin and Chang-sheng Deng
Zhong-nan Hospital of Wuhan University
Hu-bei Province, P.R. China

Introduction

Crohn's disease (CD) is a chronic, relapsing inflammatory disorder of the alimentary canal with involvement anywhere from the mouth to the anus, which arising from an interaction between genetic and environmental factors [1]. The precise etiology is unknown and therefore a causal treatment is not yet available.

Clinical Manifestations

CD can affect any part of the gastrointestinal tract; as a result, the symptoms of CD vary among afflicted individuals (heterogeneous), but commonly include diarrhea, abdominal pain, and/or weight loss. These symptoms should raise the suspicion of CD, especially in patients at young age (table 20-1) [2,3]. The usual onset is between 15 and 30 years of age but can occur at any age. Because of the patchy nature of the gastrointestinal disease and the depth of tissue involvement, initial symptoms can be vaguer than with ulcerative colitis (UC).

Chronic diarrhea is the most common presenting symptom [4.5], a definition of a decrease in faecal consistency for more than six weeks may be adequate to differentiate this from self limited infectious diarrhea[5.6]. The nature of the diarrhea in CD depends on the part of the small intestine or colon that is involved. Ileitis typically results in large-volume watery feces. Colitis may result in a smaller volume of feces of higher frequency. Fecal consistency may range from solid to watery. In severe cases, an individual may have more than 20 bowel movements per day and may need to awaken at night to defecate. Visible bleeding in the feces, or even hematochezia is less common in CD than in UC, but may be seen in the setting of Crohn's colitis. Bloody bowel movements are typically intermittent, and may be bright or dark red in color. In the setting of severe Crohn's colitis, bleeding may be copious.

Table 20-1. Clinical features of Crohn's disease

Clinical presentation (pediatric onset versus adult onset)		
Clinical findings	children	adults
Abdominal pain	62%-95%	60%
Diarrhea	66%-77%	60%-100%
Feve	22%-83%	34%
Rectal bleeding	14%-60%	26%-51%
Weight loss	80%-92%	20%
Arthritis/arthralgia	15%-25%	4%-7%
Other common complaints Fatigue Anorexia Nausea		
Common physical examination findings Abdominal tenderness Palpable mass		
Common laboratory abnormalities Mild anemia; Reduced serum iron; Decreased hematocrit; Mild leukocytosis; Thrombocytosis; Hyperglobulinemia; Hypoalbuminemia; Guaiac-positive stool; Elevated erythrocyte sedimentation rate		
Common radiographic findings Small bowel involvement Fistulas Strictures		

Abdominal pain may be the initial symptom of CD. The pain is commonly cramp-like (intermittent pain), which often periumbilical in location, and initiated by meals and may be relieved by defecation. It is often accompanied by diarrhea, which may or may not be bloody, though diarrhea is not uncommon especially in those who have had surgery. People who have had surgery or multiple surgeries often end up with short bowel syndrome of the gastrointestinal tract. The pain may evolve into a constant dull ache as the disease progresses.

Symptoms caused by intestinal stenosis are also common in CD. Abdominal pain is often most severe in areas of the bowel with stenoses. In the setting of severe stenosis, vomiting and nausea may indicate the beginnings of small bowel obstruction. CD may also be associated with primary sclerosing cholangitis, a type of inflammation of the bile ducts.

Perianal fistulas are present in 10% of patients at the time of diagnosis [4,7]. Perianal discomfort may also be prominent in CD. Itchiness or pain around the anus may be suggestive of inflammation, fistulization or abscess around the anal area or anal fissure. Perianal skin tags are also common in CD. Fecal incontinence may accompany perianal CD.

At the opposite end of the gastrointestinal tract, the mouth may be affected by non-healing sores (aphthous ulcers). Rarely, the esophagus, and stomach may be involved in CD. These can cause symptoms including difficulty swallowing, upper abdominal pain, and vomiting.

Systemic Symptoms

CD, like many other chronic, inflammatory diseases, can cause a variety of systemic symptoms [3-5]:

Among children, growth failure is common. Many children are first diagnosed with CD based on inability to maintain growth. As CD may manifest at the time of the growth spurt in puberty, up to 30% of children with CD may have retardation of growth.

Fever may also be present, though fevers greater than 38.5 °C (101.3 °F) are uncommon unless there is a complication such as an abscess.

Among older individuals, CD may manifest as weight loss. This is usually related to decreased food intake, since individuals with intestinal symptoms from CD often feel better when they do not eat and might lose their appetite.

People with extensive small intestine disease may also have malabsorption of carbohydrates or lipids, which can further exacerbate weight loss.

Extraintestinal Manifestations and Complications

Extraintestinal manifestations are most common when CD affects the colon section (table 20-2) [3].

Table 20-2. Extra-intestinal manifestations of Crohn's disease

Joint manifestations 25%)	Skin manifestations (15%)	Ocular manifestations (5%)
Arthralgia	Erythema nodosum	Episcleritis
Arthritis	Pyoderma gangrenosum	Uveitis
	Aphthous ulcers of the mouth	Recurrent iritis

The transmural involvement in CD predisposes to intestinal narrowing and obstruction, fistulas, abscesses, and perforation. In patients with intestinal obstruction, .intestinal stasis and bacterial overgrowth result in malabsorption of vitamin B12. Fistulous communications may develop between loops of small or large intestine as well as the urinary bladder, vagina, or overlying skin. Perianal complications may range from anal fissures, fistulas, and abscesses to anal strictures. The risk of small intestinal malignancy is substantially increased in CD beginning in childhood [1,4,5]. There also is an increased risk of colorectal carcinoma necessitating subsequent colonoscopic surveillance.

CD increases the risk of cancer in the area of inflammation. Similarly, people with Crohn's colitis have an increased risk of developing colon cancer. Screening for colon cancer with colonoscopy is recommended for anyone who has had Crohn's colitis for eight years, or more.

Pseudopolys are commonly seen in chronic stage of CD. They are a little different from nodular form of cobblestoning lesion, usually multiple nodules. They may present as nodular erythema on normal-colored mucosa or myriads of finger-like mucosal projections. Occasionally, pseudopolyps are sufficiently large or numerous to cause narrowing of the lumen.

Fibrotic stenoses in the later term of the disease are induced by extensive fibrosis of colon wall. Stenosed lumina are usually roundly deformed. Any stricture should raise the suspicion of carcinoma. Smooth, inactive-looking strictures are usually benign.

Fistulas are only seen in CD. The fistulous opening may not be readily apparent, and is often surrounded by marked focal edema and erythema.

In addition, CD can cause significant complications including bowel obstruction, abscesses, free perforation and hemorrhage.

Diagnosis

A single gold standard for the diagnosis of CD is not available [1,3,4]. The diagnosis is confirmed by clinical evaluation and a combination of endoscopic, histological, radiological, and/or biochemical investigations. Colonoscopy with multiple biopsy specimens is well established as the first line procedure for diagnosing colitis [1]. The most useful endoscopic features of CD are discontinuous involvement, ulcerations (erosions, linear, deep), cobblestone appearance, strictures/stenoses /fistulas, and granulomas. Focal (discontinuous) chronic (lymphocytes and plasma cells) inflammation and patchy chronic inflammation, focal crypt irregularity (discontinuous crypt distortion), and granulomas (not related to crypt injury) are the generally accepted microscopic features that permit a diagnosis of CD. Radiographic studies of the small bowel may show lumina narrowing, skip areas, nodular contour linear ulcers, or fistulas. EUS, CT, and/or MRI may help to identify abscesses and other complications.

References

[1] Baumgart DC, Sandborn WJ. Inflammatory bowel disease: clinical aspects and established and evolving therapies. *Lancet.* 2007; 369: 1641-1657

[2] Stange EF, Travis SP, Vermeire S, et al. European evidence based consensus on the diagnosis and management of Crohn's disease: definitions and diagnosis. *Gut.* 2006; 55 Suppl 1:i1-15.

[3] Hanauer SB, Sandborn W. The management of Crohn's disease in adults. *Am. J. Gastroenterol.* 2001; 96:635-643

[4] Sands BE From symptom to diagnosis: clinical distinctions among various forms of intestinal inflammation. *Gastroenterol.* 2004; 126:1518-1532.

[5] Stephen BH. Inflammatory Bowel Disease: epidemiology, pathogenesis, and therapeutic Opportunities. Inflamm Bowel Dis 2006; 12:S3–S9 Gearry RB, Roberts RL, Burt MJ, et al. Effect of inflammatory bowel disease classification changes on NOD2 genotype-phenotype associations in a population-based cohort. *Inflamm. Bowel Dis.* 2007; 13(10):1220-7.

[6] Cho JH. Inflammatory bowel disease: genetic and epidemiologic considerations. *World J. Gastroenterol.* 2008 21; 14(3):338-47.

[7] Gearry RB, Roberts RL, Burt MJ, et al. Effect of inflammatory bowel disease classification changes on NOD2 genotype-phenotype associations in a population-based cohort. *Inflamm. Bowel Dis.* 2007; 13(10):1220-7.

Chapter XXI

Severity Assessment of Ulcerative Colitis

Xiao-ping Wu
The Second Xiang Ya Hospital of Central South University,
Hu-nan Province, P.R. China

Ulcerative colitis (UC) is defined as continuous idiopathic inflammation of the colonic or rectal mucosa. Assessment of disease severity of UC is important for prognostication and therapeutic decision making. The first randomized controlled trial in UC dates back to 1955 when cortisone was shown to be effective for the treatment of active disease. Further experience in clinical trial design for UC during the last 50 years has led to the creation of a large number of disease-specific measures of disease activity.

Truelove and Witts' Severity Index

Several instruments have been developed to evaluate the severity of UC based on clinical features. The most commonly used one among them is Truelove and Witts' severity index, which is based on clinical and biochemical disease activity in 1955[1] (table 21-1). It is reliable and simple to use in clinical practice, although it is most applicable for patients with extensive colitis and may not adequately reflect disease severity in patients with limited colitis.

Lichtiger Index

In 1990, Lichtiger Index (also known as the Modified Truelove and Witts' Severity Index, MTWSI) which included 8 variables was reported: diarrhea (number of daily stools), nocturnal stools, visible blood in stool (percentage of movements), fecal incontinence, abdominal pain/cramping, general well-being, abdominal tenderness, and need for antidiarrheals. The scores range from 0 to 21 points [2] (table 21-2).

Also, there are some other indexes in published literatures: Powell-Tuck Index (also known as the St. Mark's Index), Clinical Activity Index (also known as the Rachmilewitz Index), Activity Index (also known as the Seo Index), Physician Global Assessment, Ulcerative Colitis Clinical Score.

In China, a modified standard for diagnosis and treatment of inflammatory bowel disease (IBD) based on clinical symptoms was established in Cheng-du, Si-chuan Province, in the First National IBD Meeting in 2000[3]. The main schedule was as listed below: (1) Mild-Less than four stools daily, with or without blood, with no systemic disturbance and a normal ESR, (2) Moderate-Intervenient mild and severe, (3) Severe-More than six stools daily with blood and grume, with evidence of systemic disturbance as shown by fever (more than 37.5°C), tachycardia (more than 90 pulse per minute), anemia (less than 100g/dl), or an ESR of more than 30 mm/h.

All the criteria listed above are based on the clinical features and laboratory findings. The main shortage is lack of markers from endoscopic disease activity.

Table 21-1. Truelove-Witts' classification of ulcerative colitis

	Mild	Severe
Times of stools (times/d)	<4	≥6
Blood in stools	+/-	+++
Temperature(°C)	No fever	>37.5 of 2 days per 4 days
Heart rate (beats/min)	No tachycardia	>90
Hemoglobin (g/L)	No or mild anemia	<75
ESR (mm/h)	<30	>30

Table 21-2. Lichtiger Index (also known as the Modified Truelove and Witts' Severity Index, MTWSI)

Variable	Scores					
	0	1	2	3	4	5
Diarrhea (number of daily stools)	0-2	3 or 4	5 or 6	7-9	>10	
Nocturnal diarrhea	No	Yes				
Visible blood in stool (% of movement)	0	<50	>50	100		
Fecal incontinence	No	Yes				
Abdominal pain or cramping	None	Mild	Moderate	Severe		
General well-being	Perfect	Very good	Good	Average	Poor	Terrible
Abdominal tenderness	No	Mild and localized	Mild to moderate and diffuse	Severe or rebound		
Need for antidiarrheal drugs	No	Yes				

Mayo Score

Other instruments for measuring severity of UC incorporate both clinical and endoscopic parameters into a composite index. The most common used composite indexes are Mayo Score (also known as the Mayo Clinic Score and the Disease Activity Index) and Sutherland Index (also known as the Disease Activity Index and the UC Disease Activity Index).

Mayo Score consists of 4 items: (1) stool frequency (normal stool frequency), (2) rectal bleeding (no rectal bleeding), (3) patient's functional assessment score (generally well), (4) endoscopyic findings [4] (table 21-3).

Table 21-3. Mayo Score

Stool frequency*
0=Normal number of stools for this patient
1= 1-2 stools more than normal
2= 3-4 stools more than normal
3= 5 or more stools more than normal
*Each patient served as his or her own control to establish the degree of abnormality of the stool frequency.
Rectal bleeding**
0= No blood seen
1= Streaks of blood with stool less than half the time
2= Obvious blood with stool most of the time
3=Blood alone passed
* The daily bleeding score represented the most severe day of bleeding.
Finding of flexible proctosigmoidoscopy
0=Normal or inactive disease
1=Mild disease (erythema, decreased vascular pattern, mild friability)
2=Moderate disease (marked erythema, absent vascular pattern, friability, erosions)
3=Severe disease (spontaneous bleeding, ulceration)
Physician's global assessment*
0=Normal (there are no symptoms of colitis, the patient feels well, and the flexible proctosigmoidoscopy score is 0) (stool frequency = 0, rectal bleeding = 0,patients functional assessment = 0, flexible proctosigmoidoscopy findings = 0)
1=Mild disease (mild symptoms and proctoscopic findings that were mildly abnormal) (the subscores should be mostly 1's: stool frequency = 0 or 1; rectal bleeding = 0 or 1; patients functional assessment = 0 or 1;sigmoidoscopy findings = 0 or 1)
2=Moderate disease (more serious abnormalities and proctosigmoidoscopic and symptom scores of 1 to 2) (the subscores should be mostly 2's: stool frequency = 1or 2; rectal bleeding = 1or 2; patients functional assessment = 1or 2; sigmoidoscopy findings = 1or 2)
3=Severe disease (the proctosigmoidoscopic and symptom scores are 2 to 3 and the patient probably requires corticosteroid therapy and possibly hospitalization) (the subscores should be mostly 3's: stool frequency = 2 or 3; rectal bleeding = 2 or 3; patients functional assessment = 2 or 3; sigmoidoscopy findings = 2 or 3)
*The physician's global assessment acknowledged the three other criteria, the patient's daily record of abdominal discomfort and general sense of well-being, and other observations, such as physical findings and the patient's performance status.
Patient's functional assessment (this variable is not included in the 12 point index calculation but is considered as a measure of general sense of well-being when determining the physician's global assessment score)
0 = Generally well
1 = Fair
2 = Poor
3 = Terrible

Sutherland Index

Sutherland Index was reported in 1987 based on the results of a placebo-controlled trial of mesalamine enemas for the treatment of active distal UC. Four variables determine the Sutherland Index: stool frequency, rectal bleeding, mucosal appearance, and physician's rating of disease activity. Clinical improvement was defined as a reduction in the Sutherland score ≥3 points from baseline. a score of <2.5 points has been shown to correlate with Patient-Defined Remission[5] (table 21-4).

Table 21-4. Sutherland Index

Stool frequency 0=Normal 1= 1-2 stools/day > normal 2= 3-4 stools/day > normal 3= > 4 stools/day > normal
Rectal bleeding 0= None 1= Streaks of blood 2= Obvious blood 3=Mostly blood
Mucosal appearance 0=Normal 1=Mild friability 2=Moderate friability 3=Exudation, spontaneous hemorrhage
Physician's rating of disease activity 0=Normal 1=Mild 2=Moderate 3=Severe

Rutgeerts Index

Another composite index in UC is Rutgeerts index [6] (table 21-5), which is used by a lot of investigators.

Instruments for measuring quality of life have been used recently as a secondary end point in relatively few clinical trials in patients with UC, though it has been used and validated extensively for Crohn's disease. Disease-specific quality-of-life instruments for patients with UC include the Rating Form of IBD Patient Concerns and the Inflammatory Bowel Disease Questionnaire (IBDQ). The IBDQ is a 32-item questionnaire with 4 dimensions (bowel function, emotional function, systemic symptoms, social function); the total score on this index ranges from 32 to 224, with higher scores indicating better quality of life. The scores of patients in remission usually range from 170 to 190.

Table 21-5. Rutgeerts index

	Score
1. Clinical activity index	
(1) Number of stools weekly	
<18	0
18~35	1
36~60	2
>60	3
(2) Blood in stools(based on weekly average)	
None	0
Little	2
A lot	4
(3) Investigator's global assessment of symptomatic state	
Good	0
Average	1
Poor	2
Very poor	3
(4) Abdominal pain/cramps	
None	0
Mild	1
Moderate	2
Severe	3
(5) Temperature due to colitis	
37~38°C	0
>38°C	3
(6) Extraintestinal manifestations	
Iritis	3
Erythema nodosum	3
Arthritis	3
(7) Laboratory findings	
Sedimentation rate>50 mm in 1st hour	1
Sedimentation rate>100 mm in 1st hour	2
Hemoglobin<100g/l	4
2. Endoscopic index	
(1) Granulation scattering reflected light	
No	0
Yes	2
(2) Vascular pattern	
Normal	0
Faded/disturbed	1
Completely absent	2
(3) Vulnerability of mucosa	
None	0
Slightly increased (contact bleeding)	2
Greatly increased (spontaneous bleeding)	4
Mucosal damage (mucus,fibrin,exudates,erosions,ulcer)	
None	0
Slight	2
Pronounced	4

The Geboes Index

Instruments for measuring histologic disease activity are generally recommended to be included as a secondary end point for the assessment of the therapeutic efficacy. Features for consideration include the presence of polymorphonuclear leukocytes, the formation of crypt abscesses and ulceration, and the intensity of the mononuclear cell infiltrate in the lamina propria as well as structural abnormalities of the crypts and surface. Correlations between histologic disease activity and other assessments of disease activity are fair. In general, a good correlation is found between endoscopy and histology, especially when the samples are obtained during active inflammation. However, microscopic features of activity may persist in macroscopically inactive disease. The correlation between the clinical indices of activity and histology is variable. At present, no single histology score is considered optimum. The commonly used histologic disease activity index is Geboes Index. It has been validated and tested for reproducibility and has 6 domains: structural (architectural) change, chronic inflammatory infiltrate, lamina propria neutrophils and eosinophils, neutrophils in epithelium, crypt destruction, and erosions or ulceration (table 21-6). Scores range from 0 to 5.4, with higher scores indicating more severe histologic inflammation. The Geboes Index has been used as a secondary end point in relatively few clinical trials in UC. [7]

In summary, severity evaluation based on clinical symptoms can dominate in the judgement of the severity of UC. Though there are some limitations in judging disease by symptoms only. There are also many criteria of histological and endoscopic classification in UC abroad. However, the severity of clinical symptoms sometimes does not correlate with histologic and endoscopic features well. For example, some UC patients in remission only have irritable bowel syndrome (IBS) like symptoms (called IBS-like UC). The IBD meeting of Asia and the Pacific area in 2004 have achieved a common opinion[8] that the clinical features assessment from clinicians is enough to judge the activity of the disease, and simplified disease activity index (DAI) is helpful to quantifying assessment of disease activity and response to treatment. The Sutherland index (Mayo Index) is recommended in clinical practice. Different physician may have his own understanding about different classifications, resulting in different views about severity of the same patient. However, one physician's judgment of the severity changes (such as reaction to therapy) on an identical patient at different stages can be considered referential, though some scoring systems may be too complicated to be widely used in clinic. The severity of UC can be evaluated based on a combination of clinical symptoms, endoscopic appearances, and laboratory parameters. So far, none is accepted universally as standard. It is recommended that, in the future, more stringent definitions be discussed and developed.

Table 21-6. Geboes Index

Grade	Structural (architectural) changes
0.0	No abnormality
0.1	Mild abnormality
0.2	Mild or moderate diffuse or multifocal abnormalities
0.3	Sever diffuse or multifocal abnormalities
Grade 1	Chronic inflammatory infiltrate
1.0	No increase
1.1	Mild but unequivocal increase
1.2	Moderate increase
1.3	Marked increase
Grade 2	Lamina propria neutrophils and eosinophils
2A Eosinophils	
2A.0	No increase
2A.1	Mild but unequivocal increase
2A.2	Moderate increase
2A.3	Marked increase
2B Neutrophils	
2B.0	No increase
2B.1	Mild but unequivocal increase
2B.2	Moderate increase
2B.3	Marked increase
Grade 3	Neutrophils in epithelium
3.0	None
3.1	< 5% crypts involved
3.2	< 50% crypts involved
3.3	> 50% crypts involved
Grade 4	Crypt destruction
4.0	None
4.1	Probable-local excess of neutrophils in part of crypt
4.2	Probable-marked attenuation
4.3	Unequivocal crypt destruction
Grade 5	Erosion or ulceration
5.0	No erosion, ulceration, or granulation tissue
5.1	Recovering epithelium + adjacent inflammation
5.2	Probable erosion –focally stripped
5.3	Unequivocal erosion
5.4	Ulcer or granulation tissue

References

[1] Truelove SC, Witts LJ. Cortisone in ulcerative colitis: Final report on a therapeutic trial. *Br. Med. J.* 1955; 2: 1041-82.

[2] Lichtiger S, Present DH. Preliminary report: cyclosporine in treatment of severe active ulcerative colitis. *Lancet.* 1990; 336: 16-19.

[3] Chinese Society of Gastroenterology. Suggested guideline for the diagnosis and treatment of inflammatory bowel disease. *Chinese J. Dig.* 2001; 21(4): 236-239.(Chinese)

[4] Schroeder KW, Tremaine WJ, Ilstrup DM. Coated oral 5-aminosalicylic acid therapy for mildly to moderately active ulcerative colitis. *N. Engl. J. Med.* 1987; 317:1625-1629.

[5] Sutherland LR, Martin F, Greer S, et al. 5-aminosalicylic acid enema in the treatment of distal ulcerative colitis, proctosigmoiditis, and proctitis. *Gastroenterology.* 1987; 92:1894-1898.

[6] Rutgeerts P. Medical therapy of inflammatory bowel disease. *Digestion,* 1998; 59: 453~469.

[7] Geboes K, Riddle R, Ost A, et al. A reproducible grading scale for histological assessment of inflammation in ulcerative colitis (comment). *Gut.* 2000; 47:404-409.

[8] Ouyang Q, Rakesh Tandon, KL Goh,et al.. Asia and the pacific area common opinion on the management of inflammatory bowel disease. *Chinese J. Gastroenterology.* 2006; 11(4):233-238.(Chinesae)

In: Inflammatory Conditions of the Colon
Editor: Jia-ju Zheng

ISBN: 978-1-60692-240-8
© 2008 Nova Science Publishers, Inc.

Chapter XXII

Clinical and Endoscopic Assessments of Activity and Severity of Crohn's Disease

Yi Li[1] and Bing Xia[2]
[1]Department of Computer Science and Engineering
University of Washington, Seattle, United States
[2]Wu-han University Zhong-nan Hospital
Wu-han, Hu-bei Province
P.R. China

Crohn's disease is a chronic intestinal inflammation characterized by frequent relapses. In order to clarify the disease behavior and evaluate the therapeutic effects, we need to design criteria for assessment of activity and severity of Crohn's disease. Owing to various manifestations of Crohn's disease, efforts to quantify disease activity have been more complex than in ulcerative colitis.

Clinical Assessment of Activity of Crohn's Disease

The most frequently used index for the assessment of disease activity is the Crohn's Disease Activity Index (CDAI) (table 22-1), which is preferred by Best et al. [1], with the multiple regression analysis. It contains eight variables on patient situation. The outcome of the CDAI varies between 0 and 600 points. A score below 150 is associated with clinical remission, 150 to 219 with mildly active disease, 220 to 450 with moderately active disease and above 450 with very severe disease. This index is used to select groups of patients based on activity of the disease and to evaluate therapeutic response in clinical trials. The calculation of CDAI is shown in table 22-1. Major weak of CDAI is related to a 7-day observation, high inter-observer variability and difficult calculation.

Table 22-1. Crohn's Disease Activity Index (CDAI)

Variables	Sum of 7 Days	Factors	Subtotal
Number of liquid or soft stools	_ _ _	2	_ _ _
Abdominal pain (0 = none, 1 = mild, 2 = moderate, 3 = severe)	_ _ _	5	_ _ _
General well-being (0 = generally well, 1 = slightly under par, 2 = poor, 3 = very poor, 4 = terrible)	_ _ _	7	_ _ _
Number of complications (presence or absence): Arthritis or arthralgia; Iritis or uveitis; Anal fissure, fistula or abscess; Erythema nodosum, pyoderma gangrenosum, aphthous stomatitis; Other fistula; Fever over 37.8°C (Total number of complications from the list that are present)	_ _ _	20	_ _ _
Loperamide or diphenoxylate for diarrhoea (none = 0, yes = 1)	_ _ _	30	_ _ _
Abdominal mass (none = 0, questionable = 2, definite = 5)	_ _ _	10	_ _ _
Hematocrit (males 47- Ht (%), females 42- Ht (%))	_ _ _	6	_ _ _
Body weight (1 − Body weight/standard weight) x 100=	_ _ _	1	_ _ _
		CDAI total	_ _ _

Remission: CDAI < 150;
Mildly active disease: CDAI 150 – 219;
Moderately active disease: CDAI 220 – 450;
Severe activity: CDAI > 450.

A simplified clinical index has been proposed by Harvey and Bradshaw [2], which is known as the Harvey and Bradshaw index or simplified CDAI. It includes five of the main variables of the CDAI and is easier to calculate. The simplified CDAI has good linear correlation with CDAI and is shown in table 22-2.

If the total score is 4, the activity of this case is considered as catabasis; and if between 5 and 8, moderate active stage; if more than 9, severe active stage.

The van Hees index [3] does not correlate well with the indexes mentioned above; it is probably more appropriate for trials in which disease activity should be assessed and correlated with the inflammatory parameters. van Hees index consists mainly of objective data such as albuminemia, erythrocyte sedimentation rate (ESR), body weight, sex, body temperature, intestinal resection, and extraintesinal lesions. Further more, possible abdominal masses and diarrhea as subjective symptoms are recorded. The calculation of van Hees index (VHI) is shown in table 22-3.

Table 22-2. Harvey and Bradshaw Index

1. General state of health	0=generally well	1=slightly poor	2=poor	3=very poor	4=terrible
2. Abdominal pain	0=none	1=mild	2=moderate	3=severe	
3. Diarrhea	1 score if per loose stools everyday				
4. Abdominal mass (concluded by doctor)	0=none	1=questionable	2=definite	3=with haphalgesia	
5. Complications (arthralgia, uveitis, erythema nodosum, pyoderma gangrenosum, aphthae, fissure, new fistula, abscess etc.)	1 score per item				

Table 22-3. van Hees Index (VHI)

Variables	Regression coefficient	
Serum albumin g/l	× —5.48	---
ESR mm/h	× 0.29	---
Quetelet index (weight /height ^{2})	× —0.22	---
Abdominal mass (1 = 0, 2 = questionable, 3 = <6 cm, 4 = 6-12 cm, 5 = >12 cm)	× 7.83	---
Sex (1 = male, 2 = female)	× —12.3	---
Temperature °C	× 16.4	---
Consistency of the stools (1 = normal, 2 = soft, 3 = liquid)	× 8.46	---
Resection (1 = none, 2 = yes)	× —9.17	---
Extraintestinal manifestations (1 = none, 2 = yes)	× 10.7	---
	Total	---
Subtract		- 209
	Activity index	---

^{2}square of height.

Endoscopic Scoring of Crohn's Disease Activity

Endoscopy has become extremely valuable in the diagnosis, assessment, and management of Crohn's disease. The endoscopic lesions typical of Crohn's disease are described as aphthous or fissure ulcers, cobblestone appearance, stenosis and segmental distribution. The management of Crohn's disease largely depends on the location and the severity of the inflammation. However, the activity and severity of inflammatory lesions in Crohn's disease observed colonoscopically are difficult to score.

The scoring systems which have been published in the literature can be divided into two groups: stepwise systems and numerical (quantitative) systems. In stepwise systems, the disease activity and/or severity is divided into different grades or phases for which different grades such as 1, 2 and 3 or names such as normal mucosa, quiescent, inactive disease, chronic persistent and active disease are used. Active disease can further be subdivided into mildly, moderately or severely active disease [4, 5]. In numerical systems, different variables or lesions are scored and to each of these a subjective numerical value is given [6, 7]. The final score is the result of the sum of the scores of different variables. Some of the scoring systems are elaborate and contain many variables while others are extremely simple.

On the basis of the evaluation on the inflammation of colon and terminal ileitis, the French GETAID (groupe d'etudes therapeutjques des affections inflamrnatoiaes du tube digestif) [8] developed an endoscopic scoring system, named CDEIS (Crohn's disease endoscopic index of severity) based on: (1) the nature of the inflammatory lesions in each colonic segment and terminal ileum and (2) a global severity assessment. Parameters were selected by means of regression analysis and included four types of mucosal lesions: superficial ulcerations, deep ulcerations, ulcerated stenosis and non-ulcerated stenosis. This index has been shown to be reproducible between different medical centers. However, the index score is complex and has failed to show significant correlation with patient symptoms or other objective indicators of disease activity, such as ESR and C reactive protein (CRP) [9]. An example of DCEIS is shown in table 22-4.

Table 22-4. Example of CDEIS scoring form

	Rectum	Sigmoid and left colon	Transvers colon	Right colon	Ileum	Total	
Deep ulceration (12=present, 0= absent)	0	0	0	12	--	12	Total 1
Superficial ulceration (6=present, 0=absent)	6	6	6	6	--	24	Total 2
Surface involved by the disease (/10cm)*	4.7	4.2	3.7	5.6	--	18.2	Total 3
Ulcerated surface (/10cm)*	0.6	0.5	0.4	0.9	--	2.4	Total 4
	Total 1 + total 2 + total 3 + total 4 =					56.6	Total A
	Number (n) of segments totally or partially explored (1-5)					4	n
Total A divided by n						14.15	Total B
	Quote 3 if ulcerated stenosis anywhere, 0 if not					3	C
	Quote 3 if non ulcerated stenosis anywhere, 0 if not					0	D
C + D =	Total B +					17.15	CDEIS

* Analogue scales to be converted into numeric values.

The Simplified Endoscopic Activity Score for Crohn's Disease (SES-CD)

It was recently developed and validated as a simpler, more rapid endoscopic scoring system for Crohn's disease [10]. SES-CD selected endoscopic parameters, ulcer size, ulcerated and affected surfaces and stenosis, and scored from 0 to 3. The simplest score is highly correlated with CDEIS, CDAI and serum CRP level. SES-CD definitions and an example of calculation are shown in table 22-5 and table 22-6, respectively.

Table 22-5. Definitions of simple endoscopic Score for Crohn's disease (SES-CD)

Variable	SES-CD values			
	0	1	2	3
Size of ulcers	None	Aphthous ulcers (⌀ 0.1 to 0.5cm)	Large ulcers (⌀ 0.5 to 2cm)	Very large ulcers(⌀ >2cm)
Ulcerated surface	None	<10%	10-30%	>30%
Affected surface	Unaffected segment	<50%	50-75%	>75%
Presence of narrowings	None	Single, can be passed	Multiple, can be passed	Cannot be passed

⌀, Diameter.

Table 22-6. Example of SES-CD scoring form (same case scored with CDEIS in table 22-4)

	Ileum	Right colon	Transverse colon	Left colon	Rectum	Total
Presence and size of ulcer (0-3)	--	2	1	1	1	5
Extent ulcerated surface (0-3)	--	1	1	1	1	4
Extent of effected surface (0-3)	--	2	1	1	1	5
Presence and type of narrowings (0-3)	--	3	0	0	0	3
SES-CD =						17

Rutgeerts et al. [11] also developed an endoscopic score system to describe the severity of lesions on the ileal side of the ileocolonic anastomosis: Grade i0=no lesions; Grade i1 =fewer than five aphthous ulcers; Grade i2=more than five aphthous ulcers with normal mucosa in between or lesions confined to the ileocolonic anastomosis; Grade i3 =diffuse aphthous ileitis; Grade i4=large ulcers, without normal mucosa and with stenosis. This scoring system is not only a valuable tool for clinical studies, it is also to predict the clinical course of the disease in the years ahead. Patients with grade 3 or 4 recurrence after 1 year suffer from a more aggressive course of their recurrent disease than patients with grade 1 or 2.

Scoring system for children according to Nicholls et al., and another scoring system according to D'Haens et al are shown in table 22-7 and table 22-8.

Table 22-7. Scoring system according to Nicholls et al. for children [12, 13, 14]

Blind assessment in pairs of biopsies (two specimens from the ileum and four to six throughout the colon) of the degree of inflammation before and after treatment:	
0=	normal
3=	severe inflammation (ulceration, acute and chronic inflammation, crypt distortion, goblet cell depletion, villous atrophy)
Post-treatment	-worse -no change
	- improvement -resolution of inflammation

Table 22-8. Scoring system according to D'Haens et al [15]

Histological variable	Grading
1. Epithelial damage	0 = normal; 1 = focal; 2 = extensive
2. Architectural changes	0 = normal; 1 = moderate (>50%); 2 = severe (>50%)
3. Mononuclear cells in lamina propria	0 = normal; 1 = moderate increase; 2 = severe increase
4. Polymorphonuclear cells in lamina propria	0 = normal; 1 = moderate increase; 2 = severe increase
5. Neutrophils in epithelium	0 = normal; 1 = moderate increase; 2 = severe increase
6. Erosion or ulceration	0 = no; 1 = yes
7. Granuloma	0 = no; 1 = yes
8. Number of biopsies affected (total: n = 6 or more)	0 = none; 1 = >33%; 2 = 33±66%; 3 = >66%

Each variable is scored independently. The total score is the sum of all individual scores (maximum = 16).

Other Indexes on Assessment of the Activity of Crohn's Disease

ESR and CRP are often used to predict the activity of Crohn's disease [16] CT and magnetic resonance imaging (MRI) are advantaged to diagnose inflammatory complications, such as ileocolonic thickening, stenosis, fistula and abscesses, but insensitive to disease activity [17]. 99mTc (V) DMSA scintigraphy was shown a noninvasive, practical, and accurate method for the assessment of disease activity of Crohn's disease [18].

Correlation with Endoscopy and Clinical Indices of Crohn's Disease

The correlation between endoscopy and histology in IBD is not perfect. When the extent of disease needs to be defined, biopsies may double the yield of pathology when compared with the endoscopically visible amount of inflammation and may be three-fold more informative than the barium enema radiographic examination [19, 20, 21]. A good correlation has been reported between microscopic and macroscopic scores for Crohn's colitis (r=0.68, P < 0.05) and for post-operative recurrent ileal CD (E=0.54, P=0.004) [22, 23]. Yet, endoscopic assessment of inflammation in CD had a better correlation with transmural inflammation than mucosal biopsy and thus with the severity and extent of inflammation [24]. In CD, endoscopy was superior when compared with mucosal biopsies. The correlation between the clinical indices of activity and endoscopy or histology is variable. This is partly explained by the type of endoscopic and microscopic scores used. Clinical and laboratory indices and endoscopy are the main indicators of disease activity initially and during relapse [25].

References

[1] Best WR, Bectel JM, Singleton JW, et al. Development of Crohn's disease activity index. *Gastroenterology.* 1976; 70: 439-444.

[2] Harvey RF, Bradshaw JM. A simple index of Crohn's disease activity. *Lancet.* 1980; 315: 514-519.

[3] van Hees PAM, van Elteren PH, van Lier HJJ, et al. An index of inflammatory activity in patients with Crohn's disease. *Gut.* 1980; 21: 279-286.

[4] Odze R, Antonioli D, Peppercorn M, Goldman H. Effect of topical 5-aminosalicylic acid (5-ASA) therapy on rectal mucosal biopsy morphology in chronic ulcerative colitis. *Am. J. Surg. Pathol.* 1993; 17: 869-875.

[5] Danielsson A, Hellers G, Lyrenas A et al. A controlled randomized trial of budesonide versus prednisolone retention enemas in active distal ulcerative colitis. *Scand. J. Gastroenterol.* 1987; 22: 987-992.

[6] Riley SA, Mani V, Goodman MJ, et al. Comparison of delayed release 5 aminosalicylic acid (mesalazine) and sulfasalazine in the treatment of mild to moderate ulcerative colitis relapse. *Gut.* 1988; 29: 669-674.

[7] Riley SA, Mani V, Goodman MJ, et al. Microscopic activity in ulcerative colitis: what does it mean? *Gut.* 1991; 32: 174-178.

[8] Modigliani R, Mary JY, Simon JF, et al. Clinical, biological, and endoscopic pictures of attacks of Crohn's disease. Evolution of prednisolone. *Gastroenterology.* 1990; 98: 811-818.

[9] Landi B, Anh T, Cortot A, et al. Endoscopic monitoring of Crohn's disease treatment: a prospective, randomized clinical trial. *Gastroenterology.* 1992;102:1647-1653.

[10] Daperno M, D'Haens G, van Assche G, et al. Development and validation of a new, simplified endoscopic activity score for Crohn's disease: the SES-CD. *Gastrointest. Endosc.* 2004; 60: 505-512.

[11] Rutgeerts P, Geboes K, Vantrappen G, et al. Predictability of the postoperative course of Crohn's disease. *Gastroenterology.* 1990; 99: 956-963.

[12] Beatie RM, Schiffrin EJ, Donnet-Hughes A et al. Polymeric nutrition as the primary therapy in children with small bowel Crohn's disease. *Aliment Pharmacol. Ther.* 1994; 8: 609-615.

[13] Nicholls S, Domizio P, Williams CB, et al. Cyclosporin as initial treatment for Crohn's disease. *Arch. Dis. Child.* 1994; 71: 243-247.
[14] Breese EJ, Michie CA, Nicholls SW, et al. The effect of treatment on lymphokine-secreting cells in the intestinal mucosa of children with Crohn's disease. *Aliment Pharmacol. Ther.* 1995; 9: 547-552.
[15] D'Haens G, Geboes K, Peeters M, et al. Early lesions caused by infusion of intestinal contents in excluded ileum in Crohn's disease. *Gastroenterology.* 1998; 114: 262-267.
[16] Solem CA, Loftus EV, Tremaine WJ, et al. Correlation of C reactive protein with clinical, endoscopic, histologic and radiographic activity in inflammatory bowel disease. *Inflamm. Bowel. Dis.* 2005;11:707-712.
[17] Schreyer AG, Seitz J, Feuerbach S, et al. Modern imaging using computer tomography and magnetic resonance imaging for inflammatory bowel disease (IBD). *Inflamm. Bowel. Dis.* 2004;10: 45-54.
[18] Koutroubakis IE, Koukouraki SI, Dimoulios PD, et al. Active inflammatory bowel disease: evaluation with 99mTc (V) DMSA scintigraphy. *Radiology.* 2003; 229: 70–74.
[19] Geboes K, Riddell R, OÈ st A, et al. A reproducible grading scale for histological assessment of inflammation in ulcerative colitis. *Gut.* 2000; 47: 404-410.
[20] Waye JD. Endoscopy in inflammatory bowel disease: indications and differential diagnosis. *Med. Clin. North Am.* 1990; 74: 51-65.
[21] Holdstock C, DuBoulay C, Smith C. Survey of the use of colonoscopy in inflammatory bowel disease. *Dig. Dis. Sci.* 1984; 29: 731-734.
[22] Gomes P, Du Boulay C, Smith CL, et al. Relationship between disease activity and colonoscopic findings in patients with colonic inflammatory bowel disease. *Gut.* 1986; 27: 92-95.
[23] D'Haens G. Clinical and immunopathological characteristics of early recurrent Crohn's disease: in search of the pathogenesis. Thesis, K.U. 1996; Leuven: 51-63.
[24] Smedh K, Olaison G, FranzeÂn L, et al. The endoscopic picture reflects transmural inflammation better than endoscopic biopsy in Crohn's disease. *Eur. J. Gastroenterol. Hepatol.* 1996; 8: 1189-1193.
[25] Geboes. K. Pathology of inflammatory bowel diseases (IBD): variability with time and treatment. *Colorectal Dis.* 2001; 3: 2-12.

In: Inflammatory Conditions of the Colon
Editor: Jia-ju Zheng

ISBN: 978-1-60692-240-8
© 2008 Nova Science Publishers, Inc.

Chapter XXIII

Perianal Crohn's Disease

Zhi Pang
Nan-jing Medical University, Jiang-su Province, P.R. China

Definition and Spectrum of Perianal Crohn's Disease

Perianal Crohn's disease (perianal CD) is a distinct phenotype of CD. It can manifest as skin tags, hemorrhoids, fissures, anal ulcer, low fistula, high fistula, rectovaginal fistula, perianal abscess, anorectal stricture or cancer. The various types of perianal lesions that occur in patients with CD are shown in table 23- 1[1-7].

Perianal Anatomy

The anal canal consists of an inner layer of circular smooth muscle extending downward from the rectum called the internal anal sphincter, the intersphincteric space, and an outer layer of skeletal muscle extending downward from the puborectalis and levator ani muscles called the external anal sphincter (see chapter one, figure 1-4) [1-4]. The dentate line, located in the midportion of the anal canal, separates the transitional and columnar epithelium of the rectum from the squamous epithelium of the anus. Anal crypts are located at the dentate line, and anal glands are found at the base of these crypts.

Etiology and Classification of Fistula-in-Ano

In patients without CD, perianal fistulas (often called fistula-in-ano or cryptogenic fistulas) usually arise from infected anal glands. In 1934, Milligan and Morgan classified fistula-in-ano according to their relationship to the anorectal ring (formed by the puborectalis muscle) as subcutaneous, low anal (below the dentate line), high anal (above the dentate line but below the anal ring formed by the puborectalis muscle), anorectal below the levator ani muscle (ischiorectal or infralevator), anorectal above the levator ani muscle (pelvirectal or supralevator), and submucous (high intermuscular between the internal and external anal sphincters). Most fistulas-in-ano originate below the dentate line, and many colorectal surgeons simply classify them as low or high. In 1976, Parks et al. proposed a more anatomically precise classification system for fistula-in-ano that uses the external sphincter as a central point of reference. The Parks classification describes 5 types of perianal fistulas: intersphincteric, transsphincteric, suprasphincteric, extrasphincteric, and superficial (figure 23-1)[1-6]. The presence of any branching or horseshoeing (crossing the midline anteriorly or posteriorly) and its location (intersphincteric, infralevator, and supralevator) must also be noted.

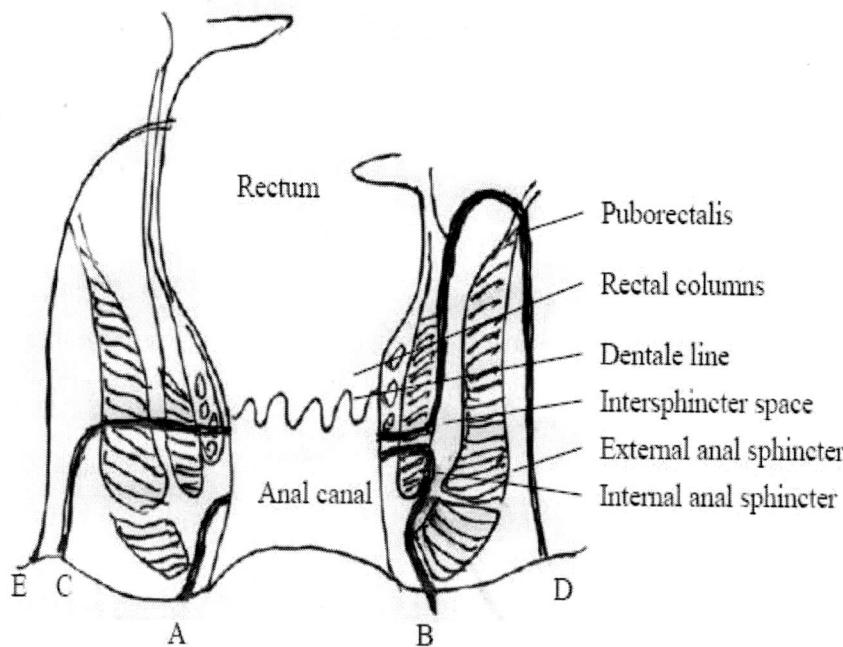

Figure 23-1. The Parks classification. (A) A superficial fistula tracks below both the internal anal sphincter and external anal sphincter complexes. (B) An intersphincteric fistula tracks between the internal anal sphincter and the external anal sphincter in the intersphincteric space. (C) A transsphincteric fistula tracks from the intersphincteric space through the external anal sphincter. (D) A suprasphincteric fistula leaves the intersphincteric space over the top of the puborectalis and penetrates the levator muscle before tracking down to the skin. (E) An extrasphincteric fistula tracks outside of the external anal sphincter and penetrates the levator muscle into the rectum.

Table 23-1. The various types of perianal lesions in patients with CD

type of lesion	description
skin tag	two types: 1. Large, edematous, hard, cyanotic skin tags. Typically arising from a healed anal fissure or ulcer. Excision contraindicated due to problems with wound healing. 2. "Elephant ear" tags that are flat and broad or narrow, soft painless skin tags. May cause perianal hygiene problems and can be safely excised.
hemorrhoids	Prolapsing internal hemorrhoids. Uncommon in CD. Often present as large external skin tags.
fissure	Anal fissures are broad based and deep with undermining of the edges. There may be associated large skin tags and a cyanotic hue to the Surrounding skin. They tend to be multiple and may be placed either eccentrically around the anal canal or in the midline in contrast to idiopathic fissure-in-ano, which tend to lie in the midline. Typically painless (pain should raise suspicion for perianal abscess or acute/chronic conventional anal fissure). Conventional anal fissures occasionally are treated by conventional fissure treatment, including lateral sphincterotomy.
anal ulcer	Anal ulcers are usually associated with rectal inflammation and may lead to destruction of the anorectum, anorectal strictures, complex anorectal fistulas, and perianal abscess.
low fistula	Superficial, low intersphincteric, or low transsphincteric fistulas. May arise from either the anal glands (cryptogenic) or from penetrating ulceration of the anal canal or rectum.
high fistula	High intersphincteric, high transsphincteric, suprasphincteric, extrasphincteric fistulas. Arise from penetrating ulceration of the anal canal or rectum.
rectovaginal fistula	Superficial, intersphincteric, transsphincteric, suprasphincteric, extrasphincteric fistulas. Arise from penetrating ulceration of the anal canal or rectum into the vagina.
perianal abscess	Potential anorectal spaces may become infected with an abscess, including perianal, ishiorectal, deep postnatal, intersphincteric, and supralevator.
anorectal stricture	May be short annular diaphragm-like strictures <2 cm in length or longer tubular strictures arising from rectal inflammation. May arise from either the anal glands (cryptogenic) or from penetrating ulceration of the anal canal or rectum.
cancer	Squamous cell carcinoma, basal cell carcinoma, or adenocarcinoma arising from malignant degeneration of nonhealing perianal fistulas or sinus tracts.

Etiology and Classification of Perianal Crohn's Disease

In patients with CD, a variety of perianal manifestations may occur, including perianal skin lesions (anal skin tags, hemorrhoids), anal canal lesions (anal fissures, anal ulcers, anorectal strictures), perianal fistulas and abscesses, rectovaginal fistulas, and cancer. The etiology of Crohn's perianal fistulas may be a fistula-in-ano arising from inflamed or infected anal glands and/or penetration of fissures or ulcers in the rectum or anal cana [1-8]. In 1978, Hughes proposed an anatomic and pathologic classification for perianal CD (the Cardiff classification) in which each major manifestation of perianal CD (ulceration, fistula, and stricture) is graded on a scale of 0 to 2 (0, absent; 2, severe); fistulas are also classified as low (not extending above the dentate line) or high (extending above the dentate line, sometimes to the levator muscles), and other associated anal conditions, the intestinal location of other sites of CD, and a global assessment of the activity of the perianal disease are noted (tables 23-2 and 23-3). Despite its descriptive accuracy and comprehensiveness, the Cardiff classification system has never gained widespread acceptance because of the perception by clinicians that it is of limited clinical relevance. Neither the Cardiff classification nor a more recent perianal CD Activity Index score have been reproduced or prospectively validated using clinically meaningful end points. These perianal disease classifications or indices of activity have yet to be standardized or used in clinical practice. The Parks classification system can be used to classify and describe perianal fistulas, but it does not address the other perianal manifestations of CD.

Epidemiology

The cumulative frequency of perianal fistulas in patients with CD in referral centers has been reported [1-9]. It is ranged from 13% to 38%. Two population based studies have reported that perianal fistulas occurred in 23% and 21% of patients. Our recent report has showed that 33.3% patients suffered from perianal fistulas or a history of perianal fistulas [9]. Perianal fistulas occurred in 12% of patients with ileal CD, 15% of patients with ileocolonic disease, 41% of patients with colonic disease with rectal sparing, and 92% of patients with colonic disease and rectal involvement. Anal fissure or perianal fistula or abscess precedes or presents simultaneously with the diagnosis of intestinal disease in 36%–81% of patients with CD who develop perianal disease. A small proportion of patients with CD may persist in having only isolated perianal involvement.

Table 23-2. Hughes/Cardiff 1979 classification of anal CD (U.F.S.)

Ulceration (U)	Fistula/abscess (F)	Stricture (S)
not present-0	not present-0	not present-0
Superficial fissures-1 a. Posterior and/or anterior b. Lateral c. With gross skin tags	Lower/superficial-1 a. Perianal b. Anovulval, anoscrotal c. Intersphincteric d. Anovaginal	Reversible stricture (spasm/membranous) -1 a. Anal canal-spasm b. Low rectum-membranous c. Spasm with severe pain, no sepsis identified
Cavitating ulcers-2 a. Anal canal b. Lower rectum c. With extension to perineal skin	High/complex-2 a. Blind supralevator b. High direct (anorectal) c. High complex(aggressive ulceration) d. Rectovaginal e. Ileoperineal	Irreversible stricture (severe fibrotic)-2 a. Anal stenosis b. Extrarectal stricture

Table 23-3. 1992 Addition to the Hughes/Cardiff classification (A.P.D.)

Associated anal conditions (A)	Proximal intestinal disease (P)	Disease activity (in anal locations) (D)
None-0	No proximal disease-0	Active-1
Hemorrhoids-1	Contiguous rectal disease-1	Inactive-2
Malignancy-2	Colon (rectum spared)-2	Inconclusive-3
Other (specify)-3	Small intestine-3	
	Investigation incomplete-4	

Diagnosis

Modalities used to diagnose and classify Crohn's perianal fistulas include examination under anesthesia (EUA), pelvic magnetic resonance imaging (MRI), and anorectal endoscopic ultrasonography (EUS) [1-6,10-13]. EUA consists of visual inspection, palpation, and the passage of malleable probes into fistula tracks under general anesthesia. EUA performed by an experienced colorectal surgeon is approximately 90% accurate in detecting and correctly classifying perianal fistulas, sinuses, and abscesses. The diagnostic accuracy of older imaging modalities such as fistulography and computed tomography for the classification of fistula- in-ano and perianal CD is too low to be clinically useful. The diagnostic accuracy of pelvic MRI with phased-array or endoanal coils and anorectal EUS for classifying fistula- in-ano and perianal Crohn's fistulas is quite high, ranging from 56% to 100%. A number of studies have reported that pelvic MRI or anorectal EUS findings combined with EUA change surgical management in 10%– 15% of cases.

Medical Treatment [1-8,13-16]

1. Steroids and Aminosalicylates

Although steroids are commonly used in the treatment of CD there is less evidence to suggest a benefit in perianal disease where they may prevent the healing of fistulas and lead to abscess formation [5]. Interestingly, patients with perianal CD are resistant to steroids. Similarly, it is unclear whether oral aminosalicylates are effective, but topical aminosalicylates, given as enemas, may provide a targeted treatment.

2. Antibiotics

There are no controlled trials showing that antibiotics are effective in the treatment of Crohn's perianal fistulas. The current clinical practice of using metronidazole or ciprofloxacin is based on uncontrolled case series. Clinicians prescribing antibiotics for fistulas typically use metronidazole at doses ranging from 750 to 1500 mg/day or ciprofloxacin 1000 mg/day for up to 3–4 months.

3. Azathioprine and 6-Mercaptopurine

There are no controlled trials with fistula closure as the primary end point showing that the antimetabolites azathioprine (Aza) and 6-mercaptopurine (6-MP) are effective in the treatment of Crohn's perianal fistulas. The current clinical practice of using these medications is based on a meta-analysis of 5 controlled trials in which fistula closure was examined as a secondary end point and uncontrolled case series in adults and children. Controlled trials indicate that Aza at doses of 2.0–3.0 mg/kg/day and 6-MP at a dose of 1.5 mg/kg/day is effective for the treatment of CD. Adverse events associated with Aza and 6-MP includes leucopenia, allergic reactions, infection, pancreatitis, drug-induced hepatitis, and possibly non-Hodgkin's lymphoma.

4. Infliximab (IFX)

Two controlled trials have shown that IFX 5 mg/kg administered as a 3-dose induction regimen at 0, 2, and 6 weeks is effective for reducing the number of draining fistulas in patients with CD and for closure of all fistulas and that maintenance therapy with IFX 5 mg/kg every 8 weeks prolongs the time to loss of response. Adverse events observed in patients treated with IFX include infusion reactions, delayed hypersensitivity reactions, formation of human antichimeric antibodies, formation of antinuclear antibodies and anti–double-stranded DNA antibodies, and rarely drug-induced lupus. There is also an increased overall rate of infection and, rarely, serious infections including pneumonia, sepsis, tuberculosis, histoplasmosis, coccidioidomycosis, listeriosis, pneumocystis carinii pneumonia, and aspergillosis occur. Because of the risk of reactivating latent tuberculosis, it is recommended that patients undergo purified protein derivative skin testing before treatment with IFX.

5. Cyclosporine

There are no controlled trials showing that cyclosporine is an effective therapy for Crohn's perianal fistulas. The current clinical practice of using intravenous cyclosporine is based on uncontrolled case series. Cyclosporine is administered as a continuous intravenous infusion at a dose of 4 mg/kg/day. Responding patients are converted to oral cyclosporine. Adverse events observed in patients treated with cyclosporine include renal insufficiency, hirsutism, hypertension, paresthesias, headache, seizure, tremor, gingival hyperplasia, hepatotoxicity, and an increased incidence of infection (including P. carinii pneumonia).

6. Tacrolimus

A single small controlled trial showed that tacrolimus (FK506) 0.20 mg/kg/day for 10 weeks reduced the number of draining fistulas in patients with Crohn's disease but did not result in complete closure of all fistulas. Adverse events observed in patients treated with tacrolimus include headache, increased serum creatinine level, insomnia, leg cramps, paresthesias, and tremor, typically resolved with dose reduction. The major toxicity observed in patients treated with tacrolimus is nephrotoxicity.

Surgical Treatment [1-7,15-18]

1. Skin Tags

A high rate of postoperative complications, including poor wound healing and subsequent proctectomy, has been reported following excision of typical CD skin tags; therefore, excision is not recommended.

2. Hemorrhoids

Simple hemorrhoidectomy, the newer procedure for prolapsing hemorrhoids, or banding of hemorrhoids in patients with CD are usually contraindicated due to the frequent occurrence of postoperative complications, including poor wound healing, anorectal stenosis, and a high rate of proctectomy.

3. Anal Fissures

Anal fissures in patients with CD are usually painless and spontaneously heal in more than 80% of patients. Operative intervention with lateral sphincterotomy should be limited to patients who have pain due to the fissure itself (not to local sepsis) and who do not have macroscopic evidence of rectal inflammation. Fissurectomy is contraindicated.

4. Anorectal Strictures

Anal or rectal strictures may arise as complications of ulceration of the anal canal or rectum, perianal abscesses, and perianal fistulas. Asymptomatic patients do not require treatment. Symptomatic patients can be treated with dilation. Repeat dilations are often required.

5. Perianal Abscess

The presence of perianal pain, tenderness, or fluctuation in a patient with CD requires EUA to exclude the presence of a perianal abscess. Perianal abscesses must be drained surgically.

6. Perianal Fistulas

Patients who have low fistulas may be treated by laying open the fistula tract through 1- or 2-stage fistulotomy. In general, there is a trend toward greater healing rates following fistulotomy for low fistulas in patients without macroscopic evidence of inflammation of the rectum when compared with patients with active proctocolitis. Thus, many experts advocate the use of a noncutting seton rather than fistulotomy in patients with low fistulas and active inflammation of the rectosigmoid colon. High fistulas involving a significant portion of the external anal sphincter require a more conservative surgical approach to reduce the risk of incontinence. Noncutting setons are the treatment of choice in patients with high fistulas who have active inflammation of the rectosigmoid colon (figure 23-2). A noncutting seton is a suture or drain that is threaded into the cutaneous orifice of a perianal fistula, through the fistula tract, across the mucosal orifice of the fistula into the rectum, and then out the anal canal. A noncutting seton maintains drainage of the fistula, thereby reducing the risk of perianal abscess formation.

An endorectal advancement flap can be used as an alternative to noncutting setons in patients with high fistulas who do not have macroscopic evidence of rectal inflammation. An advancement flap consists of incising a flap of tissue (mucosa, submucosa, circular muscle) around the internal opening of a fistula, excising the internal opening of the fistula tract, and pulling the flap down to cover the opening. Placement of a temporary diverting ileostomy or colostomy has been used to treat severe perianal CD. These procedures are now only rarely performed after a number of studies showed that most patients who undergo placement of a temporary diverting ileostomy or colostomy for perianal CD never have intestinal continuity restored. Historically, proctectomy rates for patients with perianal CD managed conservatively range from 10% to 18%.

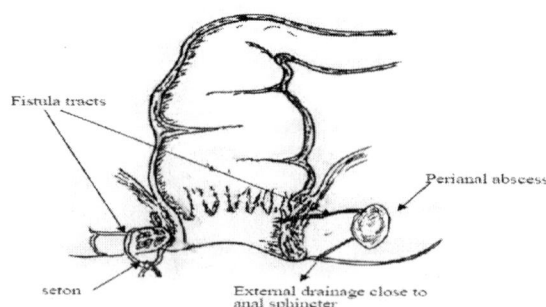

Figure 23-2. Noncutting setons are the treatment of choice in patients with high fistulas who have active inflammation of the rectosigmoid colon.

7. Rectovaginal Fistulas

Surgical treatment of rectovaginal fistulas in patients with perianal CD should only be attempted in the absence of active inflammation of the rectosigmoid colon. Fistulotomy should rarely, if ever, be used to treat low rectovaginal fistulas due to sphincter injury risk. Patients with rectovaginal fistulas may be treated by a number of other approaches, including primary closure, transanal advancement flap, sleeve advancement flap, and transvaginal advancement flap. In general, the success rates for primary closure and advancement flaps in patients with rectovaginal fistulas range from approximately 50% to 100%.

8. Obstetric Surgical Procedures (Vaginal Delivery and Episiotomy)

One study suggested that vaginal delivery led to an exacerbation of perianal disease in patients with a history of perianal disease independent of the activity of the perianal disease at the time of delivery, whereas another study suggested that worsening of perianal disease was limited to those women with active perianal disease at the time of vaginal delivery. Based on these studies, it is recommended that pregnant female patients with active perianal CD at the time of delivery undergo cesarean section. Patients with no history of perianal disease and those with inactive perianal disease can undergo vaginal delivery in the absence of other indications for cesarean section.

9. Cancer

Case reports and case series have identified patients with Crohn's perianal disease in whom squamous cell carcinoma, basal cell carcinoma, and adenocarcinoma have developed in chronic perianal fistula or sinus tracts.

Conclusions (figure 23-3)

1. Perianal disease occurs frequently in patients with CD.
2. Diagnostic evaluation with physical examination and rectosigmoid endoscopy, combined in some cases with EUA and anorectal ultrasonography or pelvic MRI, is required to determine the location and type of fistulas and the presence of absence or macroscopic rectal inflammation.
3. Skin tags and hemorrhoids should not be operated on. Most anal fissures should not be operated on.
4. Lateral sphincterotomy can be considered in selected cases.
5. Anorectal strictures should be dilated, and perianal abscesses drained.
6. Simple fistulas can be treated with antibiotics, IFX, or fistulotomy. The treatment goal is cure without suppressive maintenance therapy.

7. Complex perianal disease should be treated initially with IFX and Aza or 6-mercaptopurine, followed by maintenance therapy with Aza or 6-MP, in some cases combined with IFX. Antibiotics may be used as an adjunctive therapy during the induction phase of treatment.
8. EUA and placement of noncutting setons, or performing endorectal advancement flap procedures is reserved for patients who fail a trial of medical therapy.
9. Tacrolimus or cyclosporine can rarely be considered in selected patients who fail multimodality treatment with other medical and surgical therapies, including IFX, before proceeding to fecal diversion or proctectomy.

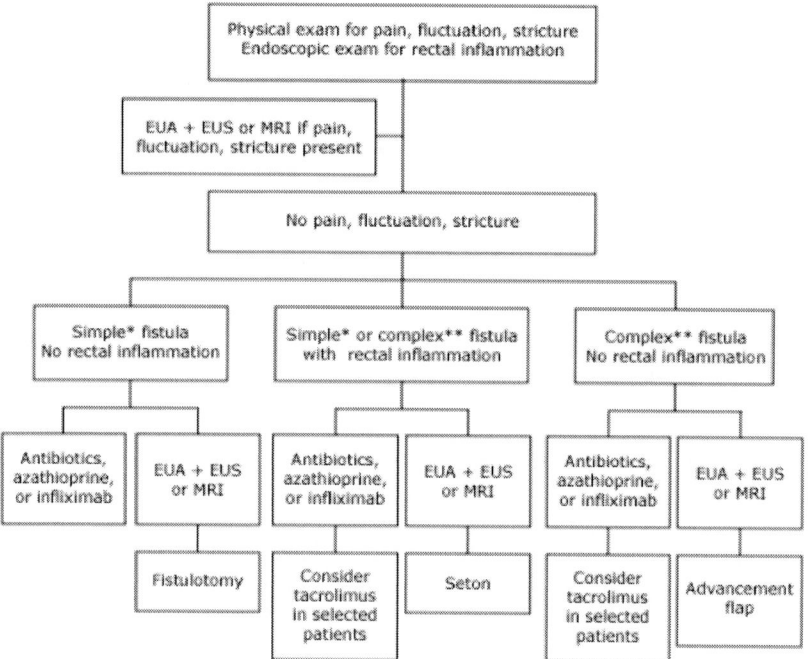

Figure 23-3. Approaches and treatment algorithm for managing patients with Crohn's perianal fistulas. EUA: examination under anesthesia; EUS: anorectal EUS; MRI: pelvic MRI. A simple fistula (*) is low, has a single external opening, and does not have associated perianal abscess, rectovaginal fistula, anorectal stricture, or macroscopically evident rectal inflammation. A complex fistula (**) is high and/or has multiple external openings, perianal abscess, rectovaginal fistula, anorectal stricture, or macroscopic evidence of rectal inflammation.

References

[1] Ardizzone S and Porro GB. Perianal Crohn's disease: overview. *Dig. Liver Dis.* 2007; 39(10):957-958.
[2] Ingle SB, Loftus EV Jr. The natural history of perianal Crohn's disease. *Dig. Liver Dis.* 2007; 39(10):963-969.

[3] Wise PE and Schwartz DA. Management of perianal Crohn's disease. *Clin. Gastroenterol. Hepatol.* 2006; 4:426-430.

[4] American Gastroenterological Association. AGA Technical Review on Perianal Crohn's Disease. *Gastroenterology.* 2003; 125:1508–1530.

[5] American Gastroenterological Association.American Gastroenterological Association Medical Position Statement: Perianal Crohn's Disease. *Gastroenterology.* 2003; 125:1503–1507.

[6] Galandiuk S, Kimberling J, Al-Mishlab TG, et al. Perianal Crohn disease: predictors of need for permanent diversion. *Ann. Surg.* 2005; 241: 796–802.

[7] Singh B, McC.Mortensen NJ, Jewell DP and George B. Perianal Crohn's disease. *Br. J. Surg.* 2004; 91:801 – 814.

[8] Vermeire S, van Assche G, Rutgeerts P. Perianal Crohn's disease: classification and clinical evaluation. *Dig. Liver Dis.* 2007; 39(10):959-962.

[9] Zheng JJ, Shi XH, Chu XQ. Crohn's disease and its diverse clinical presentations. *Chin. J. Dig. Dis.* 2002; 22(4): 226-229 (Chinese).

[10] Ardizzone S, Maconi G, Cassinotti A, et al. Imaging of perianal Crohn's disease. *Dig. Liver Dis.* 2007; 39(10):970-978.

[11] Horsthuisl K and Stoker J.MRI of perianal Crohn's disease. *AJR,* 2004; 183:1309-1315.

[12] Essary B, Kim J, Anupindi S, et al. Pelvic MRI in children with Crohn disease and suspected perianal involvement. *Pediatr. Radiol.* 2007; 37:201-208.

[13] Schwartz DA, Pemberton JH, Sandborn WJ. Diagnosis and treatment of perianal fistulas in Crohn disease. *Ann. Intern. Med.* 2001; 135:906–918.

[14] Griggs L, Schwartz DA. Medical options for treating perianal Crohn's disease. *Dig. Liver Dis.* 2007; 39(10):979-987.

[15] Lichtenstein GR. Treatment of fistulizing Crohn's disease. *Gastroenterology.* 2000; 119:1132–1147.

[16] Mendoza JL, Taxonera C, Lanal R, et al. Diagnostic and treatment recommendations on perianal Crohn's disease. *Rev. Esp. Enferm. Dig.* 2005; 97: 46-56.

[17] Hyder SA, Travis SP, Jewell DP, et al. Fistulating anal Crohn's disease: results of combined surgical and infliximab treatment. *Dis. Colon Rectum.* 2006; 49:1837-1841.

[18] Singh B, George BD, Mortensen NJ. Surgical therapy of perianal Crohn's disease. *Dig. Liver Dis.* 2007; 39(10):988-992.

Chapter XXIV

Surveillance and Prevention of Colorectal Cancer in Inflammatory Bowel Disease

Zhi-hua Ran
Ren-ji Hospital, Shang-hai Jiao-tong University School of Medicine,
Shang-hai, P.R. China

Introduction

Patients with ulcerative colitis (UC) and Crohn's disease (CD) are at increased risk for developing colorectal cancer (CRC). To date, no known genetic basis has been identified to explain colorectal cancer predisposition in these inflammatory bowel diseases (IBD). Instead, it is assumed that chronic inflammation is what causes cancer. This is supported by the fact that colon cancer risk increases with longer duration of colitis, greater anatomic extent of colitis, the concomitant presence of other inflammatory manifestations such as primary sclerosing cholangitis (PSC), and the fact that certain drugs used to treat inflammation, such as 5-aminosalicylates and steroids, may prevent the development of colorectal cancer. As a consequence of this increased risk, surveillance strategies have been proposed to prevent colorectal carcinoma through early detection of dysplasia, which may herald malignant disease. Cancer prevention in inflammatory bowel disease depends on the detection of precancerous dysplasia during scheduled screening and surveillance colonoscopy, but the detection and diagnosis of dysplasia remain challenging. [1]

Mechanism Underlying IBD Related Carcinogenesis

It has been suggested that various risk factors including extent of colonic involvement, long disease duration, severity of inflammation, young age at disease onset, geographical location, treatment with aminosalicylates, folic acid supplementation, presence of stricture, presence of primary sclerosing cholangitis and positive family history of sporadic CRC be important in the development of cancer in inflammatory bowel diseases.

Many of the molecular alterations responsible for sporadic CRC development also play a role in colitis-associated colon carcinogenesis. In fact, the emerging evidence suggests that the two major pathways of chromosomal instability (CIN) and microsatellite instability (MSI) also apply to colitis-associated CRCs and with roughly the same frequency.[2-4] Colitic mucosa progresses in a systematic fashion in the following way: no dysplasia, indefinite dysplasia, low grade dysplasia (LGD), high grade dysplasia (HGD), and, finally, carcinoma. Although this is a useful paradigm that facilitates the study of cancer risk markers in IBD, it is important to realize that the natural history of dysplasia in IBD is often unpredictable. [5-9] For example, LGD may progress to cancer without demonstrating HGD, and cancers can arise in colitic colons without any apparent prior dysplasia. These caveats should be kept in mind when interpreting the results of studies describing the predictive value of dysplasia or molecular markers in IBD.

Surveillance of IBD Related CRCS

Colonoscopic Surveillance

Dysplasia surveillance remains the standard approach to minimize colorectal cancer risk and morbidity in inflammatory bowel disease. Approaches to treatment in Crohn's disease are generally similar to those for ulcerative colitis. Recently, the addition of dye spraying onto the colon to facilitate targeted biopsy has become increasingly associated with enhanced dysplasia surveillance; however, random biopsies are mostly still undertaken, even by those endoscopists who use chromoendoscopy. The prevailing literature continues to support colectomy for any degree of dysplasia. However, for those with adenoma-like masses, ongoing surveillance after polypectomy could still be considered appropriate. Certain endoscopic features are associated with increased incidence of neoplasia. These include not only strictures but also pseudopolyps. [10]

Colonoscopic Surveillance in Ulcerative Colitis

Based on the concept of a dysplasia-to-cacinoma sequence in UC and on the development of flexible fibre-endoscope, programs for surveillance of high-risk patients were introduced in the early 1970s. By performing colonoscopies with multiple biopsies from different parts of the colon and rectum at regular intervals, those programs were aimed at detecting mucosal dysplasia, or carcinoma in early stages. The ultimate goal has been to decrease CRC morbidity and mortality in UC. Some of the larger studies have confirmed the association between colorectal dysplasia and carcinoma in UC, as well as the sequential development of lower grades of dysplasia into high-grade dysplasia (HGD) and, ultimately, to invasive carcinoma. The need for total colonoscopies has been underlined by the frequent initial finding of dysplasia or dysplasia associated lesion or mass (DALM) only in the proximal colon. It must also be remembered that dysplasia is not always found in association with a carcinoma. Studies of resected colonic specimens and studies in large surveillance programs show that no dysplasia is detected in up to 25% of the patients. The sensitivity of dysplasia as a marker for CRC-development is thus only 75%, but if the endoscopic examinations are performed at regular intervals the risk of missing a carcinoma before it becomes incurable by surgical resection is small.

Colonoscopic Surveillance in Colonic Crohn's Disease

Only limited experience exists from prospective colonoscopic surveillance of patients with longstanding, extensive colonic CD. In fact, the only study published so far reported on 259 patients with chronic Crohn's colitis of duration of 8 years or more who were followed for 18years by colonoscopic surveillance. The screening and surveillance program detected dysplasia or CRC in 16% of the patients. Furthermore, age more than 45 years at the time of colonoscopy was associated with increased risk of neoplasia. After a negative colonoscopy, the probability of finding neoplasia by the fourth surveillance examination was 22% and comparable to those reported for UC-patients undergoing surveillance. The authors recommended that all patients with extensive Crohn's colitis of long duration should undergo colonoscopic surveillance. Colonoscopy in CD-patients, with colorectal involvement, may be difficult because of colonic strictures. Thinner caliber pediatric colonoscope may help to improve the percentage of complete examinations. Besides technical difficulties with structuring, there is up to 12% chance that the stricture is of malignant nature. Ongoing prospective programs are needed to determine guidelines regarding surveillance examinations in CD. Based on the discussion above, it would be wise to apply a UC-based colonoscopic strategy at least in patients with Crohn's colitis of long duration.

Screening Colonoscopic Schedule

A screening colonoscopy should be performed in UC patients to rule out colonic neoplasia (dysplasia or cancer) 8 to 10 years after the onset of UC symptoms. At the time of this examination, extent of disease should also be evaluated, with possible reclassification of extent if there is significant change. Patients with extensive colitis or left-sided colitis who have a negative screening colonoscopy should begin surveillance within 1 to 2 years. This interval is based on studies reporting that interval cancers can develop within 2 years after a surveillance examination. With a negative surveillance colonoscopy, subsequent surveillance examinations should be performed every 1 to 2 years. With 2 negative examinations, the next surveillance examination may be performed in 1 to 3 years until UC has been present for 20 years. At that time, consideration should be given to performing surveillance every 1 to 2 years, based on the concept that CRC risk increases with longer duration of colitis. Patients with PSC should undergo surveillance yearly. Patients with other risk factors, such as positive family history of CRC, may require shorter surveillance intervals. Patients with proctosigmoiditis, who have little or no increased risk of CRC compared with the population at large, should be managed according to standard CRC prevention measures. Despite a lack of data, the presence of a so-called 'cecal patch' of erythema with microscopic inflammation in patients with proctosigmoiditis should not alter this recommendation. However, if biopsies are positive for colitis proximal to 35 cm, even though macroscopic disease is limited to the distal sigmoid and rectum, it is suggested that the patient follow a UC-type surveillance approach. Patients with major colonic involvement (at least one third of the colon involved) who have harbored disease for 8 to 10 years from onset of CD should undergo a screening colonoscopy. If no dysplasia or cancer is found, a surveillance examination protocol should be started within 2 years. After a negative surveillance colonoscopy, subsequent surveillance should be performed every 1 to 2 years. With 2 negative examinations, the next surveillance examination may be performed in 1 to 3 years until Crohn's disease has been present for 20 years. At that time, surveillance should be performed every 1 to 2 years. The recommendations for management after an abnormal finding in Crohn's disease are identical to those for UC. For patients with segmental Crohn's disease, if a dysplastic or cancerous lesion is detected and surgery is planned, it is not known whether a segmental resection alone is sufficient or whether a UC-based approach of total proctocolectomy should be considered. [11]

Recent studies indicate that chromoendoscopy can greatly enhance the endoscopic detection of dysplastic lesions in colitic colons. Other techniques that have been proposed (but not yet carefully studied) include laser fluorescence spectroscopy for in-situ dysplasia diagnosis and fecal DNA testing. Whether these or other tests will complement or replace conventional white light colonoscopy remains to be seen.

Surveillance Biomarkers

To date, only four molecular markers - aneuploidy, p53, MSI, and the mucin-associated sialyl-Tn (STn) antigen - have been evaluated in a chronologic context, and each has been demonstrated to be a harbinger of subsequent risk of developing dysplasia or cancer. An advantage to studying patients with IBD is that they typically undergo periodic surveillance colonoscopies with repeated tissue sampling. IBD is one of the few clinical settings in which multiple repetitive sampling of colonic tissue is routinely performed. This provides a unique opportunity to study histologic and molecular changes chronologically. There is no consensus as to how, or even whether, these markers of cancer risk should be incorporated into clinical management of patients with longstanding IBD. Given our current knowledge, no one is likely to recommend colectomy to a patient solely on the basis of marker positivity without some evidence of dysplasia, even if the patient's tissue demonstrated marker positivity on several colonoscopies. Perhaps more intensive surveillance should be offered to such patients. These issues should be considered as more research is conducted in this field.

Protective Factors for CRCs in IBD

5-Amino Salicylic Acid

Most data regarding the role of mesalamine in the prevention of dysplasia have been derived retrospectively, although some data have been collected prospectively. Potentially confounding factors, such as family history of sporadic CRC, smoking history, presence of PSC, use of 6-mercaptopurine/azathioprine, frequency and extent of colonoscopic surveillance, degree of mucosal inflammation and folate intake, were considered in some but not all studies. Studies analyzing sulfasalazine are potentially confounded by its effect on folate metabolism as some series have suggested there may be dose-related chemoprevention with folate. The chemoprotective effect of mesalamine has been described as being dose-dependent in at least 3 series. Population-based data suggested that there was a reduced relative cancer risk in patients who were taking at least 2 g/day of an aminosalicylate.

Several retrospective correlative studies [12-14] have suggested that the long-term use of 5-ASA in IBD patients may significantly reduce the risk of development of colorectal cancer. Pinczowski et al.[12] found that in a population-based cohort of 3 112 patients with UC, pharmacological therapy, especially sulfasalazine, lasting for at least 3 mo was associated with a significant protective effect on colon cancer by calculating relative risk through conditional logistic regression. Eaden et al. [13] designed a retrospectively matched case-control investigation study. They collected medical records of suitable patients in England and Wales. One hundred and two cases met the inclusion criteria and were matched with controls from the Leicestershire IBD patient database. A suitable model was developed to assess the contribution of the variables in a forward selection procedure. Conditional logistic regression was used to compute estimates of odds ratio (OR) as a measure of association between various exposures and colorectal cancer. The most significant finding was the strong protective association of regular 5-ASA therapy, reducing cancer risk by 75% (OR 0.25, 95% CI: 0.13-0.48, P<0.00001). When individual 5-ASA drugs and their doses were analyzed, mesalamine at a dose of 1.2 g/d or greater reduced colorectal cancer risk by 91% compared to no treatment (OR 0.09, 95 CI: 0.03-0.28, P<0.00001) and was also protective when taken at lower doses (OR 0.08, 95% CI: 0.08-0.85, P = 0.04). The benefits of sulfasalazine were less pronounced and the effect was only evident at a dose of 2 g/d or greater (OR 0.41, 95% CI: 0.41, 95% CI: 0.18-0.92, P = 0.03). Other 5-ASA medications also had a non-significant protective effect. They concluded that the benefit of regular consumption of 5-ASA was equal to frequent visits to a hospital physician.

Ursodeoxycholic Acid

Ursodeoxycholic acid (UDCA) has been noted to decrease the prevalence of colonic dysplasia in both a retrospective and a prospective study. By reducing the colonic concentration of the secondary bile acid-deoxycholic acid, UDCA inhibited carcinogenesis in animal models. The hypothesis that UDCA, a drug with relatively few side effects, may reduce colorectal neoplasia in patients with inflammatory bowel diseases and without PSC or in those at risk of colorectal neoplasia in the general population remains intriguing and still unproven.

Ursodeoxycholic acid is being increasingly used by hepatologists to treat patients with PSC to improve liver function tests, but the purported effect of slowing the rate of progression of disease has not been demonstrated.[15] Only 23% of patients in our study were taking UDCA, and now a vast majority takes the medication. UDCA has not been shown to improve mortality in PSC. For patients with UC and PSC, UDCA could have several beneficial effects. Two studies have examined the effectiveness of UDCA as a chemopreventive agent in UC patients with PSC. Tung et al [16] studied 59 patients with UC and PSC and found that UDCA was associated with a lower frequency of colorectal dysplasia. Dysplasia was found in 32% of the 41 patients treated with UDCA and 72% of the 18 patients not treated with UDCA. The main difference in results between our two studies is the extremely high rate of dysplasia among controls in the Tung study, which may be explained by their classification of patients who were indefinite for dysplasia as having dysplasia. Pardi et al [17] found UDCA to be chemopreventive for CRC or dysplasia. The data for their study were obtained from a prior randomized, placebo-controlled trial on 52 patients with PSC and UC designed to evaluate the effect of UDCA on liver function. The relative risk of UDCA treated patients for developing CRC or dysplasia was 0.26.

Folic Acid

In the case of folic acid, efficacy has not been established and is probably a borderline effect. [18] In the setting of sporadic CRC, low folate intake has been associated with an increased risk for developing colorectal adenomas and carcinomas [19, 20]. Patients with chronic IBD are predisposed towards folate deficiency because of inadequate nutritional intake, excessive intestinal losses with active disease, and reduced intestinal absorption from competitive inhibition from sulfasalazine use. Results of two studies suggest a trend towards protection against CRC in folate users, although neither study demonstrated statistical significance [21, 22]. Nonetheless, since it is rather safe and inexpensive, folate supplementation should be considered for CRC risk reduction in patients with longstanding IBD.

Immunomodulating Agents

6-Mercaptopurine and azathioprine are probably not chemopreventive. However, the use of these agents did not increase malignant transformation in patients with long-standing UC.

In addition, CRC risk in patients with IBD increases to 18% after 30 years. New methods to reduce this risk are required. Prevention strategies such as surveillance, drug treatment and regular doctor visits are warranted and probably effective. There are also indirect lines of evidence suggesting that surveillance colonoscopy is beneficial for patients with IBD, particularly patients with long-standing pancolitis or PSC-associated IBD. [23] Different agents show controversial results, and their benefit in chemoprevention has not been established. However, the accumulated evidence favors a role for 5-aminosalicylic acid in the primary prevention of dysplasia and CRC in IBD. Preliminary data also suggested that 5-aminosalicylic acid might be of greater benefit than sulfasalazine. An expanded role for the use of 5- aminosalicylic acid in chronic extensive UC is suggested. Together with other prevention strategies, this could lead to a reduction of CRC risk in IBD patients.

References

[1] Rubin DT, Turner JR. Surveillance of dysplasia in inflammatory bowel disease: The gastroenterologist-pathologist partnership. *Clin. Gastroenterol. Hepatol.* 2006; 4: 1309-1313

[2] Willenbucher RF, Aust DE, Chang CG, et al. Genomic instability is an early event during the progression pathway of ulcerative colitis-related neoplasia. *Am. J. Pathol.* 1999; 154: 1825–1830.

[3] Suzuki H, Harpaz N, Tarmin L, et al. Microsatellite instability in ulcerative colitis-associated colorectal dysplasias and cancers. *Cancer Res.* 1994; 54:4841–4.

[4] Tarmin L, Yin J, Harpaz N, et al. Adenomatous polyposis coli gene mutations in ulcerative colitis-associated dysplasias and cancers versus sporadic colon neoplasms. *Cancer Res.* 1995; 55:2035–8.

[5] Redston MS, Papadopoulos N, Caldas C, et al. Common occurrence of APC and K-ras gene mutations in the spectrum of colitis-associated neoplasias. *Gastroenterology.* 1995; 108:383–92.

[6] Aust DE, Terdiman JP, Willenbucher RF, et al. The APC/b-catenin pathway in ulcerative colitis-related colorectal carcinomas. *Cancer.* 2002; 94:1421–7.

[7] Burmer GC, Rabinovitch PS, Haggitt RC, et al. Neoplastic progression in ulcerative colitis: histology, DNA content, and loss of a p53 allele. *Gastroenterology.* 1992; 103:1602–10.

[8] Brentnall TA, Crispin DA, Rabinovitch PS, et al. Mutations of the p53 gene: an early marker of neoplastic progression in ulcerative colitis. *Gastroenterology.* 1994; 107: 369–78.

[9] Klump B, Holzmann K, Kuhn A, et al. Distribution of cell populations with DNA aneuploidy and p53 protein expression in ulcerative colitis. *Eur. J. Gastroenterol. Hepatol.* 1997; 9: 789–94.

[10] Bernstein CN. Neoplasia in inflammatory bowel disease: surveillance and management strategies. *Curr. Gastroenterol. Rep.* 2006; 8(6): 513-518

[11] Itzkowitz SH, Present DH. Consensus conference: Colorectal cancer screening and surveillance in inflammatory bowel disease. *Inflamm. Bowel Dis.* 2005; 11(3): 314-321

[12] Pinczowski D, Ekbom A, Baron J, et al. Risk factors for colorectal cancer in patients with ulcerative colitis: a case-control study. *Gastroenterology.* 1994; 107: 117-120.

[13] Eaden J, Abrams K, Ekbom A, et al. Colorectal cancer prevention in ulcerative colitis: a case-control study. *Aliment Pharmacol. Ther.* 2000; 14: 145-153.

[14] Moody GA, Jayanthi V, Probert CS, et al. Long-term therapy with sulphasalazine protects against colorectal cancer in ulcerative colitis: A retrospective study of

colorectal cancer risk and compliance with treatment in Leicestershire. *Eur. J. Gastroenterol. Hepatol.* 1996; 8: 1179-1183.
[15] Lindor KD. Ursodiol for primary sclerosing cholangitis. Mayo PSC-UDCA Study Group. *N. Engl. J. Med.* 1997; 336: 691–5.
[16] Tung BY, Edmond MJ, Haggitt C, et al. Ursodiol use is associated with lower prevalence of colonic neoplasia in patients with ulcerative colitis and primary sclerosing cholangitis. *Ann. Intern. Med.* 2001; 134: 89–95.
[17] Pardi DS, Loftus EV, Kremers WK, et al. Ursodeoxycholic acid acts as a chemopreventive agent in patients with ulcerative colitis and primary sclerosing cholangitis. *Gastroenterology.* 2003; 124: 889–93.
[18] Stange EF. Review article: the effect of aminosalicylates and immunomodulation on cancer risk in inflammatory bowel disease. *Aliment Pharmacol. Ther.* 2006; 24 Suppl 3: 64-67
[19] Freudenheim JL, Graham S, Marshall JR, et al. Folate intake and carcinogenesis of the colon and rectum. *Int. J. Epidemiol.* 1991; 20: 368-374.
[20] Giovannucci E, Stampfer MJ, Colditz GA, et al. Folate, methionine, and alcohol intake and risk of colorectal adenoma. *J. Natl. Cancer Inst.* 1993; 85: 875-884.
[21] Lashner BA, Heidenreich PA, Su GL, et al. Effect of folate supplementation on the incidence of dysplasia and cancer in chronic ulcerative colitis. A case-control study. *Gastroenterology.* 1989; 97: 255-259.
[22] Lashner BA, Provencher KS, Seidner DL, et al. The effect of folic acid supplementation on the risk for cancer or dysplasia in ulcerative colitis. *Gastroenterology.* 1997; 112: 29-32
[23] Munkholm P, Loftus EV Jr, Reinacher-Schick A, et al. Prevention of colorectal cancer in inflammatory bowel disease: value of screening and 5-aminosalicylates. *Digestion.* 2006; 73: 11-19

Section Five: Medical Treatment in Inflammatory Bowel Disease

In: Inflammatory Conditions of the Colon
Editor: Jia-ju Zheng

ISBN: 978-1-60692-240-8
© 2008 Nova Science Publishers, Inc.

Chapter XXV

Treatment of Inflammatory Bowel Disease with Aminosalicylates

Zhan-ju Liu
The Second Affiliated Hospital, Zheng-zhou University,
He-nan Province, P.R. China

Introduction

Inflammatory bowel disease (IBD) encompassing Crohn's disease (CD) and ulcerative colitis (UC), are chronic inflammatory disorders of the gastrointestinal tract. Increasing evidences have demonstrated that dysregulation of the mucosal immune response toward commensal bacterial flora together with genetic and environmental factors plays an important role in the pathogenesis of human IBD [1,2]. Importantly, differentiation and activation of lamina propria $CD4^+$ T cells, macrophages and dendritic cells as well as secretion of large amount of proinflammatory cytokines contribute to the tissue damage in gut.

Currently, therapeutic strategies for the management of IBD include aminosalicylates, corticosteroids, antibiotics, immunosuppressants, probiotics, biologics and curative surgery [3]. Sulfasalazine was the first aminosalicylate used for the treatment of IBD, although it was initially developed for the treatment of rheumatoid arthritis in the 1940s. Sulfasalazine is comprised of sulfapyridine linked to 5-aminosalicylate (5-ASA) by an azo bond and was intended to provide antibacterial (salfapyridine) and anti-inflammatory (5-ASA) effects to arthritic joints. Since some rheumatoid arthritis patients have clinical symptoms of UC, sulfasalazine treatment also demonstrates to be effective in the management of UC. Once salfasalazine enters the colon, the azo bond is cleared by bacterial azo-reductase, releasing sulfapyridine and 5-ASA. The sulfapyridine is absorbed systemically and accounts for most of the drug's toxicity and intolerance.

The 5-ASA is the active anti-inflammatory compound and ultimately is excreted into the feces. It is generally accepted that aminosalicylates or 5-ASA (namely mesalamine or mesalazine) represents a drug of first choice in the treatment of IBD, particularly in UC [4-6].

As a topical agent, the local availability of 5-ASA at the inflamed areas of intestinal tract has been assumed to be an important determinant of its clinical efficacy [7]. In the past few years it has been appreciated that absorption and oral bioavailability of many drugs can be affected to a large extent by metabolic enzymes and efflux transporters present in the epithelial cells of the intestine [8]. Recent years, the recognition that 5-ASA component is the active moiety in UC has allowed the development of numerous oral, and rectal, better-tolerated 5-ASA formulations [9], which lack the sulfapyridine moiety and are classified into an azo bond or delayed or sustained release (table 25-1). The topical 5-ASA preparations are delivered rectally as a suppository or enema and have minimal systemic absorption.

Table 25-1. 5-ASA preparations

Preparations	Constituents	Formulation	Delivery
Azo-bond			
Sulfasalazine	Sulfapyridine+5-ASA	Sulfapyridine carrier	Colon
Olsalazine	5-ASA dimmer	Gelatin capsule	Colon
Basalazide	5-ASA+4-ABBA	Capsules	Colon
Delayed-release mesalamine			
Asacol	5-ASA	Eudragit S (pH7)	Ileum to colon
Claversal/Mesasal/Salofalk	5-ASA	Eudragit S (pH6)	Ileum to colon
Sustained-release mesalamine			
Pentasa	5-ASA	Ethylcellulose granules	Stomach to colon
Topical therapy			
Mesalamine suppository	5-ASA		Rectum
Mesalamine	5-ASA	Suspension	Rectum to splenic flexure

Mechanism of Action

The precise mechanism of action of 5-ASA is not known, but is likely due to a local anti-inflammatory effect from the luminal site in the diseased parts of gut [10]. Absorption of 5-ASA is followed by extensive metabolism to the major inactive N-acetyl-5-aminosalicylate (N-acetyl-5-ASA) by the N-acetyl-transferase 1 enzyme in intestinal epithelial cells and the liver. Oral or rectal administration of 5-ASA the released active agent is taken up by intestinal epithelial cells in the small and large bowel. In earlier clinical studies it has been shown that absorbed 5-ASA and intestinally inactivated N-Ac-5-ASA are partly secreted back into the intestinal lumen [11,12]. The exact role of 5-ASA in the prevention of intestinal mucosal inflammation remains unknown, but it is generally accepted that 5-ASA acts locally by a combination of anti-inflammatory properties in the gastrointestinal mucosa [8]. Following oral ingestion, 5-ASA is rapidly absorbed from the upper gastrointestinal tract and prevented from reaching the inflamed regions in the terminal ileum, ileo-caecal region and ascending colon.

Evidences have shown that 5-ASA could affect on eicosanoid metabolism and inhibit prostanglandin production in intestinal mucosa. It may interfere with the production of arachidonic acid by affecting the thromboxane and lipoxygenase synthsis pathway, function as "scavengers" of free oxygen radicals and inhibitors of reactive oxygen metabolite production. Moreover, 5-ASA may play a role in regulating mucosal lymphocyte and macrophage activities and inhibiting proinflammatory cytokine production such as IL-1 and IL-2.

Regular 5-ASA intake may also reduce the risk of colorectal cancer [13]. 5-ASA is a derivative of aspirin, which has been shown to have a modest chemo-preventive effect for sporadic colorectal cancer. 5-ASA therapies are attractive as potential chemo-preventive agents since they are very safe, relatively inexpensive, and are effective as maintenance therapy. 5-ASA may reduce cancer risk by mechanism other that by simple controlling inflammation, such as by increasing apoptosis, decreasing cellular proliferation, inactivating reactive oxygen species, and activating the peroxisome proliferator-receptor-gamma (PPAR gamma) [14].

Pharmacokinetics

Orally administered sulfasalazine is largely unabsorbed in the small intestine and mostly passes into the colon. Sulfasalazine itself is poorly absorbed (3% to 12%) and its elimination half-life of about 5-10h is probably affected by the absorption process. The major part of sulfasalazine is split by bacterial azo-reduction in the colon into 5-ASA and sulfapyridine, the latter accounting for most of the agent's adverse effects. The effective cleavage of sulfasalazine depends on an intact colon and transit time. Sulfapyridine is almost completely absorbed from the colon and it is then metabolized by hydroxylation, glucuronidation and polymorphic acetylation and excreted in the urine.

Pharmacokinetic studies have also demonstrated that, when given orally, the active moiety of mesalazine is delivered mainly to the distal ileum and proximal large bowel thus ensuring a higher mucosal drug concentration in the right than in the left colon, with only negligible amounts of the drug reaching the rectal mucosa [15,16]. Topical mesalazine administration (e.g., suppositories, enema) assures considerable drug availability in the recto-sigmoid sites and, to a lower extent, also in the descending colon [17,18].

As all formulations are metabolized by the same pathway to N-acetyl-5-ASA, a meta-analysis have assessed whether plasma levels and/or urinary excretion of 5-ASA or N-acetyl-5-ASA varied between formulations [19]. However, it remains to be determined whether differences translate into clinically significant variations in efficacy or safety [19,20]. Sulfasalazine and Olsalazine showed similar pharmacokinetic properties in patients with active UC, although the data for other aminosalicylates have not been identified in patients with active disease [19]. The range of urinary excretion for the azo-bond compounds and

Asacol ranges between 10% and 35%, for Pentasa, between 15% and 53%, and for Salofalk/ Claversal/ Mesasal, between 27% and 56%. The meta-analysis have demonstrated that all compounds show comparable ranges of systemic absorption of total 5-ASA based on plasma pharmacokinetics, 24-96 h urinary excretion of total 5-ASA and fecal excretion of 5-ASA. The selection of a 5-ASA formulation for UC should be based on factors other than pharmacokinetics, such as efficacy, dose response, toxicity of the parent compound, compliance issues and cost [19,20].

Clinical Efficacy

Sulfasalazine has an established role in the treatment of UC, being effective in controlling mild-to-moderate disease and in maintaining the remission in approximately 70% of patients. The recommended dose for sulfasalazine is 4 g/d in active UC, although some work suggests increased efficacy at 6 g/d. The side-effects are dose dependent, and many patients do not tolerate higher doses of sulfasalazine. Although it was first used in clinic for decades, a recent review has argued that the additional costs of newer preparations cannot be justified in most patients, and has concluded that sulfasalazine may still be the drug of choice for active UC [21].

Currently, mesalazine (5-ASA), the therapeutically active moiety of sulphasalazine, is a first-line drug for the treatment of patients with IBD [4, 22,23], since lower frequencies of side effects appear. Mesalazine has a topical effect, which means that the drug may significantly concentrate into the intestinal mucosa only during its absorptive process. Thus, if it is absorbed by inflamed mucosa it may concentrate in the inflamed tissue, but if the drug is absorbed by normal mucosa it is almost completely lost for its therapeutic use Thus, the goal of treatment is not only to achieve an optimal dosage, but especially to take the drug where it needs [24]. The delayed and sustained formulations (as shown in table 25-1) have a dose response between 1.5 g/d and 4.8 g/d. Previous data demonstrated that balsalazide had a faster onset of action at 6.75 g/d over 12 weeks and improved tolerance compared to a pH-release mesalazine formulation of Asacol 2-4 g/d in patients with active UC [25-29]. Post hoc analysis also suggested that patients with left-sided disease might have responded better to basalazide. However, direct comparison studies are needed to determine whether left-sided disease responds better to an azo-bond compound than to alternative delivery systems of mesalazine. Olsalazine may increase small bowel secretion and thus limit the upward dosing of azo-compound in active disease because of increasing loosening of stools at doses greater than 2 g/d (similar to basalazide at 6 g/d). Recently, mesalazine with MMX Multi Matrix System (MMX) technology was developed. This high-strength formulation of 5-ASA (1.2 g/tablet) utilizes MMX technology comprising lipophilic and hydrophilic excipients enclosed within a gastro-resistant, pH dependent coating. The gastro-resistant film, covering the tablet core, delays the initial release of 5-ASA until the tablet is exposed to pH 7 or higher, normally in the terminal ileum. As the gastroresistant coating disintegrates, it is thought that intestinal fluids interact with the hydrophilic excipient causing the tablet to swell (much like a sponge in water) and form an outer viscous gel mass. The viscous gel mass is believed to slow diffusion of the 5-ASA from the tablet core into the colonic lumen. As the tablet core and its surrounding gel mass progress through the colon, it is thought that pieces of the gel mass gradually break away from the core, releasing 5-ASA. It is supposed that the lipophilic excipient slows the penetration of aqueous fluids into the tablet core, reducing the rate of dissolution and thus prolonging therapeutic activities. MMX mesalazine 2.4 g (given once daily or 1.2 g twice daily) has been shown to be effective, safe and tolerant in the maintenance of remission of UC [30].

The issue of optimal therapy for left-sided disease with varied formulations of oral aminosalicylates is made less relevant by the well-defined superiority of topical (rectal) mesalazine in distal colitis. Topical 5-ASA administration is higher effective for the management of mild-to-moderate distal UC and proctitis. The suppository preparations reach the upper rectum, and the enema formulations reach the splenic flexure and distal transverse colon. The dose of 5-ASA enema varies from 1 to 4 g/d, but there is no proven benefit of topical doses greater than 1 g/d. Rectal formulations are superior to oral administration for the treatment of distal colitis and proctitis with remission rates of 76% versus 46% for oral 5-ASA.

Clinical data have also indicated that sulfasalazine and the newer 5-ASA formulation are effective to the maintenance of remission of UC. When the active disease is controlled, the dose required to maintain remission is the same as that used to induce remission. It is recommended that 2-4 g/d of sulfasalazine and 0.7-4.8 g/d of the newer 5-ASA formulations are necessary to maintain the remission. Importantly, 75% patients maintain long-term remission if continuous 5-ASA administration. There is evidence from randomized controlled studies that sulfasalazine is not effective for the maintenance of remission of Crohn's disease.

Side Effects

Sulfasalazine and the newer 5-ASA formulations are well-tolerated for mild-to-moderate UC, and have a dose-effect in the maintenance of remission in UC. Unfortunately, dose-related side effects are seen in as many as 20% of patients, and dose-reduction to 2 g daily for sulfasalazine (or more likely switching to a non-sulfa containing mesalamine) may be necessary in those patients. As many as 30% of patients taking sulfasalazine report side effects that correlate closely with the amount of sulfapyridine moiety and the individual's acetylator status (i.e. how fast sulfasalazine is metabolized) [31]. Generally, adverse effects include common and dose-dependent reactions such as headache, nausea, vomiting, and diarrhea; idiosyncratic symptoms such as rashes and itching; rare manifestations such as toxic hepatitis, pancreatitis, leukopenia, haemolytic anemia, and agranulocytosis; and extremely rare side effects such as neurotoxicity, pulmonary fibrosis and fetal hyperbilirubinemia. Nephrotoxic reactions reported in animal studies are dose-dependent, and nephrotoxicity has been reported repeatedly in patients taking sulfasalazine and 5-ASA [32].

References

[1] Podolsky DK. Inflammatory bowel disease. *N. Eng. J. Med.* 2002; 347:417-29.
[2] Sartor RB. Mechanisms of disease: pathogenesis of Crohn's disease and ulcerative colitis. *Nat. Clin. Pract. Gastroenterol. Hepatol.* 2006; 3:390-407.
[3] Tamboli CP. Current medical therapy for chronic inflammatory bowel disease. *Surg. Clin. North. Am.* 2007; 87:697̄725.
[4] Klotz U. The role of aminosalicylates at the beginning of the new millennium in the treatment of chronic inflammatory bowel disease. *Eur. J. Clin. Pharmacol.* 2000; 56:353-62.
[5] Zheng J-j. Clinical phatmacology of aminosalicylate in treatment of inflammatory bowel disease. *Chin. Phatmacy.* 2005;16(13):1025-1028 (Chinese).
[6] Chinese Medical Association Digestive Disease Branch. Collaboration Group on Inflammatory Bowel Disease, A consensus for the management of inflammatory bowel disease in China. *Chin. J. Dig.* 2007; 27(5):545-550 (Chinese).
[7] Klotz U, Schwab M. Topical delivery of therapeutic agents in the treatment of inflammatory bowel disease. *Adv. Drug. Delivery Rev.* 2005; 57:267-79.
[8] Suzuki H, Sugiyama Y. Role of metabolic enzymes and efflux transporters in the absorption of drugs from the small intestine. *Eur. J. Pharm. Sci.* 2000; 12:3-12.
[9] Hanauer SB, Meyers S, Sachar DB. The pharmacology of anti inflammatory drugs in inflammatory bowel disease. In: Kirsner JB, Shorter RG, eds. Inflammatory Bowel Disease, 4th ed. Baltimore: Williams and Wilkins, 1995: 643-63.
[10] Cohen RD. Review article: evolutionary advances in the delivery of aminosalicylate for the treatment of ulcerative colitis. *Aliment Pharmacol. Ther.* 2006; 24:465-74.
[11] Goebell H, Klotz U, Nehlsen B, et al. Oroileal transit of slow release 5-aminosalicylic acid. *Gut.* 1993; 4:669-75.
[12] Layer PH, Goebell H, Keller J, et al. Delivery and fate of oral mesalamine microgranules within the human small intestine. *Gastroenterology.* 1995; 108:1427-33.
[13] Eaden J. Review article: the data supporting a role for aminosalicylates in the chemoprevention of colorectal cancer in patients with inflammatory bowel disease. *Aliment Pharmacol. Ther.* 2003;8(suppl 2):15-21.
[14] Allgayer H. Review article: mechanisms of action of mesalazine in preventive colorectal carcinoma in inflammatory bowel disease. *Aliment Pharmacol. Ther.* 2003; 18 (Suppl.2):10-4.
[15] Hebden JM, Blackshaw PE, Perkins AC, et al. Limited exposure of the healthy distal colon to orally-dosed formulation is further exaggerated in active left-sided ulcerative colitis. *Aliment Pharmacol. Ther.* 2000; 14:155-61.
[16] De Vos M, Verdievel H, Shoonjans R, et al. Concentrations of 5-ASA and Ac-5-ASA in human ileo-colonic biopsy homogenates after oral 5-ASA preparations. *Gut.* 1992; 33:1338-42.
[17] Campieri M, Corbelli C, Gionchetti P, et al. Spread and distribution of 5-ASA colonic foam and 5-ASA enema in patients with ulcerative colitis. *Dig. Dis. Sci.* 1992; 37:1890-7.

[18] Frieri G, Pimpo MT, Palumbo GC, et al. Rectal and colonic mesalazine concentration in ulcerative colitis: oral vs. oral plus topical treatment. *Aliment Pharmacol. Ther.* 1999; 13:1413-7.

[19] Sandborn WJ, Hanauer SB. The pharmacokinetic profiles of oral mesalazine formulations and mesalazine pro-drugs used in the management of ulcerative colitis. *Aliment Pharmacol. Ther.* 2003; 17:29-42.

[20] Sandborn WJ. Rational selection of oral 5-aminosalicylate formulations and prodrugs for the treatment of ulcerative colitis. *Am. J. Gastroenterol.* 2002; 97:2939-41.

[21] Sutherland L, Roth D, Beck P, May G, Makiyama K. Oral 5-aminosalicylic acid for inducing remission in ulcerative colitis (Cochrane Review). In: The Cochrane Library, Issue 4. Oxford: Update Software, 2000.

[22] Hanauer SB. Review article: aminosalicylates in inflammatory bowel disease. *Aliment Pharmacol. Ther.* 2004; 20(Suppl 4):60-5.

[23] Gearry RB, Ajlouni Y, Nandurkar S, et al. 5-aminosalicylic acid (mesalazine) us in Crohn's disease: a survey of the options and practice of Australian gastroenterologists. *Inflamm. Bowel. Dis.* 2007; 13:1009-15.

[24] Klotz U. Colonic targeting of aminosalicylates for the treatment of ulcerative colitis. *Dig. Dis. Liver.* 2005; 37:3818.

[25] Cooperative Group of 5-ASA Clinical Trial. A multicenter study of 5-aminosalicylic acid treatment for ulcerative colitis *Chin. J. Dig.* 2002; 22(6):379-380 (Chinese)

[26] Coordinate Group of homemade 5-aminosalicylic acid enteric-coated tablets. Efficacy evaluation of homemade enteric-coated tablets of 5-aminosalicylic acid in the treatment in ulcerative colitis: a multi center randomized controlled trial. *Chin. J. Dig.* 2004; 24(7):399-402.(Chinese)

[27] Cai J-t, Wu L-f, Du Q, et al. Olsalazine versus sulfasalazine in the treatment of ulcerative colitis: randomized controlled clinical trial. *Chin. J. Dig.* 2001, 21(10).593-595 (Chinese).

[28] Green JRB, Mansfield JC, Gibson JA, et al. A double-blind comparison of balsalazide, 6.75 g daily, and sulfasalazine, 3 g daily, in patients with newly diagnosed or relapsed active ulcerative colitis. *Aliment. Pharmacol. Ther.* 2002; 16:618.

[29] Cooperative Group of Balsalazide in Hen-an Province. The efficacy of balsalazide in the treatment of acute ulcerative colitis. *Chin. J. Dig.* 2007; 27(5):295-298 (Chinese).

[30] Kamm MA, Lichtenstein GR, Sandborn WJ, et al. Randomised trial of once- or twice-daily MMX mesalazine for maintenance of remission in ulcerative colitis. *Gut.* 2008; 57:893902.

[31] Taffet SL, Das KM. Sulfasalazine. Adverse effects and desensitization. *Dig. Dis. Sci.* 1983; 28:833-42.

[32] Ishag S, Green JR. Tolerability of aminosalicylates in inflammatory bowel disease. *BioDrugs.* 2001; 15:33949.

In: Inflammatory Conditions of the Colon
Editor: Jia-ju Zheng

ISBN: 978-1-60692-240-8
© 2008 Nova Science Publishers, Inc.

Chapter XXVI

Glucocorticosteroid Therapy in Inflammatory Bowel Disease

Zhi-hua Ran

Ren-ji Hospital, Shang-hai Jiao-tong University School of Medicine,
Shang-hai, P.R. Chin

Glucocorticosteroids (GCS) are the most commonly used agents for the treatment of moderately to severely active inflammatory bowel disease (IBD) [1-3]. GCS affects many aspects of the immune and inflammatory cascades involved in the tissue responses of IBD.

Mechanism of Action

1. The actions of glucocorticoids are mediated by specific intracytoplasmic glucocorticoid receptors [1]. Hormone-receptor binding to DNA leads to activation and expression of a number of different genes and eventual anti-inflammatory effect.
2. Glucocorticoids impair specific and nonspecific immune reactions, affecting both early and late inflammatory events [2,3] through direct effects on lymphocytes, monocytes and macrophages, and neutrophils.
3. Glucocorticoids also have effects on eosinophils, basophils, and mast cells glucocorticoids also affect nonimmune cells, such as endothelial cells and mesenchymal cells influencing microvascular permeability and adhesion [4].
4. A highly increased activation of nuclear factor kβ (NFkβ) has been found in the intestinal mucosa of patients with IBD. GCS may induce inhibitor kβ (Ikβ) to downregulate this reaction.
5. "Downstream" mediators of inflammation also are suppressed by GCS.
6. Numerous cellular effects of steroids have been delineated that impact on tissue responses in IBD. Induced cytokine inhibition also may account for defective T- and

B-cell function, including reduced suppressor cell function, cellular cytotoxicity, and inhibited immunoglobulin production.
7. In addition to the anti-inflammatory effects of GCS, symptomatic benefits in IBD include reduction of diarrhea via enhanced sodium and water absorption.
8. Other effects include the systemic impact on intermediate metabolism of glucose metabolism, the well-known (but poorly understood) impacts on the central nervous system (CNS) and sense of well-being, and stimulation of the "stress response".

Synthetic GCS and Its Application in IBD [4,5]

Synthetic GCS, such as prednisone or prednisolone, are the most commonly used corticosteroids in the treatment of IBD (table 26-1). The systemic bioavailability of these compounds is 50 to 80% after oral ingestion. Prednisone requires hepatic activation by 11-β-hydroxydehydrogenase to prednisolone. Although absorption has been reduced among some Crohn's disease patients, conversion to prednisolone is normal.

Ninety percent of plasma steroids are protein bound either to albumin or transcortin (α-1-glycoprotein corticosteroid-binding protein). The pharmacologic effect depends on the free plasma steroid concentration and is diminished by hypoalbuminemia. Oral contraceptives delay steroid clearance by increasing GCS binding protein, and conversely drugs that induce hepatic enzymes can increase GCS clearance.

The modification of hydrocortisone to prednisolone increases its glucocorticoid activity fourfold, and decreases its mineralocorticoid activity. Further modification to methylprednisolone increases glucocorticoid activity another 20%.

Budesonide is a novel synthetic corticosteroid structurally related to 16ahydroxyprednisolone. Budesonide has a very strong affinity for the glucocorticoid receptor, giving it potent local anti-inflammatory activity.

Budesonide capsules are designed to delay the release of budesonide until reaching the ileum and ascending colon. The capsules start releasing their content at a pH of over 5.5. Systemic availability is approximately 10%.

Adrenocorticotrophic hormone (ACTH) has also been used to treat UC by stimulating endogenous corticosteroid production, and has the advantage of avoiding adrenal suppression. Despite controlled evidence favoring intravenous ACTH over hydrocortisone, particularly in patients not previously treated with corticosteroids, ACTH is now rarely used

Table 26-1. Commonly available glucocorticoid preparations

Dreg	Route of administration	Strength
Hydrocortisone	IV, p.o, suppository, enema	1×
Prednisone	IV, p.o	4×
Methylprednisolone	IV, p.o	5×
Dexamethasone	IV, p.o	10×
Budesonide	Po, enema	16×

Adverse Effects

The adverse effects of GCS are related to the dose and duration of therapy. Steroids can be expected to have an impact on every organ system and on most metabolic activities of the body (table 26-2).

1. The metabolic effects of steroid therapy include hyperglycemia and an unmasking of a genetic predisposition to diabetes mellitus, hyperlipidemia, alteration of fat distribution with development of a Cushingoid appearance and hepatic steatosis.
2. Glaucoma and cataracts have been described in both adults and children and correlate with the intensity and duration of treatment [6].
3. Wound healing is impaired after steroid therapy, and corticosteroids are associated with increased postoperative infectious complications [7].
4. Steroid-induced subcutaneous tissue atrophy causes striae, and predisposes to purpura and ecchymoses.
5. Corticosteroid-induced neuropsychiatric complications occur in approximately 25% of patients and are severe in up to 6% of patients, with symptoms including psychosis, depression, mania, and delirium [8].
6. Osteopenia and osteoporosis are common complications of IBD.
7. Steroid-related osteonecrosis, particularly of the femoral head, is a less common musculoskeletal complication of IBD [9].
8. Patients treated with high doses of steroids for prolonged periods of time are at an increased risk of infectious complications [10].

Table 26-2. Side effects of corticosteroid therapy [21]

Metabolic
Hyperglycemia, diabetes mellitus
Hypertension
Hypercholesterolemia
Hypokalemia
Edema
Adrenal suppression
Growth retardation in children
Musculoskeletal
Osteoporosis
Aseptic necrosis of bone
Proximal myopathy
Dermatologic
Acne
Plethora
Striae
Ocular
Cataracts
Glaucoma
Neuropsychiatric
Neuropathy

Table 26-2. (Continued).

Psychosis
Insomnia
Immunologic
Increased risk of infection, impaired wound healing
Miscellaneous
Cushingoid appearance ("moon face," "buffalo hump")
Increased appetite, weight gain
Ulcer disease

Recommendations for GCS Use

Corticosteroids may be administered topically as suppositories or enemas, orally, or intravenously. In the United States, most physicians use hydrocortisone or methylprednisolone for intravenous administration and prednisone for oral administration.

1. Mild to Moderate IBD

1. Ileal-release preparations of budesonide (Entocort) 9 mg/d are indicated for the treatment of patients with ileal and right-sided colonic CD [11], are not effective in patients with UC. (Grade A).
2. Topical therapy with either hydrocortisone (Grade A) or budesonide enemas and foams (Grade B) is effective for distal colonic inflammation.
3. 10% hydrocortisone foam or 100 mg hydrocortisone enema also induces remission for distal UC and may be tolerated better; however, compared with topical mesalamine
4. Oral corticosteroids at dosages equivalent to prednisone 20–60 mg/d can be prescribed [11] followed by a slow taper, with no obvious benefit from higher oral doses [12,13]. A comparison of once a day dosing at 40 mg versus 10 mg four times a day showed no difference in response [14].
5. Split-dosing two to four times a day may be helpful in patients who remain symptomatic after a trial of once daily dosing, particularly if they are bothered by nocturnal bowel movements. It may also be useful for hospitalized patients transitioning from parenteral steroids to oral therapy [15].
6. Rectally administered steroids have lower systemic absorption than oral, and therefore may provide a therapeutic advantage by acting locally in distal UC.

2. Moderate to Severe IBD

1. GCS such as prednisone are effective in both patients with CD and patients with UC. (Grade A).
2. GCS are not effective for the treatment of patients with perianal fistulas (Grade C).

3. Parenteral corticosteroids are the treatment of choice for hospitalized patients with severe UC [16].
4. The use of conventional GCS such as prednisone is generally reserved for patients with moderate to severe disease who failed to respond to first-line therapies for IBD such as mesalamine (UC) or budesonide (CD) (Grade B).
5. Budesonide controlled ileal release is almost as efficacious as prednisolone for the treatment of active CD
6. Once the decision has been made to initiate oral steroid therapy for the treatment, no rationale exists for starting at lower doses to prevent steroid side effects [15].
7. Prednisone, 0.5 to 0.75 mg/kg/d, or 6-methylprednisolone, 48 mg/d (dosage equivalent 60 mg/d prednisone) for at least 4 months. Remission rates in moderate-severe CD with inductive systemic corticosteroids approach 80% [17].
8. Cortisone beginning at 100 mg/day was effective in inducing remission in patients with mildly to severely active UC
9. A typical induction regimen used in North America is oral prednisone, 40 to 60 mg/d, with tapering to discontinuation over 8 to 16 weeks. Other investigators recommend 12 weeks as the maximal extent of steroid induction therapy.
10. If the presentation is more fulminate with hypovolemia or other indications for hospitalization, intravenous (IV) steroids usually are administered (e.g., methylprednisolone, 48–60 mg/d, or hydrocortisone, 300–400 mg).

3. Severe and Fulminate IBD

1. Hospitalization for parenteral GCS is indicated for patients failing to respond to oral GCS or for patients with severe disease with UC (Grade A) or CD (Grade B)
2. Most treatment regimens use methylprednisolone, 60 mg/d, or its equivalent [18], and there is little evidence to support the use of higher doses [19].
3. Although a continuous infusion of ACTH was superior to intermittent infusions of hydrocortisone for patients never before treated with corticosteroids, ACTH is frequently used [4].
4. Most practitioners treat severe colitis with 7 to 10 days of intravenous corticosteroid before moving to other medical treatments or surgery.

4. Maintenance Therapy

1. Conventional GCS are not efficacious in maintenance treatment of patients with CD (Grade A) or patients with UC (Grade B).
2. Budsonide therapy is effective in the maintenance of short-term (3 months) but not long-term (1 year) remission compared with placebo in patients with mild to moderate ileocecal CD. (Grade A).
3. Oral corticosteroids are neither effective nor indicated in preventing relapse of UC.
4. Budesonide does not prevent relapse in patients with quiescent CD.

Dosing and Tapering for IBD

1. Corticosteroids should be continued at full dose until clinical remission has been obtained, typically within 2 weeks, but occasionally longer, followed by gradual dose tapering.
2. Dosages in the range of 40-60 mg/day or 1 mg .kg -1 .day -1 of prednisone or equivalent are effective for induction of remission. (Grade A).
3. Induction of response averages 7-14 days. A gradual taper by 5 mg/wk of prednisone (or equivalents GCS) to a dose of 20 mg and then 2.5-5 mg/wk below 20 mg is recommended (Grade B).
4. Budesonide may be tapered gradually from the initial induction dose of 9 mg to dose suppress the adrenocortical axis; clinicians should evaluate for adrenal insufficiency as warranted by clinical symptoms (Grade C).
5. An inability to taper GCS is an indication for antimetabolite and/or infliximab therapy (Grade A).
6. For patients failing to respond to 7-14 days of high-dose oral prednisone or equivalent GCS therapy, parenteral GCS are indicated. (Grade C).
7. Dosages for parenteral GCS typically are in the range of methylprednisolone 40-60 mg/day or hydrocortisone 200-300 mg/day. (Grade A).
8. Patients unable to taper off of corticosteroids need to be evaluated for alternative medical therapy or surgical intervention.

Monitoring for Complications

1. Periodic bone mineral density assessment (dual-energy X-ray absorptiometry scanning) is recommended for patients on long-term GCS therapy (>3 months). (Grade).
2. Annual ophthalmologic examinations are recommended for patients on long-term GCS therapy. (Grade C).
3. Patients with GCS use within the past year are at greater risk for adrenal insufficiency, especially following surgery, and may need stress-dose GCS perioperatively. (Grade C).
4. Patients who are using GCS should be monitored for glucose intolerance and other metabolic abnormalities. (Grade B).
5. Patients being treated with GCS are at increased risk for infectious complications. (Grade B).
6. Patients with osteoporosis should receive calcium and vitamin D supplementation and a bisphosphonate compound, such as alendronate or risedronate [20].
7. The most important side effect of corticosteroid therapy in childhood is growth retardation. Alternate-day corticosteroids have been shown to reduce this complication,
8. If steroids must be used during pregnancy it makes sense to use one more extensively metabolized by the placenta, such as prednisone or prednisolone.

9. The newer high-potency, low-bioavailability steroids such as budesonide may be associated with less risk of inducing bone disease. Newer oral and topical formulations (e.g., budesonide and fluticasone) that have less systemic absorption and/or more first-pass hepatic clearance have been developed [11].

References

[1] Gustafsson JA, Carlstedt-Duke J, Poellinger L, et al. Biochemistry, molecular biology, and physiology of the glucocorticoid receptor. *Endocr. Rev.* 1987; 8:185-234.

[2] Schleimer RP. Effects of glucocorticoids on inflammatory cells relevant to their therapeutic applications in asthma. *Am. Respir. Dis.* 1990; 141:S59-69.

[3] Zheng J-j Application of glucocorticosteroids for the treatment of inflammatory bowel disease. *J. Clin. Dig. Dis.* 2005; 17(4):185-187 (Chinese).

[4] Williams TJ, Yarwood H. Effect of glucocorticoids on microvascular permeability. *Am. Rev. Respir. Dis.* 1990; 141:S39-43.

[5] Meyers S, Sachar DB, Goldberg JD et al. Corticotropin versus hydrocortisone in the intravenous treatment of ulcerative colitis. *Gastroenterology.* 1983; 85:351-357.

[6] Tripathi RC, Kirschner BS, Kipp M, et al. Corticosteroid treatment for inflammatory bowel disease in pediatric patients increases intraocular pressure. *Gastroenterology.* 1992; 102:2164-2165.

[7] Allsop JR, Lee EC. Factors which influenced postoperative complications in patients with ulcerative colitis or Crohn's disease of the colon on corticosteroids. *Gut.* 1978; 19:729-34.

[8] Ismail K, Wessely S. Psychiatric complications of corticosteroid therapy. *Br. J. Hosp. Med.* 1995; 53:495-499.

[9] Vakil N, Sparberg M. Steroid-related osteonecrosis in inflammatory bowel disease. *Gastroenterology.* 1989; 96:62-67.

[10] Stuck A, Minder CE, Frey FJ. Risk of infectious complications in patients taking glucocorticosteroids. *Rev. Infect. Dis.* 1989; 11:954-963.

[11] Greenberg GR, Feagan BG, Martin F, et al. Oral budesonide for active Crohn's disease. The Canadian Inflammatory Bowel Disease Study Group. *N. Engl. J. Med.* 1994: 331(13):836-841.

[12] Hanauer SB, Meyers S. Management of Crohn's disease in adults. *Am. J. Gastroenterol.* 1997; 92(4):559-566.

[13] Baron JH, Connell AM, Kanaghinis TG, et al. Out-patient treatment of ulcerative colitis: comparison between three doses of oral prednisone. *BMJ.* 1962; 2:441-443.

[14] Powell-Tuck J, Brown R, Lennard-Jones JE. A comparison of oral prednisolone as single or multiple daily doses for active proctocolitis. *Scand. J. Gastroenterol.* 1987; 13:833-837.

[15] Hanauer SB. Medical therapy for ulcerative colitis. In: Kirsner JB, editor. Inflammatory bowel disease. 5th edition. Philadelphia: WB Saunders; 2000. P.529-556.

[16] Katz JA. Medical and surgical management of severe colitis. *Semin. Gastrointest. Dis.* 2000; 11:18-32.

[17] Malchow H, Ewe K, Brandes JW, et al. European Cooperative Crohn's Disease Study (ECCDS): results of drug treatment. *Gastroenterology.* 1984; 86(2):249-266.
[18] Truelove SC, Jewell DP. Intensive intravenous regimen for severe attacks of ulcerative colitis. *Lancet.* 1974; 2:1067-1070.
[19] Rosenberg W, Ireland A, Jewell DP. High-dose methylprednisolone in the treatment of active ulcerative colitis. *J. Clin. Gastroenterol.* 1990; 12:40-41.
[20] Valentine JF, Sninsky CA. Prevention and treatment of osteoporosis in patients with inflammatory bowel disease. *Am. J. Gastroenterol.* 1999; 94:878-883.
[21] Cyrus P. Tamboli, MD, FRCPC. Current Medical Therapy for Chronic Inflammatory Bowel Diseases. *Surg. Clin. N. Am.* 87 (2007) 697-725.

Chapter XXVII

Chemical Immunomodulator Therapy in Inflammatory Bowel Disease

Jia-ju Zheng

Su-zhou Institute for Digestive Disease and Nutrition, Su-zhou Municipal Hospital,
Nan-jing Medical University, Su-zhou, Jiang-su Province, P.R. China

Purine analigues azathioprine (AZA) and 6-mercaptopurine (6-MP) are chemically related immunomodulators (table 27-1). AZA is nonenzymatically converted to 6-MP. Their onset of full activity is slow and may take 3 months. 6-MP and AZA are members of the thiopurine class of medications and are commonly used to treat patients with Crohn's disease (CD and ulcerative colitis (UC) who are corticosteroid dependent in an attempt to withdraw corticosteroids and maintain patients in remission off corticosteroids. AZA and 6-MP have also been shown in some studies to reduce clinical and endoscopic postoperative recurrence of CD table 27-2).

Table 27-1. Summary of man immunosuppressive and immunomodulatory agents and their use in IBD

Drug type	Use (CD and UC)	Dosage/toxicity
Purine analogues (6-MP/AZA)	CD: indicated for chonic active disease, particularly in steroid-dependent patients; some efficacy against perianal fistulas. Proven efficacy after medically and surgically induced remissions.UC: use similar to that of CD. Used most commonly for chronic active/recurrent proctitis.	Starting dose (range) 50 mg/day for 6-MP (1.5 mg·kg^{-1}·d^{-1}); 100 mg/day (1-2.5 mg·kg^{-1}·d^{-1}) for AZA. See text for toxicity and monitoring
Methotrexate	CD: effective at 25 mg/wk IM for chronic active disease, including steroid-dependent patients: effective at 15 mg/wk IM in patients responding to the higher dose; uncertain it applies to all patients in remission.UC: evidence for efficacy is established	Dose 15-25 mg/wk IM but full dose/response range not yet defined; toxicity: relatively minor in reported trials, but significant toxicities include hepatic fibrosis, cirrhosis, pneumonitis, gastrointestinal upset, and pancytopenia; teratogenic

Table 27-1. (Continued).

Drug type	Use (CD and UC)	Dosage/toxicity
Mycophenolate	CD: reported to be as effective as azathioprine in an unblended study of steroid-treated chronic moderately active disease; tolerated well and may be an option for patients intolerant of purine analogues and/or methotrexate; long-term efficacy not yet studied; UC:insufficient data to recommend use here	Dose 1.5 $mg \cdot kg^{-1} \cdot day^{-1}$, but dose-response range not studied yet; toxicity is dose related, includes diarrhea, vomiting, leukopenia, and opportunistic infections; teratogenic in animals.
Cyclosporine	CD: conflicting evidence for efficacy, controlled studies failed to confirm efficacy with oral cyclosporine, although uncontrolled studies have claimed efficacy when administered IV; UC:main indication is acute severe colitis unresponsive to steroids as a bridge to other immunosuppressive therapy and/or where surgery is not desirable; long-term (maintenance) not advised because of toxicity	≤ 4 $mg \cdot kg^{-1} \cdot day^{-1}$ IV for acute disease and should be monitored with blood levels; toxicity; renal impairment, neurotoxicity, hepatotoxicity, hypertension, electrolyte imbalance; dosage should also be reduced by about 50% if cholesterol level is low to minimize risk of seizures

Table 27-2. Indications of AZA/6-MP Treatment for IBD [3,4]

disease	AZA	6-MP
1. Crohn's disease		
- Mild to moderate inflammation (steroids refractory)	yes	yes
- Severe inflammation (steroids refractory)	No	No
- Steroids dependent	yes	yes
- Fistula	yes	yes
- Maintenance of remission	yes	yes
2. Ulcerative colitis		
- Mild tomoderate inflammatory (steroids refractory)	?, No	?, No
- Severe inflammation (steroids refractory)	No	No
- Steroids dependent	yes	yes
- Maintenance of remission	yes	yes

Recommendation for AZA or 6-MP Use

When initiating therapy with either 6-MP or AZA, measurement of complete bleed count with differential is advocated at least every other week as long as doses of medications are being adjusted. Thereafter, the measurement of complete blood count with differential should be performed as clinically appropriate at least once every 3 months. Periodic measurement of liver-associated chemistries is also advocated. (Grade C).

Current Food And Drug Administration (FDA) recommendations suggest that individuals should have thiopurine methyltransferase (TPMT) genotype or phenotype assessed before initiation of therapy with AZA or 6-MP in an effort to detect individuals who have low enzyme activity (or who are homozygous deficient in TPMT) in an effort to avert AZA or 6-MP therapy and thus avoid potential adverse events. Individuals who have intermediate or normal TPNT activity (wild type or heterozygotes) need measurement of frequent complete blood counts (as above) in addition to TPMT assessment because these individuals may still develop myelosuppression subsequent to use of AZA or 6-MP. (Grade B).

Long-term treatment with corticosteroids is undesirable. Patients with chronic active corticosteroidependent disease (either CD or UC) should be treated with AZA 2.0-3.0 $mg \cdot kg^{-1} \cdot d^{-1}$ or 6-MP 1.0-1.5 $mg \cdot kg^{-1} \cdot d^{-1}$ in an effort to lower or preferably eliminate corticosteroid use. Infliximab is another option in this situation, as is combination infliximab/antimetabolic therapy. (Grade A).

Individual patients with either CD or UC who experience severe flare of disease requiring corticosteroid treatment or require re-treatment during the year with another course of corticosteroids should be considered for initiation therapy with AZA 2.0-3.0 $mg \cdot kg^{-1} \cdot d^{-1}$ or 6-MP 1.0-1.5 $mg \cdot kg^{-1} \cdot d^{-1}$ in an effort to avoid future corticosteroid use (Grade C). Infliximab is another option in this situation, as is combination infliximab/antimetabolite therapy.

6-MP (and likely AZA) is modestly effective for decreasing postoperative recurrence in CD both endoscopicaly and clinically. Use of this agent should be considered for patients at high risk for postoperative recurrence or in whom postoperative recurrence would have deleterious effects (Grade B).

Some studies have shown AZA 2.0-3.0 $mg \cdot kg^{-1} \cdot d^{-1}$ or 6-MP 1.0-1.5 $mg \cdot kg^{-1} \cdot d^{-1}$ to have some efficacy in treating and healing perianal and enteric fistulae. (Grade C).

Thiopurione metabolite monitoring in the treatment of patients with 6-MP or AZA is useful when attempting to determine medical noncompliance and may be helpful for optimizing dose and monitoring for toxicity (table 27-3). (Grade C).

Table 27-3. Adverse events[1]

Types	AZA (%)	6-MP (%)
1. Allergic reaction (not dose dependent)		
- Pancreatitis	yes NA	yes 3
- Others		
fever	yes NA	yes 2
rash	yes NA	yes NA
arthralgia	yes NA	yes NA
malaise	yes NA	yes NA
nausia	yes NA	yes NA
diarrhea	yes NA	yes NA
2. non-allergic reaction (may be dose dependent)		
mucositis	No	No 1
bone marrow suppression	yes 5.3	yes 2
macrocytosis	yes NA	yes NA
opperturity infection	yes NA	yes NA
hepatitis	yes NA	yes 0.3
malignancies	?, No 3	?, No 3
lymphoma	?, No NA	?, No 1.5

[1]occur at very high dose. [2]may occur from 2 weeks to 11 years after treatment [5,6]. [3]NA: data not available.

AZA 2.0-3.0 mg·kg^{-1}·d^{-1} or 6-MP 1.0-1.5 mg·kg^{-1}·d^{-1} is effective for maintenance of remission in patients with CD regardless of disease distribution. (Grade A).

AZA 2.0-3.0 mg·kg^{-1}·d^{-1} or 6-MP 1.0-1.5 mg·kg^{-1}·d^{-1} is effective for reducing corticosteroid dose in patients with UC regardless of disease distribution (Grade A). These drugs may also be effective in maintaining remission in patients with UC, but data are conflicting and this has not been confirmed by large well-controlled studies.

IBD patients with gastrointestinal intolerance (except for fever, pancreatitis, or hypersensitivity reactions) to AZA may be cautiously tried on 6-MP before being considered for other therapy or surgery (Grade C). Similarly, patients with gastrointestinal intolerance (except for fever, pancreatitis, or hypersensitivity reactions) to 6-MP may be cautiously tried on AZA before being considered for other therapy or surgery (Grade C).

Cyclophosphamide

Cyclophosphamide is a potent suppressor of immune function, at high doses resulting in a sustained decrease in both the number and function of T and B cells. Based on its established efficacy of intravenous cyclophosphamide in systemic vasculitis, and with the positive result of intravenous application of 750 mg cyclophosphamide which induced a rapid clinical improvement in a severely ill women with steroid resistant indeterminate colitis, cyclophosphamide was reported safe and effective in acute steroid refractory IBD patients (treatment with prednisone 50 mg/day or more for at least seven days).

Dosing and method: cyclophosphamide 750 mg (independent of body weight) is given during a 12 hour hospital stay combined with intravenous fluids at a rate known to produce a urine output of 2 ml/kg/h. Mesna (2-mercatoethansulphonic acid, total dose equal to 50% of the dose of cyclophosphamide to prevent hemorrhagic cystitis) is administered in three equal doses, during and after cyclophosphamide treatment, for 12 hours. Follow up white blood cell (WBC) counts with differential is performed on post-cyclophosphamide day 7, 10, 14, and 21 to detect WBC nadir and rebound levels. Each patient received between four and six monthly treatments. A daily regimen of prednisolone is continued and a daily dose of prednisolone is decreased according to individual clinical activity. Azathioprine (2.5 mg·kg^{-1}·d^{-1}) is initiated orally to maintain remission following cyclophosphamide treatment after the onset of remission.

Discussion: The remarkable clinical benefit of intravenous pulse cyclophosphamide therapy has been reported by open label study. This may be a safe and effective treatment in patients with severe IBD unresponsive to steroid treatment and merits evaluation in a controlled trial. Prolonged use of daily cyclophosphamide has been associated with toxic effects such as gonadal dysfunction (approximately 70%), bone marrow suppression, hemorrhagic cystitis (17-34%), and increased risk of neoplasms. Studies have demonstrated that intermittent pulse cyclophosphamide in systemic lupus erythematasus is at least as efficacious as daily therapy while utilizing lower cumulative doses and producing less toxicity.

Methtrexate

Methotrexate has been used in clinical medicine for nearly half a century. This agent induces clinical response more rapid than 6-MP or AZA in patients with IBD. Over the course of the past decade, evidence has shown that methotrexate has an emerging role for the treatment of patients with CD.

Recommendations for Methotrexate Use [1]

Parenteral methotrexate is indicated for induction of remission in patients with active CD. (Grade B).

Parenteral methotrexate is indicated for maintenance of remission in patients with inactive CD. (Grade B).

The currently available evidence supports the use of methotrexate for induction of remission with corticosteroid withdrawal in patients with active CD who are corticosteroid dependent. (Grade B).

Methotrexate maintenance therapy (15-25 mg intramuscularly weekly) is effective for patients whose active CD has responded to intramuscular methotrexate (Grade A).

Methotrexate 25 mg intramuscularly weekly for up to 16 weeks followed by 15 mg intramuscularly weekly is effective in patients with chronic active CD. (Grade A).

Methotrexate is absolutely contraindicated in pregnancy. (Grade B).

The currently available evidence is insufficient to support the use of methotrexate for the induction of maitenance of remission in patients with active UC. (Grade B).

Routine monitoring of laboratory parameters, including complete blood counts and liver-associated laboratory chemistries, is recommended In patients who are treated with methotrexate. (grade C).

Patients with persistently abnormal liver-associated chemistries should either discntinue therapy with methotrexate or undergo liver biopsy. (Grade C).

Cyclosporine

Cyclosporine has a rapid onset of action (more rapid than AZA, 6-MP, or methotrexate) and when administered intravenously has been shown to be efficatice in the management of patients with severe UC. It often demonstrates clinical efficacy wirhin 1 week when administered intravenously. Oral cyclosporing has a possible role in the induction of a clinical response in UC and short term in the maintenance of an intravenous cyclosporine-induced response, allowing time for the slow-acting purine analogues to become effective. Its efficacy in patients with luminal CD has only been shown for higher doses, and the risk of therapy may not warrant its use. Intravenous cyclosporine is effective for the treatment of patients with fistulizing CD; however, toxicity has limited its applicability, and when administered orally, disease often reflares.

Mycophenolate Mofetil

Mycophenolate mofetil inhibits lymphocyte proliferation by selective blocking the synthesis of guanosine nuceotide in T cells. Its use in IBD was first proposed as an alternative immunosuppressive in patients intolerance to AZA or 6-MP. Early enthusiasm over the use of mycophenolate mofetil has been tempered by studies that showed lower efficacy rates and a higher incidence of patient intolerance.

This lack of convincing evidence of efficacy, couipled with concerning safety data, make it difficult to justify the use of mycophenolate mofetil in the treatment of patients with IBD at this time.

Crohn's Disease in Remission

1) 6-MP and AZA are the benchmark drugs for the maintenance of long-term symptomatic remission in Crohn's disease[1,8]. Among Crohn's disease patients in remission for at least 42 months, withdrawal of AZA leads to an 18-month relapse rate of 21% compared with 8% among the group randomized to continue active treatment[1]. However, 6-MP and AZA are not universally effective, require regular toxicity monitoring, and have significant adverse event profile.

2) Immunomodulates: one year prognosis following parenteral cyclosporine A (2 mg/kg or 4 mg/kg dosing, alone or in conjunction with steroids) and maintained on AZA is superior to that of the steroid-treated patients maintained on aminosalicylates (78% vs 37% remission), and has become an acceptable therapy for severe steroid-refractory ulcerative colitis [2,6,7]. However, oral cyclosporine agents have not been widely accepted because of their potential toxicity and requisite evaluation in a controlled setting.

There have been few new data regarding the utility of purine antimetabolites (AZA and 6-MP) for ulcerative colitis [1]. Despite their general acceptance for steroid-dependent ulcerative colitis, there remain limited evidence-based data to support the overall efficacy or to delineate a dose response in ulceratic colitis. The most convincing controled trial to date evaluated the maintenance benefits of AZA for patients who had required AZA to achieve remission: the 12-month relapse rate was 36% for patients maintained on AZA, compared with 59% for patients randomized to placebo. An area of consistency has been the general acceptance that a purine antimetabolite is useful to prolong remission after induction with cyclosporine.

References

[1] Lichtenstein GR, Abreu MT, Cohen R, et al. American gastroenterological association institute medical position statement on corticosteroids, immunomodulators, and inflixinmab in inflammatory bowel disease. *Gastroenterol.* 2006;130(3):935-939; 940-987.

[2] Shanahan F. Inflammatory bowel disease: immunodiagnostics, immunotherapeutics, and ecotherapeutics. *Gastroenterol.* 2001;*120(3)*:622-635.

[3] Sandborn WJ. A review of immune modifier therapy for inflammatory bowel disease: azathioprine, 6-mercaptopurine, cyclosporine and methotrexate. *Am. J. Gastroenterol.* 1996;91(3):423-433.

[4] Hanauer S. Medical therapy of ulcerative colitis. In: Kirsner JB (ed). Inflammatory Bowel disease. W.B. Saunders Company. Philadelphia, London, New York. St. Louis. Syd. 2000;P.529-556.

[5] Su A, Lichtenstein GR. Treatment of inflammatory bowel disease with azathioprine and 6-mercaptopurine. *Gastroenterol. Clin. N. Am.* 2004;33(2):209-304.

[6] Zheng J-j. Pharmacology and clinical application of purine analogues in inflammatory bowel disease. *Chin. J. Gastroenterol.* 2003; 8 (4): 253-255 (Chinese).

[7] Zheng J-j, Chu X-q, Shi X-h, et al. Efficacy and safety of azathioprine maintenance therapy in patients with Crohn's disease. *J Dig Dis* 2008;9(2):84-88.

[8] Zheng J-j. Cyclopharninde treatment for steroid refractory inflammatory bowel disease. *Chin. J. Gastroenterol.* 2004;9(4):254 (Chinese).

[9] Stallmach A, Witting BM, Moser C, et al. Safety and efficacy of intravenous pulse cyclophosphamide in acute steroid refractory inflammatory bowel disease. *Gut.* 2003;52:377-382.

In: Inflammatory Conditions of the Colon
Editor: Jia-ju Zheng

ISBN: 978-1-60692-240-8
© 2008 Nova Science Publishers, Inc.

Chapter XXVIII

Topical (Rectal) Therapy in Inflammatory Bowel Disease

Ming Zhang
Drum Tower Hospital Affiliated, Nan-jing University Medical School, Nan-jing, 210008, Jiang-su Province, P.R. China

As inflammatory bowel disease (IBD) primarily represents a local inflammation of the luminal mucosa, in addition to systemic administration of anti-inflammatory drugs for the treatment of IBD, topical (intra-rectal) agents have been widely used as an important component of medical therapy for IBD [1,2].Topical treatment targets directly to the affected areas, active drug concentrations in the mucosa can be achieved and systemic adverse effects limited. Studies have shown that there is a significant inverse correlation between the drug concentrations in the mucosa and the clinical outcome of IBD [3-5]. Topical treatments are effective for most left side colitis, even when used intermittently [6]. However, topical treatment is often thought to be uncomfortable and some patients with active disease have trouble in retaining enemas and suppositories. Thus patients' preference becomes even more important when considering long-term treatment.

There is a large choice of topical treatments with suppositories, foams, gels and liquid enemas. The choice depends largely on disease extent, ability to retain the preparations, patient preference, disease severity, previous responsiveness to therapies, profile of adverse effect and economic considerations. Liquid enemas can reach as far as the splenic flexure, foam and gel enemas typically do not reach above the sigmoid colon, and suppositories can only act on the rectum and distal sigmoid [6].Suppositories are best retained and can be accepted by most patients. Retention of foam and gel tends to be better than liquid enemas [7].

Ulcerative Colitis (UC)

The principal aims of medical therapy for UC patients are to induce remission and to maintain remission, and the most used agents to treat an acute exacerbation of colitis are 5-aminosalicylates (5-ASA) and steroids. Both the agents are available in a variety of forms, such as oral preparations, liquid and foam enemas, suppositories and gels.

The primary advantage of topical 5-ASAs in the treatment of UC is the active agents direct to inflamed mucosa, achieving up to 100 times higher mucosal concentrations of 5-ASAs and correspondingly higher efficacy with less risk of systemic side-effects than oral treatment [8]. Clinical trials and meta-analyses indicated that rectally delivered 5-ASA is more effective than oral 5-ASA and that combination of the two further improves efficacy and speed of improvement in patients with distal colitis [6,9,10]. Some recent evidence suggests that even those with extensive disease may benefit from mesalazine enemas [11].

The dose of mesalamine enema varies from 1 to 4 g/d, but in contrast to the dose response with the oral 5-ASA agents, there is no proven benefit of topical doses greater than 1 g/d [2,3]. Rectal formulations are superior to oral medications for the treatment of distal colitis and proctitis with remission rates of 76% versus 46% for oral mesalamine.

Liquid enemas distributed 5-AS within 0.5 to 2 h from the rectum and sigma up to the transverse colon and partly even to the ascending colon. During steady state urinary recovery of 5-AS indicated an absorption of approximately 25%. The volume of the enemas affected the spread: with 100-ml enemas, a better and more consistent distribution was seen than with 30- or 60-ml enemas [12].

The combination of oral and topical 5-ASA agents is superior to either alone, and one study reported an 89% remission rate for combination therapy [13,14].Topical mesalamine is effective for the maintenance of remission of distal colitis. Ultimately the dose may be reduced to an alternate-night or alternate-week schedule, which improves patient compliance without reducing efficacy.

Topical steroids have a definite role in the treatment of distal UC and have been introduced into the treatment of severe colitis as an adjunct to parenteral steroids. Studies have shown that topical steroids administered rectally are effective in the treatment of distal colitis, and can be used as adjunctive therapy in pancolitis [13,14]. Preparations are available in the form of suppository, foam, or enema. Budesonide and beclomethasone diproprionate have been the most extensively studied. Topical steroids available are shown in table 28-1.

In studies evaluating the efficacy of corticosteroid enemas, 60% of patients with distal colitis treated with topical hydrocortisone (80 to 100 mg), prednisolone (20 to 40 mg), or betamathasone (5 to 20 mg) showed an improvement [1,2]. Hydrocortisone enemas and foams are effective for active distal colitis, however have not been proved effective for maintain remission. Although the topically applied corticosteroids have less systemic absorption than the oral formulations, there is still the potential for adrenal suppression and associated side effects.

Prednisolone metasulfobenzoate, tixocortol pivalate, beclomethasone diproprionate, and budesonide are rapidly metabolized corticosteroid enemas that have been evaluated for the treatment of distal colitis [1,2]. Budesonide enema (2 mg) has the potency of high first pass metabolisation and show little systematic side effects. When administered 2 mg per day for 8 weeks, budesonide enema controlled active colitis in a similar percentage of patients as prednisolone enema (36% versus 47%) with fewer corticosteroid-like side effects.

The efficacy of topical 5-ASA has been compared with that of topical steroids. Several meta-analyses have pooled half century original data and have found 5-ASA to have efficacy superior to corticosteroid treatment [15,16]. Various end points, including clinical, endoscopic and histological features, were taken into account 5-ASA yielded consistently better results. Even though different dosages of 5-ASA used (from 1 to 4 g daily) and the various different steroids employed, most expert commentary remains convinced that 5-ASA preparations are superior, which in conjunction with avoidance of steroid-related side effects.

Table 28-1. Topical steroids[4]

Agents	Comments	Recommended dosage
Conventional agents		
Hydrocortisone	Significant side effects after long-term use	100-125 mg Q.d (suppository, enema).
Prednisolone		20-40 mg Q.d (suppository, enema).
Betamethasone		5mg Q.d. (enema)
Newly developed agents		
Hydrocortisone[1]	Poor intestinal absorption with reduced systemic side effects,	80 mg Q.d (suppository, foam).
Prednisolone-metasulfobenzoate		20 mg Q.d (enema)
Beclomethasone	Rapid hepatic first-pass effect	0.5-3 mg Q.d (enema).
Tixocortol pivalate		250 mg Q.d (enema)
Budesonide[2]	Very rapid hepatic first-pass, nearly no systemic side effects	2 mg Q.d (enema).

[1] equal efficacy to hydrocortisone enema[4].

Crohn's Disease (CD)

Although Crohn's disease is usually not involved in rectum (rectal sparing), topical preparations can be used as an adjunctive therapy in colonic CD (especially with an involvement of distal colon). Unlike UC, data derived from clinical trials of mesalazine in CD do not show clear evidence of efficacy.

Other Topical Agents

5-AS and glucocorticosteroids (e.g. budesonide) represent standard topical treatments in IBD. Any new therapeutic principle, which might be primarily developed for systemic action, should be regarded also as a candidate for topical delivery [17]. Some other agents, such as short-chain fatty acids (e.g. nbutyrate), local anaesthetics, bismuth compounds, nicotine, nitric oxide donor glyceryl trinitrate, sucralfate or enemas of immunoglobulin G, interleukin-

10 and epidermal growth factor (EGF) also can be used topically. However, so far the very limited clinical experience with all these agents is not encouraging.

References

[1] Lichtenstein GR. Infliximab maintenance treatment reduces hospitalizations, surgeries, and procedures in fistulizing Crohn's disease . *Gastroenterol.* 2005; 128(4):862-869.

[2] Travis SPL, Stang EF, Lémann M, et al. European evidence based consensus on the diagnosis and management of Crohn's disease: current management. *Gut.* 2006; 55(supple. 1):i16-i35.

[3] G. Frieri, M.T. Pimpo, A. Andreoli, et al. Prevention of postoperative recurrence of Crohn's isease requires adequate mucosal concentrations of mesalazine, *Aliment. Pharmacol. Ther.* 13 (1999) 557-582.

[4] G. Frieri, G. Giacomelli, M. Pimpo, et al. Mucosal 5-aminosalicylic acid concentrations inversely correlates with severity of colonic inflammation in patients with ulcerative colitis, *Gut.* 47 (2000) 410- 414.

[5] M. Naganuma, Y. Iwao, H. Ogata, et al. Measurement of colonic mucosal concentrations of 5-aminosalicylic acid is useful for estimating its therapeutic efficacy in distal ulcerative colitis: comparison of orally administered mesalamine and sulfasalazine, Inflamm. *Bowel Dis.* 7 (2001) 221- 225.

[6] Regueiro M, Loftus EV Jr, Steinhart AH, et al. Medical management of left-sided ulcerative colitis and ulcerative proctitis: critical evaluation of therapeutic trials. *Inflamm. Bowel Dis.* 2006; 12:979-94.

[7] Campieri M, Paoluzi P, D'Albasio G, et al. Better quality of therapy with 5-ASA colonic foam in active ulcerative colitis. A multicentre comparative trial with 5-ASA enema. *Dig. Dis. Sci.* 1993; 38:1843-50.

[8] Frieri G, Pimpo MT, Palumbo GC, et al. Rectal and colonic mesalazine concentration in ulcerative colitis: oral vs. oral plus topical treatment. *Aliment Pharmacol. Ther.* 1999; 13: 1413-7.

[9] Cohen RD, Woseth DM, Thisted RA, et al. A meta-analysis and overview of the literature on treatment options for left-sided ulcerative colitis and ulcerative proctitis. *Am. J. Gastroenterol.* 2000; 95: 1263-76.

[10] Marshall JK, Irvine EJ. Rectal aminosalicylate therapy for distal ulcerative colitis: a meta-analysis. *Aliment Pharmacol. Ther.* 1995; 9: 293-300.

[11] Marteau P, Probert CS, Lindgren S, et al. Combined oral and enema treatment with Pentasa (mesalazine) is superior to oral therapy alone in patients with extensive mild/moderate active ulcerative colitis: a randomised, double blind, placebo controlled study. *Gut.* 2005; 54: 960-5.

[12] M. Schwab, U. Klotz, Pharmacokinetic considerations in the treatment of inflammatory bowel disease, *Clin. Pharmacokinet.* 40 (2001) 723-751.

[13] Marteau P, Probert CS, Lindgren S, et al. Combined oral and enema treatment with Pentasa (mesalazine) is superior to oral therapy alone in patients with extensive

mild/moderate active ulcerative colitis: a randomised, double blind, placebo controlled study. *Gut.* 2005; 54(7):960-65.

[14] Hanauer SB, Kane S. The pharmacology of antiminflammatory drugs in inflammatory bowel disease. In: Kirsner JB (ed.) Inflammatory bowel disease (5th ed.) W.B. Saunders Company Philadelphia London New York St. Louis Syd, 2000,P.510-528.

[15] Marshall JK, Irvine EJ. Rectal corticosteroids versus alternative treatments in ulcerative colitis: a meta-analysis. *Gut.* 1997; 40:775–81.

[16] Cohen RD, Wosworth DM, Thisted RA, et al. A meta-analysis and overview of the literature on treatment for left sided colitis and ulcerative proctitis. *Am. J. Gastroenterol.* 2000; 95:1263–76.

[17] Mutlu EA, Farhadi A, Keshavarazian A, New developments in the treatment of inflammatory bowel disease, *Expert Opin. Investig. Drugs.* 11 (2002) 365–385.

Chapter XXIX

Nutritional Therapy in Inflammatory Bowel Therapy

Xue-liang Jiang
General Hospital of Ji-nan Command Area of Chinese PLA,
Shan-dong Province, P.R. China

Nutritional disturbances are commonly seen in inflammatory bowel diseases (IBD), which may lead to anemia, low serum albumin, weight loss, vitamin and trace element deficits and delay disease amelioration. Appropriate nutritional management plays an important role in IBD treatment. It may relieve symptoms, improve general conditions, elevate anabolism, and promote immune function. Enteral nutrition (EN) and total parenteral nutrition (TPN) can be used according to patient's situation.

Causes of Malnutrition in Inflammatory Bowel Disease

1. Reduced or imbalance of dietary intake: Reduction of dietary intake results from the fear of abdominal pain or diarrhea. In some patients, they would avoid or reduce their food intake such as milk, cheese, fish and fresh vegetable during active phases; imposed dietary restrictions result in imbalance of dietary intake [1].
2. Malabsorption: It is mainly because of reduced secretion of digestive juice, and dyspepsia due to intestinal mucosa injury, low absorption capacity result from extensive and severe intestinal disease as well as short bowel syndrome after resection surgery [2].
3. Increased intestinal loss: It is one of the important factors involved in the development of malnutrition in IBD. Severe inflammatory, diarrhea, pus and blood in the stool and excessive digestive excretion lead to loss of protein, water, electrolytes, vitamins and minerals [3].

4. Increased needs: IBD patients need more nutrition because of fever, inflammatory injuries and cellular restoration while it plays little roles comparably in malnutrition.
5. Side effects of medication: Some nutritional deficits can also be caused or amplified by the use of drugs, such as sulfasalazine (which may cause deficit of folates), corticosteroids (which may impair absorption of calcium and induce negative nitrogen balance), cholestyramine(which may decrease fat and lipid-soluble vitamins absorption),and antibiotic(which can cause deficit of vitamin K) etc[4].

The above mentioned factors which may contribute to malnutrition in patients with IBD can be summarized in table 29-1.

Table 29-1. Factors contributing to malnutrition in IBD

mechanisms	causes
reduced dietary intake	1. anorexia, postprandial pain and diarrhea 2. on restricted diets
malabsorption	1. diffuse small intestinal mucosal disease ↓ inadequate mucosal surface for nutrient digestion and absorption 2. medications ↓ adversely affect nutrient absorption
excessive secretion and intestinal loss of nutrients	1. active intestinal inflammation ↓ protein losing enteropathy 2. gastrointestinal bleeding
increased nutrient requirements	1. infectious complications 2. Fever ↓ increased metabolic rates

Total Parenteral Nutrition (TPN)

TPN provides nutritional requirements through parenteral route. TPN can provide enough nutritional requirements without enteral nutrition, correct malnutrition, and maintain basically normal nutritional status in many of IBD patients. In the TPN formula, hyperosmotic glucose, compound amino acid, lipoid, metals, vitamins and trace elements are included [5,6,7].

1. Aim

1).Used in active and severe IBD patients to make bowel rest;
2).As an adjuvant therapy in condition of intestinal obstruction and fistula;
3).Correct imbalanced nutritional status and improve growth;

4)Fulfill postoperative nutritional requirements and reduce postoperative mortality and complication;

5)Maintain nutritional status in extensive and severe intestinal disease or short bowel disease [8].

2. Indication

1).Patients who are intolerant oral nutrition due to intestinal obstruction or fistula, and acute, severe exacerbation,or bowel rest is necessary after operation;

2).Other cases are whose nutrition is insufficient provided only through oral or enteral nutrition, and those bear concurrent malnutrition pre- or post- operation [8] .

3. Administration

1).Nutritional assessment: based on weight loss, sustained inadequate food intake, the history of gastrointestinal symptoms, and poor functional status, coupled with a physical examination focused on the identification of muscle wasting, fat loss and edema.

2).Calculation of nutrition requirement Glucose and lipid mainly provide calories, and with amino acid to maintain weight and nitrogen balance. Adequate estimates of calories: 104.6 kJ/kg/day, nitrogen: 0.15 $g \cdot kg^{-1} \cdot d^{-1}$. In medium stress condition: calories167.4-209.2 $kJ \cdot kg^{-1} \cdot d^{-1}$, nitrogen>0.4 $g \cdot kg^{-1} \cdot d^{-1}$. Caloric : nitrogen equals 627.6~753.1 kJ : 1.0g nitrogen. Glucose should provide caloric calories, lipid 20%~25%, but should not over 30%. Total calories and nitrogen an individual needs is calculated out based on the mentioned method, then each element quantity can be decided. Water and electrolyte, vitamin, trace element needs are essential and require attention to individual needs, insulin also should be provided in special condition.

3).Transfusion Central venous catheterization makes central venous pressure estimable and hyperosmotic glucose transfusion practicable, the catheter can be reserved for more than 30-60 days. For those long-term venous nutrition cases, catheter in silica gel stuff is recommended, then catheter in polyethylene or polyflon. Catheterization is commonly used with percutaneous centesis in supraclavian, or subclavianvein, etc.

4).Technical requirements ①Fluid transfused in uniform velocity in 24 hours to avoid the quantity of water, glucose, amino acid, vitamins and trace element provides surpass metabolic ability of patient; ②For long-term use of TPN, serum trace element levels should pay careful attention in order to avoid trace element deficiency; ③Nutritional solution is given and increased gradually until to the level that patient can tolerate (e.g. 2 000~2 500 ml/d), which equal to provide water 30 ml/kg. Water supply can be calculated as 418 kJ: 100 ml; ④Water volume should be no less than 2000ml/day, adequate electrolyte supplement also needed.

4. Notice

1). TPN solutions should be prepared in sterile circumstance, and;

2). Transfusion style should be appropriately selected: solution with amino acid- high concentrate glucose-lipoid formula should be transfused through central vein, while amino acid- modest or low concentrate glucose-lipoid formula can be transfused through either central or peripheral veins;

3). Monitor periodically the changes of blood biochemistry such as serum K^+, Na^+, Cl^-, Ca^{2+}, P, Mg^{2+}, serum albumin, liver enzymes, kidney function, blood cell counts, and urea ketobodies and glucose by which to adjust ingredient in nutritional solution;

4). Attach importance to explanation to patients, especially to home TPN [9].

5. Complications and Prevention

1). Standardized procedures in central venous catheterization can remarkably decrease complication such as aerothorax, hemothorax, air embolism and thrombosis.

2). Infection management : insist strictly sterilized catheter insertion and dressing replacement, occasionally drug given and blood sample through the catheter should not be allowed.

3). To avoid hyperglycosemia, control the transfusion speed and time of hypertonic glucose, and decrease the glucose concentration, transfusion speed to avoid hypoglycemia or transfuse isoosmotic glucose for at least 6 hours before stop TPN. Test serum glucose level during TPN, if serum glucose concentration reaches to 33.3-38.9mmol/L, hyperosmolar nonketotic diabetic coma would occur.

4). Choose appropriate type of amino acid, it is recommended to select amino acid acetous salts and free amino acid, amino acid may lead to hyperchloremia while free amino acid easily lead to hyperammonemia.

5). Prevent nutritional element deficiency, such as trace element and vitamins and supply them timely and adequately.

6). Long-term TPN can induce gastrointestinal mucosa atrophy, bacterial translocation, and macrophage dysfunction, patients should be encouraged to use EN provided it is allowed based on symptom [10,11].

Total Enteral Nutrition (TEN)

EN comprises delivery of nutrients to the gastrointestinal tract through different liquid formulas administered directly by nasal or oral tube, or by enteral tube via percutaneous tubing with gastrostomies / jejunostomies [2,9,10,12].

1. Aim and clinical value Advantages are lower costs, easy administration, lower complication rates; elemental diets can be absorbed by the proximal jejunum, keeping the distal small bowel and colon at relative rest; prevent mucosa atrophy which frequently occurred during TPN, keeping integrity of intestinal mucosa and function.

2. Indication

1). Mild IBD

2). Be selected to supply nutrient after remission of severe IBD by using TPN.

3). Correct nutritional deficits by oral diets, and when the patient can tolerate, TEN is the first choice in nutritional support method.

3. Contraindications Multiple intestinal perforation; high site intestinal fistula, mechanic intestinal obstruction; extensive intestinal surgical resection. For these cases, TEN is recommended after 4-6 week TPN.

4. Formula and preparation method

1). There are variety of market diets, include non-element diets and element diets. Element diet is a kind of powder made up of variety of nutritional elements which change into liquid in suspension when added water, or liquid in suspension free of infection during preparation. Powder and fatty liquid can be packaged separately. With little residuum, element diet can be totally absorbed in the upper intestine without gastrointestinal digestion, or only with mildly water solution. As the resource of nitrogen in element diet, amino acid can also induce diarrhea. The formula and preparation method of element should be ascertained before using. Take optimum dosage based on the concentration, add water to adequate volume and blend fully. Element diets should be prepared freshly and stored in 0-4 centigrade and no longer than 24 hours.

2). Delivery method Element diets can be taken orally or delivered to the gastrointestinal tract by nasal, oral or enteral tubes, or via gastrostomies / jejunostomies. Dosage can be given once or drip continuously. Clinically continuous drip element diets firstly are isoosmotic (10%) and dripped slowly (40~60 ml/h), daily concentration increase is 5% until daily nutrition is enough and patients can tolerate.

3). Notice ①Sterilized preparation and resolved with sterilized water, ②Continuous drip container should be replaced 8 hours, and drip tubes, 24 hours, ③Add potassium triphosphate in to the prepared solution to the concentration 0.036% per Liter to inhibit intestinal bacteria growth.

5. Complication and management

Complication in IBD cases nourished by tubes may be induced by (1)EN tube insertion problems: if the tubes is wrongly inserted into the trachea, aerothorax, pneumonia, pulmonary abscess may occur, improper tubes insertion may injure mucosa of nose, throat, esophagus; (2)Gastrointestinal factor : such as nausea, vomit, diarrhea, if it happens, adjust drip speed or concentration; (3)metabolic factors : such as hyperglycemia, hypoglycemia, kalemia, hypokalemia, it is important to test the nutritional and metabolic changes regularly.

Clinical Strategy of Nutritional Therapy

For both TEN and TPN, one of the major aims is to let the injured bowel to be rest, to promote inflammation remission, and lead to a relief of symptoms during nutrition supplement. Which method should be selected, or whether combine both of them in nutritional treatment for IBD patients are based on the severity of disease. Though TPN gains more advantages, cases should be selected strictly because of the manifest complications. TEN is the first choice if oral taken nutrition catches the need of patient, and if not, partially parental nutrition should be considered. TPN can induce disease remission but it should be reserved for patients for whom enteral feeding is impossible, and if permitted, TPN should be transferred to TEN gradually as soon as possible.

The change should be gradually. If the bowel burden is suddenly increased, it will retard disease remission. The transition from TPN to TEN consists four phase to follow: ①Combined use of TPN and TEN; ②TEN (tube feeding only); ③Tube feeding combined with oral feeding, and finally ④normal oral diet [13-17].

TPN has been proved a valuable therapy in CD treatment, including obtaining an obvious symptomatic remission in cases that they showed little response to regular drug therapies [3,18]. However, the relapse rate is similarly high. There is no evidence that nutritional treatment receives a consistence efficacy of remission in patients with colitis, TPN has no significant difference in treating CD compare to treatment with oral drugs. Moreover, TPN therapy has higher cost and more complication.

References

[1] Zvirbliene A, Kiudelis G, Zalinkvicius R, et al. Dietary characteristics of patients with inflammatory bowel diseases. *Medicina. (Kaunas).* 2006; 42(11):895-9.

[2] Jiang X-l. Nutritional Therapy. In: Jiang X-l, Cui H-f (eds.) Ulcerative colitis (1st ed) Bei-jing, China Medical and Pharmacological Science and Technology Press. 2004; 275-296 (Chinese).

[3] Campos FG, Waitzberg DL, Teixeira MG, et al Inflammatory bowel diseases: principles of nutritional therapy. 2002; *Rev. Hosp. Clin. Fac. Med. Sao Paulo.* 57(4):187-198

[4] Gassull MA. Review article: the role of nutrition in the treatment of inflammatory bowel disease. *Aliment Pharmacol. Ther.* 2004; 20 Suppl 4:79-83.

[5] Konno M, Kobayashi A, Tomomasa T, et al. Guidelines for the treatment of Crohn's disease in children by the Working Group of the Japanese Society for Pediatric Gastroenterology, Hepatology and Nutrition, Pediatr Int. 2006; 48(3):349-52.

[6] Porter L, Reynolds N, Ellis JD. Total parenteral nutrition, vitamin E, and reversible macular dysfunction morphologically mimicking age related macular degeneration. *Br. J. Ophthalmol.* 2005; 89(11):1531-2

[7] Stein J. Nutrition and dietary treatment of chronic inflammatory bowel disease. *MMW Fortschr. Med.* 2004; 146(14):31-4.

[8] O'Sullivan M, O'Morain C. Nutritional Therapy in Inflammatory Bowel Disease. *Curr. Treat Options Gastroenterol.* 2004; 7(3):191-198.

[9] Jeejeebhoy KN. Total parenteral nutrition: potion or poison? *Am. J. Clin. Nutr.* 2001; 74(2):160-3.

[10] O'Sullivan M, O'Morain C. Nutritional treatments in inflammatory bowel disease. *Curr. Treat. Options Gastroenterol.* 2001; 4(3):207-213

[11] Cashman KD. Altered bone metabolism in inflammatory disease: role for nutrition. *Proc. Nutr. Soc.* 2008; 67(2):196-205.

[12] Griffiths AM. Enteral nutrition in the managment of Crohn's disease. *JREN J. Parenter Enteral. Nutr.* 2005; 29(4 Suppl):S108-12.

[13] Wild GE, Drozdowski L, Tartaglia C, et al. Nutritional modulation of the inflammatory response in inflammatory bowel disease--from the molecular to the integrative to the clinical. *World J. Gastroenterol.* 2007; 7; 13(1):1-7.

[14] Semrin G, Fishman DS, Bousvaros A, et al. Impaired intestinal iron absorption in Crohn's disease correlates with disease activity and markers of inflammation. *Inflamm. Bowel. Dis.* 2006; 12(12):1101-6.

[15] Esaki M, Matsumoto T, Nakamura S, et al, Factors affecting recurrence in patients with Crohn's disease under nutritional therapy. *Dis. Colon. Rectum.* 2006; 49(Suppl. 10):S68-74.

[16] Sido B, Seel C, Hochlehnert A, et al, Low intestinal glutamine level and low glutaminase activity in Crohn's disease: a rational for glutamine supplementation? *Dig. Dis. Sci.* 2006; 51(12):2170-9.

[17] Macdonald A. Omega-3 fatty acids as adjunctive therapy in Crohns disease. *Gastroenterol. Nurs.* 2006; 29(4):295-301.

[18] Zheng J-j. Treatment of Crohn's disease with combination of TPN and other medications – case study. *Parent Enter. Nutrit.* 2007; 14(5):317-318 (Chinese).

In: Inflammatory Conditions of the Colon
Editor: Jia-ju Zheng

ISBN: 978-1-60692-240-8
© 2008 Nova Science Publishers, Inc.

Chapter XXX

Treatment of Inflammatory Bowel Disease with Traditional Chinese Medicine

Jia-ju Zheng

Su-zhou Institute for Digestive Disease and Nutrition, Su-zhou Municipal Hospital,
Nan-jing Medical University, Su-zhou, Jiang-su Province, P.R. China

Traditional Chinese medicine (TCM) has been widely used as a fundamental medical therapy with an age-old history in China [1]. TCM also can be employed as a primary or an adjunctive therapy for inflammatory bowel disease (IBD). TCM has been reported effective in induction and maintenance of remission of IBD. One of the distinguished features of TCM therapy is relatively less adverse events occurred in practice (some herbs may be toxic to a certain extent, and should be used cautiously).

Causes and Mechanisms of IBD in TCM Theory

The main symptoms of ulcerative colitis (UC) include bloody diarrhea with mucus, abdominal pain, and tenesmus in most patients. According to TCM theories, these symptoms are caused by unclean foods or emotional factors such as excessive joy, anger, melancholy, anxiety and fear, etc.; they belong to "dampness" and "heat" in TCM theories [1]. The dampness and heat, after gathering and brewing, are accumulated in the body in particular in the "Zang and Fu" (internal organs and hollow viscera) of "the Spleen and Stomach, and the Bowel", and at last insufficiencies of the function of "Zang and Fu" occur when the patient's vital function (called Yang) and energy (called Ying) are severely impaired following a long course of disease.

TCM Principles for Diagnosis and Treatment of IBD

Based on a comprehensive review and analysis of symptoms and signs, including the four diagnostic methods of "Wàng" (inspection of patient's general condition and his or her fur of the tongue), "Wèn" (taking medical history), "Wén" (smell special ordors associated with specific diseases) and "Qiē" (palpation of the pulse) [1], a TCM diagnosis of IBD can be established and classified as followings:

1. Dampness and heat stagnancy and lingering inside of the "Zang and Fu" of the Spleen and Stomach, and the Bowel;
2. Disharmony of the functions of the "Zang and Fu" of "the Liver and Stomach";
3. Dysfunction and energy deficiency (Yin) of the "Zang" of "the Spleen and Kidney".

Treatment with Decoctions

The basic therapeutic strategy is to "remove evil heat and resolve dampness" with febrifuges and detoxifying herbs, or "warm the Kidney to cure diarrhea" in different stages of the disease [1].

The principal method of treatment with TCM for IBD is to prescribe pills, powders, soft extract (electuary), and decoctions (made of predominantly herbs, insects and/or ore powder; they are detoxified or with low-toxicity) according to TCM theories [1]. It is based on an overall analysis and consideration of symptoms and signs, including the possible cause, mechanism, location of the illness and patients' condition (called "differentiation of symptom-complexes").

Composition of the Basic Decoction

In our practice, the basic decoction contains Pilose Asiabell Root (Radix Codonopsis Pilosulae), White Atractylodes Rhizome (Rhizoma Atractylodis Macrcephalae), White Peony Root (Radix Paeoniae Alba), Evodia Fruit (Fructus Evodiae) Psoralea Fruit (Fructus Psoraleae), Nutmeg (Semen Myristicae), Coptis Root (Rhizoma Coptidis), Chinese Angelica Root (Radix Angelicae Sinensis), Pulsatilla Root (Radix Pulsatillae), etc. For individual patients with UC, the basic prescription of decoction can be modified with addition, or subtraction with other herbs depending on individual symptom-complexes of the patients.

Other Forms of TCM Therapies

Various forms of TCM therapy or TCM preparations are applied to treat UC. Fox example, Xi-lei powder for enema (contains Margarita Pearls, berberine and other herbs) [2],

Kuijie decoction (contains Radix codonopsis Pilosulae and other twelve herbs) [3], compound glycerhizin for injection [4], compound injection of Radix Salviae Miltiorrhizae [51], and Radix Angelicae Sinensis injection [6], etc. have been shown effective and useful in improving clinical symptoms or mucosal lesions in UC patients.

In addition, acupuncture and moxibustion are used to treat UC patients with symptoms of bloody diarrhea or abdominal pain. Various degrees of symptomatic improvement are reported. TCM is also indicated for extraintestinal complications including the skin lesions of Pyoderma gangrenosum etc. [7]. Further studies with randomization and controlled design are warranted in order to exactly clarify efficacy and mechanisms of TCM therapies in IBD.

It has been reported that patients with Crohn's disease (CD) may respond to TCM therapy with similar efficacy to UC patients.

TCM Effects and Mechanisms in Animal Model Studies

The reported therapeutic effects and possible mechanisms of TCM in IBD have been investigated with promising and encouraging results in a number of animal model studies [8-14]. Either male SD rats [7,8], male BALB/C mice [9], or SIL/J murine [10] have been successfully employed as animal model of experimental colitis. They were induced by dextran sulfate sodium (DSS) or oxazolone for clinicopathologic or pharmacological studies. For example the therapeutic effects of two Chinese herb extracts with potentially immunomodulatory effects, oxymatrine (OM) [8] and multi-glycosidorum triptery (MGT) [10], have been studied in these animal colitis models, and the results showed that serum levels of tumor necrosis factor (TNF)-α, interleukin (IL)-6 and expression of nuclear factor (NF)κB and intercellular adhesion molecule-1 (ICAM-1) in colonic mucosa in DSS-induced rat colitis model were significantly reduced by OM treatment [8], while IL-4 production of murine splenocytes in oxazolone-induced murine colitis model was remarkably inhibited by MGT treatment.

In a rat experimental colitis study, not only the disease activity index (DAI) of colitis was decreased, but also mucosal levels and expression of TNF-2α, IL-26 and prostaglandin (PG)-E2 were inhibited by administration of Pulsatilla root (Radix Pulsatillae) [6]. Either TNBS (trinitrobenzene sulfonic acid) or DSS-induced colitis was also improved with stomach perfusion of Ginkgo biloda extract (EGB) solution. EGB lowered serum level of TNF-a and IL-6, and inhibited TNF-α-induced reactive oxygen species generation, NF-κB and IL-6 protein and mRNA expression in colonic mucosa[13,14]. The herb for invigorating blood circulation and eliminating blood-stasis, Ligusticum Wallichii Franch (Chun-xiong Rhizoma) increased apoptosis rate of lamina propria mononuclear cells (LPMC) and attenuated mucosal damage in rat colitis model [15]. Curcumin, an anti-inflammatory herb showed therapeutic effects on trinitrobenzene sulphonic acid (TNBS)-induced colitis in rats, and the mechanisms of actrvating peroxisome proliferators - activated receptor (PPAR)-γ, regulating the balance of Th1/Th2 in colonic mucosa and inhibiting expression of cyclooxygenase-α (cox-2) were suggested [16-18]. In another animal study, tripterine (0.5 mg·kg^{-1}·d^{-1}) significantly improves TNBS-induced rat colitis macroscopically and microscopically when compared to normal control groups. Tripterine inhibits expression of nuclear factor (NF)-κB P65, IL-1β and TNF-α mRNA in inflamed mucosa [19].

Obviously, the improving effects of TCM on IBD were shown in IBD patients and experimental colitis models. However, studies focusing on enhancing their efficacy and primary mechanisms are warranted.

References

[1] Sun X-x. Treatment of ulcerative colitis with Xi-lei powder and berberine mixture solution for enema. *Chin. J. Dig.* 1987; 7(3):169 (Chinese).

[2] Chen C-h. Clinical study of KuiJie decoction in treatment of non-specific ulcerative colitis. *Chin. J. Coloproctol.* 2004; 24(7):23-25 (Chinese).

[3] Chang T-m, Han Y and Zhang C-x. Therapeutic effect of compound Glycyrrhizin on ulcerative colitis. *Chin. Pharmac.* 2004; 15(9):559-560 (Chinese).

[4] Zhang L-f and Liu J-z. Influence of compound injection of Radix Salviae Miltiorrhizae on platelet function. *Chin. J. Dig.* 2002; 22(6):383-384 (Chinese).

[5] Liu H, Huang Z-m, Liu S-p, et al. Influence of Radix Angelicae Sinensis injection on function of platlet in patients with ulcerative colitis. *Chin. J. Coloproctol.* 2004; 24(7):9-11 (Chinese).

[6] Zhang W-y, Han S-x, Yang H. Study on the activity of intestinal mucosal mast cells in rats with dextran sulfate sodium induced colitis. *Chin. J. Dig. Endosc.* 2004; 21(6):385-387 (Chinese).

[7] Zheng J-j. Treatment of Pyoderma gangrenosum complicated with ulcerative colitis with Sanguis Draconis and Steroids. *Chin. J. Dig. Endosc.* 2008; 25(5):273-274 (Chinese).

[8] Zheng P, Niu F-l, Liu W-z, et al. Study of the effects of Palsatilla Root on the anti-inflammatory mechanism of oxymatrine in dextran sulfate sodium induced colitis of rats. *Chin. J. Dig.* 2003; 23(4):207-210 (Chinese).

[9] Hu R-w, Ouyang Q, Chen D-y. Establishment of dextran sodium sulfate-induced mice ulcerative colitis. *Chin. J. Gastroenterol.* 2002; 7(6):331-334 (Chinese).

[10] Han Y, Chen G, Song Y-x, et al. Multiglycosidorum triptery suppresses production of interleukin-4 by splenocytes in oxazolone-induced murine colitis. *Chin. J. Dig.* 2002; 22(6):335-337 (Chinese).

[11] Li H-z. Clinical observative on Titanoreine and SASP suppositories for ulcerative colitis. *Chin. J. Coloproctol.* 2004; 24(7):16-17 (Chinese).

[12] Zhang Z-m. Retention enema with BeiFuJi (rbFGF) for treating Chronic non-specific ulcerative colitis. *Chin. J. Coloproctol.* 24(7):17-19 (Chinese).

[13] Zhou Y-h, Yu J-p, Lu H-s et al. Protective effect of GinKgo biloba extract (EGB) on experimental colitis in rats. *Chin. J. Dig.* 2007; 27(2):129-131 (Chinese).

[14] Kou J-g, Chi C, Yuan H-l, et al. Therapeutic effect and mechanisms of GinKgo biloba extract in DSS induced colitis in rats. *Chin. J. Dig.* 2007; 4(4):269-270 (Chinese).

[15] Chen W-x, Lu Y-m, Chen J-l, et al. Treatment of experimental colitis with Ligusticum Wallichii Franch (Chun-xiong Rhizoma) *Chin. J. Dig.* 2007; 27(3):203-205 (Chinese).

[16] Zhang M, Deng C-s, Zheng J-j, et al. Curcumin inhibits trinitrobenzene sulphonic acid-induced colitis in rats by activation of peroxisome proliferator- activated receptor gamma. *Internat. Immunopharmacol.* 2006; 6(8):1233-1242.

[17] Zhang M, Deng C-s, Zheng J-j, et al. Curcumin regulated shift from Th1 to Th2 in trinitrobenzene sulphonic acid-induced chronic colitis. *Acta Pharmacol. Sini.* 2006; 27(8):1071-1077.

[18] Jiand H, Deng C-s, Zhang M, et al. Curcumin-attenuated trinitrobenzene sulphonic acid induces chronic colitis by inhibiting expression of cyclooxygenase-2. *Worl J. of Gastroenterol.* 2006 J28; 12(24):3848-3853.

[19] Zhou J, Wu S-m, Chen X-y, et al. Protective effects of Tripterine on rat colitis induced by trintrobenzene sulfonic acid. *Chin. J. Gastroenterol.* 2007; 12(3):144-147 (Chinese).

In: Inflammatory Conditions of the Colon
Editor: Jia-ju Zheng

ISBN: 978-1-60692-240-8
© 2008 Nova Science Publishers, Inc.

Chapter XXXI

Conservative Management of Ulcerative Colitis

Fang Gu and Yu-min Lü
The Third Hospital of Peking University, Bei-jing, P.R. China

The etiology and pathogenesis of ulcerative colitis (UC) is presently unclear and there is no optimal therapy [1]. Current therapeutic goals are to induce remission, maintain remission, reduce disease and treatment related complications and to improve the quality of patients' life [1,2]. Conservative management is preferred for patients without severe complications.

General Supportive Therapy

Appropriate rest is necessary in patients with active disease [1]. Patients with severe or fulminate colitis require hospital admission. Patients with mild symptoms usually are able to take food orally. The diet should be nutritious and restricted of fiber. Milk should be avoided to some patients who cannot tolerate it. In patients with severe colitis, an elemental oral diet or nothing by mouth with total parenteral nutrition (TPN) has been recommended. Correct the acid-base imbalance, disorders of water and electrolyte, anemia and hypoproteinemia. The patients with secondary infection should be treated with antibiotics, and a broad–spectrum antibiotic regimen including anaerobic coverage should be given to patients with severe colitis. Antidiarrheal agents or anticholinergics are contraindicated in patients with severe colitis because of the risk of precipitating toxic megacolon. Psychotherapy may be indicated in some patients to help them cope with living with a chronic disease.

Drug Treatment

1. Aminosalicylates

Aminosalicylates have been the drugs of choice for the treatment of mild to moderate colitis or severe colitis alleviated with corticosteroids [1,3]. Sulfasalazine has historically been the most commonly used drug in the treatment of UC. It has been shown to be efficacious in active and remitted UC. The drug consists of sulfapyridine linked to 5-aminosalicylic acid (5-ASA) via an azo bond. When taken orally, intestinal bacteria break the azo bond by the action of bacterial azo reductase and release the two components, sulfapyridine moiety and the 5-ASA moiety. 5-ASA is the active component which appears to account for most of the therapeutic effect of this agent. 5-ASA is released primarily in the colon and acts topically by a variety of mechanisms. A therapeutic dose of 3 to 4 g (up to 6g) per day in divided is appropriate for active colitis. Clinical response is usually within 2 to 3 weeks. The dosage can be tapered to lower levels after the disease is brought under control. The usual maintenance dosage is 2 to 4g per day in divided doses, although an occasional patient may benefit from 1 g per day. A conclusive answer to the total duration of maintenance therapy has not been yielded, long term maintenance therapy is generally recommended. Side effects of sulfasalazine occur in 10-45% of sulfasalazine–treated patients and are mainly attributed to the effects of sulfapyridine. Abdominal discomfort is common and is minimized by ingestion of the sulfasalazine after meal. Patients also may become folate-deficient because of the competition between folate and sulfasalazine in absorption. Other side effects, such as skin eruptions, bone marrow suppression, hemolysis and sperm motility disorders, are less common. A blood count and liver chemistry test should be obtained before starting therapy, every 1 to 3 months initially, and every 6 to 12 months during long-term treatment.

Because the serious side effects of sulfasalazine are related to the sulfa portion, some new salicylate preparations have been developed that retain the salicylate portion but replace the sulfapyridine [1]. When administered by mouth, 5-ASA is rapidly absorbed from the jejunum and consequently does not get into the colon. Therefore, two types of delivery systems have been used to obtain high concentrations of drugs in the colonic lumen. The first method is to coat 5-ASA with a resin or a semipermeable membrane that is pH sensitive. Pentasa, Etiasa, Solofalk and Asacol are examples of this kind of new preparations. The generic name for enteric-coated or delayed-release preparations is mesalazines (mesalamines in the United States) that have substantial release of 5-ASA in the small bowel and colon. The second method is to link 5-ASA with another carrier molecule by an azo bond such as Olsalazine (Dipentum) or Balsalazide (Colazide). The pharmacodynamics of these two prodrugs are similar to those of sulfasalazine, with release of 5-ASA after splitting by bacterial enzymes in the colon. Many clinical trials showed that these new salicylate drugs are as effective as sulfasalazine, in both controlling active disease and maintaining remission. Adverse effects have been minimal and occur in fewer than 5% of patients. Furthermore, the majority of sulfasalazine-intolerant patients are able to tolerate these new preparations.

In addition to oral preparations, aminosalicylates are also available as topical formulations such as suppositories, foam or liquid enemas. Patients with distal colitis should be encouraged to use topical therapies applied per rectum once or twice daily. Choice of topical formulation should be determined by the proximal extent of the inflammation. Suppositories are for disease limited to the distal 10cm of rectum, foam enemas are for disease involving the distal 15 to 20cm of proctosigmoid. Patients with more proximal disease should be treated with liquid enemas. Table 31-1 lists the aminosalicylates that have been developed [2].

Table 31-1. Aminosalisylate preparations

Preparation	Dosage	Components	Site of action	Dosages according to literatures	
				Induction of remission	Maintenance of remission
Topical agents					
SASP Suppositories	0.5g	linked to a sulfapyridine moiety	rectum	1-2g/d in divided doses	0.5g at bed time every or every other day
Mesalazine Suppositories	0.5g or 1g		rectum	1-1.5g/d	0.5g at bed time every or every other day
Mesalazine Enemas	1-4g	60/100ml	left colon	1-4g/d at bed time	1g at bed time every or every other day
Oral Agents					
Prodrugs					
Sulfasalazine	0.5g	linked to a sulfapyridine moiety	colon and terminal ileum	4-6g/d in divided doses	2-4g/d in divided doses
Olsalazine	0.25g	dimmer of 5-ASA	colon and terminal ileum	1.5-3.0g/d in divided doses	1.5-3.0g/d in divided doses
Balsalazide	0.75g	linked to N-(p-hydroxyphenyl) glycine	colon and terminal ileum	2-6g/d in divided doses	2-6g/d in divided doses
Delayed-release manner					
Asacol	0.4g	Eudragit-S coating released when pH>7	distal ileum and colon	2.4-4.8 g/d in divided doses	0.8-4.8 g/d in divided doses
Claversal, Salofalk, Rowasa	0.25g or 0.5g	Eudragit-L coating released when pH P>6	distal jejunum ileum and colon,	1.5-4.5 g/d in divided doses	0.75-1.5 g/d in divided doses
Controlled-release manner					
Pentasa	0.25g or 0.5g	controlled-release spheres	duodenum, jejunum, ileum and colon	2-4g/d in divided doses	1.5-3g/d in divided doses

2. Corticosteroids

Corticosteroids should be used for patients with mild to moderate active ulcerative colitis unresponsive to initial therapy with an aminosalicylate, particularly in patients with severe active colitis to induce remission [3-6]. They have benefits for colitis in acute episode, but are inappropriate for maintenance therapy because of their major side effects and inefficiency in preventing relapse.

Prednisone or prednisolone, at doses of 30-40mg/d (up to 60mg/d) orally, induces remissions in 75-90% of patients with mild or moderate active colitis. In patients with active severe or fulminate colitis, parenteral administration of corticosteroids (i.e. methyllprednisolone 45-60mg/d, or hydrocortisone 200-300mg/d, or dexamethasone 10mg/d) is usually preferable. Symptoms improvement is usually noted after 7-10 days of such therapy and then patients can be shifted to oral prednisone (60mg/d). After induction of remission, corticosteroids are tapered and withdrawn according to severity and patient response over a period of several months (generally over a 8-week period). Aminosalicylates or immunomodulators should be administered concomitantly during tapering of steroids to take advantage of their "steroid-sparing" effects. Once the acutely ill patients with severe colitis is taking oral feeding, aminosalicylates should be added immediately, and immunomodulators or surgery should be considered as early as possible if the disease is poorly controlled or in exacerbation.

Corticosteroids are also effective for active distal colitis when used as topical treatment in the form of suppositories, foams or retention enemas.

Choice of topical formulations is based on proximal extent of the inflammation. Topical corticosteroids (i.e, hydrocortisone sodium succinate 100mg, prednisolone 20mg or dexamethasone 5mg dissolved in 100ml of saline) are usually administered per rectum once or twice a day. When symptoms improve, they are reduced to 2-3 times a week, with the total duration within 1-3 months. Severe side effects of steroids in long term use should not be neglected

Some newer corticosteroids such as budesonide are highly affinitive with steroid receptors, topically active and rapidly cleared by hepatic first pass metabolism, and therefore have potent therapeutic benefits with reduced systemic toxicity. Generally speaking, they are as efficacious as conventional steroids, although there are some studies with inconsistent outcomes. Many studies demonstrated that oral budesonide has comparable efficacy in the treatment of patients with mild to moderate left-sided or extensive colitis compared with prednisolone. But it is less effective for distal UC because of the low concentration in rectum and sigmoid colon. Topical budesonide of 2mg/d in the form of retention enemas are effective for distal colitis.

3. Immunomodulators

Immunosuppressive agents are indicated for the treatment of steroid-refractory or steroid-dependent UC. Their main role is steroid sparing [3,5-7]. Toxicity should be monitored carefully because they may cause severe side effects.

Purine analogues should be considered for patients with chronically active steroid-refractory or steroid-dependent UC. Azathioprine (AZA) or its active metabolite, 6-MP is effective for both controlling active disease and maintaining remission in UC. Aza is prescribed in dose of 1.5-2.5 g/kg per day and 6-MP is 0.75-1.5 mg/kg per day. The therapeutic effects of Aza and 6-MP are usually not seen until after 3 months. Long-term (at least 3-5 years) maintenance therapy is generally recommended. The major limiting factor in use of purine analogues is their toxicities, including bone marrow depression, pancreatitis, abdominal discomfort, infectious complications, or possibly increasing the incidence of lymphoma. Leukocyte count of patients receiving them must be monitored periodically to prevent leucopenia. There is no universally acceptable timetable for monitoring blood count. Monitoring every week or two weeks at the start of therapy and then every 1 to 3 months is reasonable. Patients intolerant of AZA may cautiously put on 6-MP before considering other therapy.

An alternative to purine analogues for inducing and maintaining remission in refractory or steroid-dependent UC might be methotrexate.(MTX) However, the efficacy of MTX in UC is controversial. Larger double-blind randomized studies need to be performed.

Cyclosporine A is established as a therapy in case of severely active UC refractory to steroids. To control the disease activity, intravenous cyclosporine is usually employed initially at a daily dose of 2-4mg/kg for 1 to 2 weeks and then switched to oral cyclosporine (8mg/kg.d) for 3 to 6 months. During that time, the patients begin on 6-MP. The total duration of cyclosporine therapy should not exceed 6 months. Typically, cyclosporine has been confined to patients with severe disease who fail to respond to at least 7-10 days of intravenous corticosteroids. In this patient group, intravenous cyclosporine (2-4mg/kg.d) induces a rapid remission in approximately 80% of patients within 2 weeks. However, up to 50% of these individuals ultimately require colectomy during 6 months of follow-up. If concomitant immunosuppressants such as purine analogues are used, approximately 60-70% of patients who respond to cyclosporine may achieve remission and avoid colectomy. Cyclosporine is mainly regarded as a "bridge" therapy to either long-term immunomodulatory therapy (i.e. with purine analogues) or definitive colectomy in severe steroid-refractory UC. Cyclosporine should not be used for remission maintenance for UC. Side-effects include nephrotoxicity, seizures, hypertension, bone marrow suppression, and opportunistic infections. Monitoring of cyclosporine plasma concentration and side effects especially nephrotoxicity is required. Therapeutic range of 200-400ng/ml is advisable. The dose should be adjusted downward whenever the baseline serum creatinine level increases by 30%.

Tacrolimus (FK-506) is one kind of macrolide antibiotics with immunomodulatory effect similar to cyclosporine. It has lower bioavailability with little individual difference and is relatively safe. Oral (0.1-0.2mg/kg/d) or intravenous (0.01-0.02mg/kg/d) tacrolimus can be an alternative to cyclosporine especially for those require long term therapy.

4. Other medications

Infliximab (IFX) is a chimeric monoclonal antibody to human tumor necrosis factor-α (TNF-α) with potent anti-inflammatory effects [3,5,6]. Controlled trials have demonstrated efficacy for IFX in moderate to severe active UC refractory to steroids. But the results concerning of its effectiveness in earlier studies are conflicting. Clinical response is rapid (within 1-2 weeks) and the duration of response ranges from 8-12 weeks per infusion. IFX is administered IV (5mg/ kg) over 2 hours. Infusion reactions may be minimized by pretreatment with an antihistamine and a steroid preparation. To minimize recurrence, the infusions are repeated at 8 week intervals. IFX should be used as part of a strategy, it is advisable to continue the use of other therapy during and after infusions of IFX. Side effects (IFX) include formation of human antichimeric antibodies (HACA), autoantibodies and a serum sickness-like delayed hypersensitivity reaction. The risk of development of lymphoma and cancer is reported.

Recent evidence suggests that the administration of probiotics may be beneficial in the management of UC [3,4]. Preliminary clinical studies have demonstrated that probiotics are effective in maintaining remission in ulcerative colitis and preventing and treating pouchitis. Equivalent efficacy is found between some probiotics and 1.5-2g 5-ASA in maintaining remission of patients with mild to moderate colitis. But their effectiveness in active UC needs to be confirmed.

Other new therapeutic agents and approaches include mycophenolate mofetil, anti-CD3 antibodies, anti-α4 integrin antibodies, anti-IL-2 antibodies, interferon, epidermal growth factor, heparin, nicotine, fish oil, and ω-3 fatty acid, leukocyte plasmapheresis etc [3]. Most of them should be subjected to further rigorous assessment through larger randomized, placebo-controlled trials.

Therapeutic Strategy Options

The therapeutic strategy in each case must be individualized depending on the severity, extent, activity, complications and clinical response to treatment [5,6] (table 31-2). After clinical remission of active disease is achieved, the patients should be kept on maintenance therapy to prevent relapse.

1. Management of Active Disease

Mild-moderate active left-sided colitis or pancolitis Oral aminosalicylates or glucosteroids are recommended to patients with mild-moderate active left-sided colitis (defined as disease limited to below the splenic flexure) or pancolitis(defined as disease extending proximal to the splenic flexure) [1,3,5,6].

Oral aminosalicylates (SASP 4-6g/d, mesalamine 2-4g/d, Balsalazide 6.75g/d) are effective first-line therapy [2]. Topical aminosalicylates or corticosteroids could be added to the above agents to relieve the rectal symptoms more effectively.

Oral corticosteroids (prednisolone 40mg/d, BUD 9mg/d) are appropriate for patients in whom a prompt response are required, or those unresponsive to oral aminosalicylates (with or without topical agents).

AZA (1.5-$2.5 mg \cdot kg^{-1} \cdot d^{-1}$) or 6-MP ($0.75$-$1.5 mg \cdot kg^{-1} \cdot d^{-1}$) is recommended for steroid refractory or steroid dependent patients. MTX acts more rapidly than AZA/6-MP and may be also effective for these patients, especially when they are unresponsive or intolerant of AZA/6-MP. But the efficacy needs to be confirmed by randomized controlled trials (RCTs).

Mild-moderate active distal colitis Topical agents (aminosalicylates or steroids) combined with oral agents (aminosalicylates or steroids) are effective for mild to moderate active distal colitis (defined as disease extending up to the sigmoid descending junction or limited to the rectum). Several factors such as patients' will, patients' compliance to topical agents or oral agents and economic factors should be considered in determining the therapy.

Topical aminosalicylates 1g/d (appropriate form according to the extent of disease) combined with oral aminosalicylates (SASP 4-6g/d, mesalamine 2-4g/d, Balsalazide 1.5-3g/d) are effective first-line therapy [2]. Topical aminosalicylates are usually more effective in distal colitis and should be the first choice. Topical or oral aminosalicylates alone are both less effective than combination therapy.

Topical steroids (hydrocortisone 100 mg/d or BUD 2 mg/d) are less effective than topical mesalamine, and should be reserved as second-line therapy for patients who are intolerant of topical mesalamine. Patients who have failed to improve on a combination of oral mesalamine with either topical mesalamine or topical corticosteroids should be treated with oral prednisolone 40mg daily. Topical agents may be used as adjunctive therapy in this situation.

Severe UC Intravenous corticosteroids (hydrocortisone 300-400mg/d or methyllprednisolone 45-60mg/d) are the first-line therapy of severe UC. Oral and topical aminosalicylates or steroids should be continued only if patients can tolerate.

If there is no improvement after 7-10 days, intravenous cyclosporine ($2 mg \cdot kg^{-1} \cdot d^{-1}$) or colectomy should be considered. Following induction of remission, oral cyclosporine for 3-6 months is appropriate and the addition of AZA/6-MP may enhance the long-term remission rate. Due to the side effects, cyclosporine alone is not recommended as first-line therapy.

The urgency for surgery in patients with toxic megacolon depends on the patient's condition itself. The greater the dilation and the greater the degree of systemic toxicity, the sooner surgery should be undertaken. In patients with mild dilation, conservative management could be considered, but if there is any deterioration in clinical signs, laboratory results or imaging studies, immediate colectomy should be performed.

Patients with severe UC need hospitalization and intensive investigation. Anticholinergic, antidiarrheal agents, NSAID and opioid drugs which risk precipitating colonic dilation should be withdrawn. Intravenous broad-spectrum antibiotics should be considered in patients with infection or systemic toxic symptoms, or those fail to other aggressive management. Intravenous fluid and electrolyte replacement are needed to correct and prevent dehydration or electrolyte imbalance, together with blood transfusion to maintain a hemoglobin level of > 100g/L. Nutritional support (by enteral or parenteral route) is appropriate in malnourished patients. Anticoagulation therapy is effective in reducing the risk of thromboembolism.

2. Maintenance Therapy

Long term even lifelong maintenance therapy is generally recommended for all patients, especially those with left sided or extensive disease, and those with distal disease who relapse more than once a year [1,3,5,6]. Discontinuation of medication may be reasonable for those with distal disease who have been in remission for 2 years and are averse to such medication.

Aminosalicylates are first-line therapy for maintenance. (such as SASP2-4g/d, mesalamine 1-2g/d, Balsalazide 2.5g/d or Olsalazine 1.5-3g/d for oral administration,). Topical aminosalicylates (0.5-1g/d) may be used in patients with distal colitis with or without oral mesalazine.

AZA (1.5-2.5 $mg·kg^{-1}·d^{-1}$) or 6-MP(0.75-1.5 $g·kg^{-1}·d^{-1}$) are recommended for patients who frequently relapse despite adequate doses of aminosalicylates or those who are intolerant of aminosalicylates.

Recent research revealed probiotics and mesalamine (1.2 or 1.5 g/d) have similar efficacy in preventing relapse of UC or pouchitis [4].

Steroids (including budesonide) are not recommended for maintaining remission.

Table 31-2. Therapeutic Strategies of Ulcerative Colitis

Induction of Remission	Therapeutic Protocols
Mild-morderate distal colitis	topical aminosalicylates → steroids →immunomodulators (AZA/6-MP) (combined with oral agent) (topica →oral) (refractory UC).
Mild-morderate left-sided, extensive colitis and pancolitis	oral aminosalicylates → oral steroids →immunomodulators (AZA/6-MP) (combined with topical agent) (refractory UC)
Severe or fulminate colitis	steroids i.v. + antibiotics → cyclosporine /or colectomy (combined with systemic therapy) (refractory UC+AZA etc., leukopheresis or IFX considered for unresponsive ones)
Maintenane of Remission	aminosalicylates → immunomodulators (AZA/6-MP)

Management in Pregnancy

Maintaining adequate disease control is essential for both maternal and fetal health [3,5,6]. The risks to the fetus from disease activity appear to be greater than continued therapy. If planning pregnancy, patients should obtain professional consultation to conceive during remission and continue their maintenance medication. In general, the medication for pregnant patients is the same as those who are not pregnant, but the safety to fetus must be evaluated adequately.

SASP together with other aminosalicylates are usually safe in pregnancy. Given the interference of folate absorption from SASP, folate supplements of 2mg/d are recommended in pregnancy, Sulfasalazine should be stopped if there is suspected neonatal hemolysis. Corticosteroids can be used for active disease in the same dose as not in pregnancy. It is appropriate to choose formulations which metabolize in placenta completely such as prednisone or prednisolone. Immunosuppressants should be avoided as far as possible in pregnancy. Current research suggests AZA and 6-MP are safe in pregnancy and could be continued in general if necessary when pregnant during therapy, although babies born to mothers on Aza may be lighter than normal and the risk-benefit ratio should be discussed with patients. Cyclosporine has no teratogenic effect but can impair renal tubules of fetus mouse. Related human data is deficient although preliminary use is safe. MTX is absolutely contraindicated in pregnancy. Abortion should be adopted if pregnant unexpectedly during treatment. Discontinuation for 6 weeks or longer as far as possible is necessary if planning pregnancy. IFX has limited human data although it's safe in rats. IFX has ever been reported to lead to abortion in first 3 months of pregnancy and is inappropriate to use in lactation.

Quinolones should be avoided in pregnancy [3,5,6]. Loperamide is considered safe although congenital deformities have been reported. It is inappropriate to use loperamide in large dose or use diphenoxylate for long term. Probiotics or enteral nutrition is safe and parenteral nutrition can be used if necessary, although fat emulsion should be restricted because of the risk of fat embolism of placenta.

Management of Pouchitis

Metronidazole 250-400mg tid or ciprofloxacin 250-500mg bid for 2 weeks are the first-line therapy of acute pouchitis [5,6]. Mesalamine or corticosteroids can be used for patients who do not respond to antibiotics. Long-term metronidazole or ciprofloxacin in low dose are effective in chronic pouchitis. Topical or oral aminosalicylates, topical steroids or probiotics can also be considered. Some patients have to take AZA for remission.

In conclusion, new therapeutic drugs and methods which offer clinicians more and more options are emerging unceasingly with more and more recognition of UC. It is essential to tailor an individualized therapeutic strategy suitable to his conditions in each case. During the treatment, therapeutic reaction and therapeutic complications such as drug toxicity and neoplasms should be adequately investigated. It is also important to evaluate patients' general condition and life quality. The optimal timing for surgery should be decided in time.

References

[1] Jewell DP. Ulcerative colitis. In: Feldman M, Scharsschmidt BF, Sleisenger MH. (eds). Sleisenger and Fordtran's Gastrointestinal and Liver disease. 6thed. Printed in China Harcourt Asia W.B. Saunders Company.1998 1735-1761.

[2] Zheng J-j. Drug treatmemt of ulcerative colitis. *China Prescription Drug.* 2005; 3(36)18-23.

[3] Katz S. Update in medical therapy of ulcerative colitis. Newer concepts and therapies. *J. Clin. Gastroenterol.* 2005; 39(7):557-69.
[4] Rioux KP, Fedorak RN. Probiotics in the treatment of inflammatory bowel disease. *J. Clin. Gastroenterol.* 2006; 40(3):260-3.
[5] Carter MJ, Lobo AJ, Travis SPL. Guidelines for the management of inflammatory bowel disease in adults. *Gut.* 2004; 53(suppl V): v1-v16.
[6] Kornbluth A, Sachar DB. Ulcerative colitis practice guidelines in adults (update): American college of gastroenterology, practice parameters committee. *Am. J. Gastroenterol.* 2004; 99(7):1371-85.

In: Inflammatory Conditions of the Colon
Editor: Jia-ju Zheng

ISBN: 978-1-60692-240-8
© 2008 Nova Science Publishers, Inc.

Chapter XXXII

Medical Treatment of Crohn's Disease

Zhi-hua Ran
Ren-ji Hospital, Shang-hai Jiao-tong University School of Medicine,
Shang-hai, P.R. China

Import progress has been made in recent years in the medical treatment of inflammatory bowel disease (IBD). This review will focus on the most recent advances, emphasizing the results of recent randomized clinical trials of traditional drugs and biologic agents.

Active Inflammatory Crohn's Disease (CD)

1) Corticosteroids, both prednisone or controlled ileal release budesonide have been found to be consistently superior to placebo, sulfasalazine (popularly called SASP in China), or mesalamine for the induction of remission in mild to moderately active ileal or ileocolonic CD [1-3].

2) SASP was previously established to be significantly superior to placebo for left colonic disease [1,2,4]. No other medications, when compared with SASP, have consistently been shown to be superior to placebo or to other less effective controls for induction of remission in mild to moderately active CD.

3) Infliximab (IFX) is usually reserved for patients with more active disease (the ACCENT I trial showed 58% of 573 patients responded to an initial infusion of IFX 5 mg/kg) [1].

Other anti-TNF-α agents, CDP571 (a humanized mouse monoclonal antibody against TNF-α) and CDP870 (a pegylated fragment of anti-TNF-α antibody) demonstrated induction of short-term (weeks 2-4) response. However, highly significant and longer-term benefit was observed in the subgroup of patients with elevated C-reactive protein for both CDP571 and CDP870.

The Classic-1 Trial reported that Adalimumab, the fully humanized antibody against TNF-α, was effective in the induction of remission of active disease, optimal induction dosing regimen was 160 mg at week 0 followed by 80 mg at week 2 via subcutaneous injection [4].

Recently, a better therapeutic program (called Top-Down regimen) was suggested for induction of remission in severe patients with CD (figure 32-1) [1,6]; however, long-term safety was uncertain and tong-term complications were unknown.

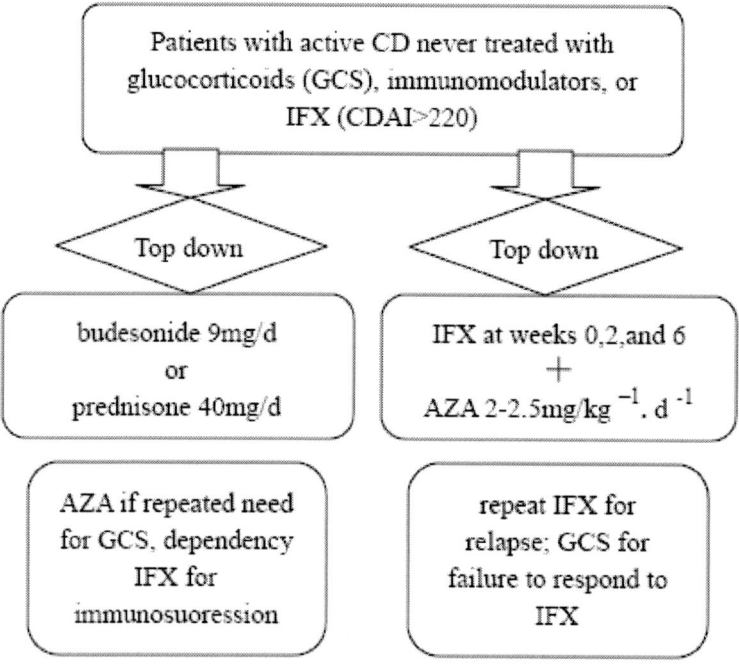

Figure 32-1. "Step-Up vs. "Top-Down" paradigm.

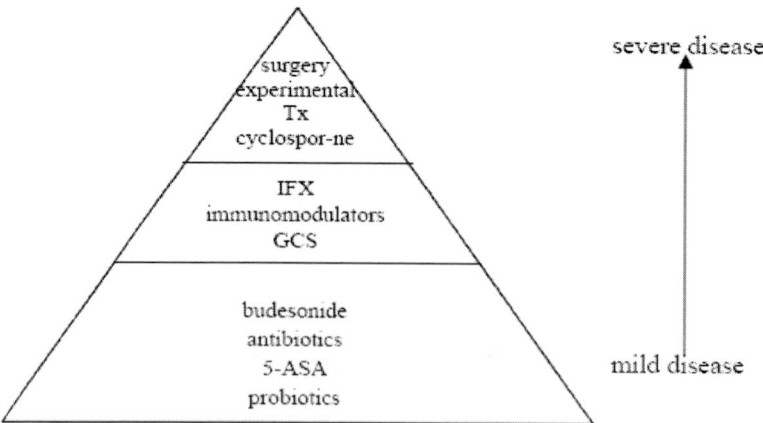

Figure 32-2. Therapeutic paramid for IBD: the "Step-Up" paradigm.

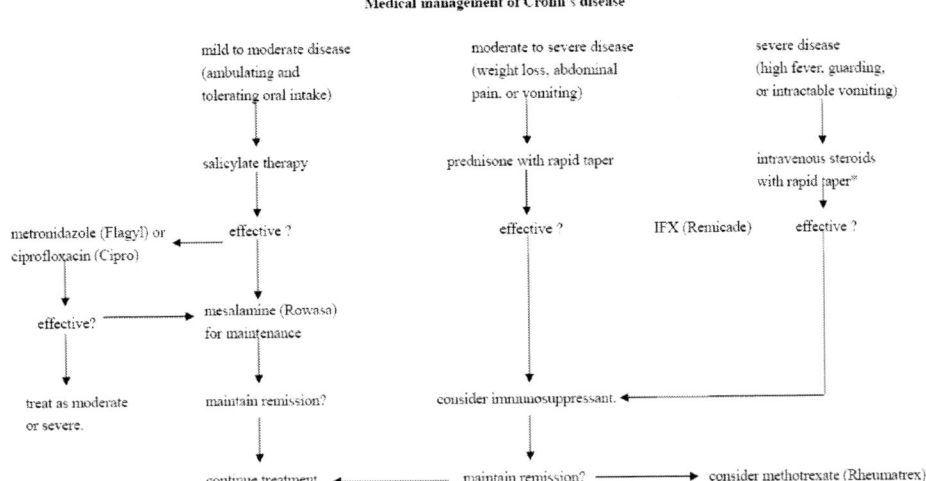

Figure 32-3. Algorithm for the medical management of Crohn's disease. (adopted from Wall GC et al. Pharmacotherapy 1999. [11,14]

Natalizumab (a humanized mouse monoclonal antibody against α4 integrin that blocks the efflux of activated lymphocytes and monocytes from the vasculature into tissues) showed similar beneficial results to the CDP571 and CDP870 [1,5,6].

4) The addition of ciprofloxacine and metronidazole to budesonide (or the addition of ciprofloxacine to prednisolone) dose not produce any additional clinical benefit.

5) Patients with less than complete response to standard doses of conventional first-line therapy with corticosteroids, budesonide or SASP call for the addition of oral 6-mercaptopurine (6-MP, 1.5 mg·kg^{-1}·d^{-1}) or azathioprine (AZA, 2.0-2.5 mg·kg^{-1}·d^{-1}), injection (subcutaneously or intramuscularly) of methotrexate (MTX, 25 mg once per week), or IFX 5 mg/kg for 3 injections at 0, 2, and 6 weeks. The time to response appears to be fastest with IFX (1-2 weeks), intermediate with MTX (4-6 weeks), and slowest with 6-MP or AZA (4-8 weeks).

6) The new therapy with intestinal helminth Trichuris suis (ingestion of 2500 live T. suis ova every three weeks for 24 weeks) has been shown effective in the treatment of patients with active Crohn's disease. At week 24, 23 patients (23/29, 79.3%) responded (decrease in CDAI>100 points or CDAI<150) and 21/29 (72.4%) remitted (CDAI<150). Mean CDAI of responders decreased 177.1 points. There were no adverse events observed.

The medical management of Crohn's disease is based on the location and severity of disease and extra-intestinal complications .Therapy has two goals—to treat the acute disease flare-ups and to maintain remission [8].

Mild To Moderate Disease

Ileal, ileocolonic, or colonic disease is treated with an oral aminosalicylate (mesalamine 3.2–4 g or sulfasalazine 3–6 g daily in divided doses) [9]. Alternatively, metronidazole 10–20 mg/kg/day may be effective in a proportion of patients not responding to sulfasalazine.

Ciprofloxacin 1 g daily is equally effective to mesalamine, and controlled ileal release budesonide may become an available alternative in the near future.

Moderate to Severe Disease

Patients with moderate–severe disease are treated with prednisone 40–60 mg daily or budesonide 9 mg daily (currently not FDA approved), until resolution of symptoms and resumption of weight gain (generally 7–28 days) [10,11]. Infection or abscess requires appropriate antibiotic therapy or drainage (percutaneuous or surgical). Infusions of IFX are an effective adjunct and may be an alternative to steroid therapy in selected patients in whom corticosteroids are contraindicated or ineffective.

Severe Disease

Patients with persisting symptoms despite introduction of oral steroids or IFX, or those presenting with high fever, frequent vomiting, evidence of intestinal obstruction, rebound tenderness, cachexia, or evidence of an abscess should be hospitalized [12-14]. Surgical consultation is warranted for patients with obstruction or tender abdominal mass. An abdominal mass should be evaluated via ultrasound or computerized tomography to exclude an abscess. Abscesses require percutaneous or surgical drainage. Once an abscess has been excluded or if the patient has been receiving oral steroids, parenteral corticosteroids equivalent to 40-60 mg of prednisone are administered in divided doses or as a continuous infusion. There is no specific role for total parenteral nutrition in addition to steroids. Nutritional support via elemental feeding or parenteral hyperalimentation is indicated, after 5-7 days, for patients unable to maintain nutritional requirements.

Crohn's Disease in Remission

Corticosteroids should not be used as long-term agents to prevent relapse of Crohn's disease. AZA/6-MP have demonstrable maintenance benefits after inductive therapy with corticosteroids. Mesalamine or AZA/6-MP should be considered after ileocolonic resections to reduce the likelihood of symptomatic recurrence.

1) 6-MP and AZA are the benchmark drugs for the maintenance of long-term symptomatic remission in CD [1,15]. Among CD patients in remission for at least 42 months, withdrawal of AZA leads to an 18-month relapse rate of 21% compared with 8% among the group randomized to continue active treatment [1]. However, 6-MP and AZA are not universally effective, require regular toxicity monitoring, and have significant adverse event profile.

2) Meta-analysis showed that 5-aminosalicylic acid, SASP and osalazine (were found to be not superior to placebo for remission maintenance) [1]. Thus, these drugs should not be prescribed to Crohn's disease patients for maintenance of remission.

3) Conventional corticosteroids are not effective for maintaining CD remission at doses low enough to avoid obvious adverse effects with long term use. However, budesonide 6 mg/day is effective for prolongation of time to relapse and maintenance of remission at 6 months but not 1 year in patients with CD in medically induced remission.

4) The role of metronidazole for postoperative maintenance of remission in clinical practice remains uncertain [1,7].

5) A 40-week trial found that, at a dose of 15-mg weekly, MTX was superior to placebo in patients who had entered symptomatic remission with MTX 25mg once weekly [1].

6) The ACCENT I Trial reported that about 25% of patients who enter into a long-term treatment program with 8 weekly 5 mg/kg or 10 mg/kg IFX infusions should remain in long-term remission [1].

Therefore, AZA, 6-MP, MTX, or IFX, and in some cases budesonide, are efficacious for maintaining medically induced remission in CD, and should be administered to avoid symptomatic relapse.

Perianal Disease

CD patients with perianal fistula and/or abscess can be treated with traditionally used antibiotics such as metronidazole and IFX (as reported by ACCENT II Trial) or 6-MP/AZA and tacrolimus for induction and maintenance of remission [1].

Antibiotics

There are no controlled trials showing that antibiotics are effective in the treatment of Crohn's perianal fistulas. The current clinical practice of using metronidazole or ciprofloxacin is based on uncontrolled case series. Clinicians prescribing antibiotics for fistulas typically use metronidazole at doses ranging from 750 to 1500 mg/day or ciprofloxacin 1000 mg/day for up to 3–4 months [16].

AZA and 6-MP

There are no controlled trials with fistula closure as the primary end point showing that the antimetabolites AZA and 6-MP are effective in the treatment of Crohn's perianal fistulas. The current clinical practice of using these medications is based on a meta-analysis of 5 controlled trials in which fistula closure was examined as a secondary end point and uncontrolled case series in adults and children. Controlled trials indicate that AZA at doses of

2.0–3.0 mg·kg^{-1}·day^{-1} and 6-MP at a dose of 1.5 mg·kg^{-1}·day^{-1} is effective for the treatment of Crohn's disease [16].

IFX

Two controlled trials have shown that IFX 5 mg/kg administered as a 3-dose induction regimen at 0, 2, and 6 weeks is effective for reducing the number of draining fistulas in patients with Crohn's disease and for closure of all fistulas and that maintenance therapy with IFX 5 mg/kg every 8 weeks prolongs the time to loss of response.

Cyclosporine

There are no controlled trials showing that cyclosporine is an effective therapy for Crohn's perianal fistulas. The current clinical practice of using intravenous cyclosporine is based on uncontrolled case series. Cyclosporine is administered as a continuous intravenous infusion at a dose of 4 mg·kg^{-1}·day^{-1}. Responding patients are converted to oral cyclosporine [16].

Tacrolimus

A single small controlled trial showed that tacrolimus 0.20 mg·kg^{-1}·day^{-1} for 10 weeks reduced the number of draining fistulas in patients with Crohn's disease but did not result in complete closure of all fistulas.

Other Sites

The same general principles apply, although there are no randomized controlled trials in the treatment of gastroduodenal or diffuse small bowel disease.

Crohn's disease of the mouth This is best managed in conjunction with a specialist in oral medicine. Topical steroids, topical tacrolimus, intra-lesional steroid injections, enteral nutrition, and IFX may have a role in management but there are no randomized controlled trials.

Gastroduodenal disease. Symptoms are often relieved by proton pump inhibitors. Surgery is difficult and may be complicated by fistulization.

Diffuse small bowel disease Stricture dilatation or strictureplasty with or without triamcinolone injection should be considered. Nutritional support before and after surgery is usually essential. Other approaches, including the combination of IFX with surgery for residual strictures, are evolving.

References

[1] Zheng J-j. Drug therapy of inflammatory bowel disease. *Chin. J. Dig.* 2005;25(11):700-701 (Chinese).

[2] Lichtenstein GR. Infliximab maintenance treatment reduces hospitalizations, surgeries, and procedures in fistulizing Crohn's disease. *Gastroenterol.* 2005; 128(4):862-869.

[3] Travis SPL, Stang EF, Lémann M, et al. European evidence based consensus on the diagnosis and management of Crohn's disease: current management. *Gut.* 2006;55(supple. 1):i16-i35

[4] Hanauer SB, Sandborn WJ, Rutgeerts P, et al. Classic-I Trial (Clinical assessment of Adalimumab Safety and efficacy Studied as Induction therapy in Crohn's disease) *Gastroerterol.* 2006;130(2):323-333

[5] Hommes D, Baert F, van Assche G, et al. Management of recent onset Crohn's disease: A controlled, randomized trial comparing step-up and top-down therapy. *Gastroenterol.* 2005;129(1):371

[6] Zheng J-j Biologic therapy of inflammatory bowel disease. *Chin. Med. Trib.* 2007;33(7):B11 （Chinese）

[7] Hanauer SB, Korelitz BI, Rutgeerts P, et al.Postoperative maintenance of Crohn's disease remission with 6-mercaptopurine, mesalamine, or placebo: a 2-year trial. *Gastroenterology.* 2004; 127(3):723-9.

[8] Hanauer SB, Sandborn W; Practice Parameters Committee of the American College of Gastroenterology.Management of Crohn's disease in adults. *Am. J. Gastroenterol.* 2001; 96(3):635-43.

[9] Kaplan MA, Korelitz BI.Narcotic dependence in inflammatory bowel disease. *J. Clin. Gastroenterol.* 1988 Jun;10(3):275-8.

[10] Tan WC, Allan RN. Diffuse jejunoileitis of Crohn's disease. *Gut.* 1993; 34:1374–8.

[11] Belaiche J, Louis E. Corticosteroid treatment in active.Crohn's disease. *Acta Gastroenterol. Belg.* 1998; 61:153–7.

[12] Bernstein CN, Shanahan F. Critical appraisal of enteral nutrition as primary therapy in adults with Crohn's disease (see comments). *Am. J. Gastroenterol.* 1996;91:2075–9

[13] Han PD, et al. Nutrition and inflammatory bowel disease. *Gastroenterol. Clin. North Am.* 1999; 28:423–43.

[14] Felder JB, Adler DJ, Korelitz BI. The safety of corticosteroid therapy in Crohn's disease with an abdominal mass. *Am. J. Gastroenterol.* 1991; 86:1450–5.

[15] Zheng J-j, Chu X-q, Shi X-h, et al. Efficacy and safety of azathioprine maintenance therapy in a group of Crohn's disease patients in China. *J. Dig. Dis.* 2008; 9(2):84-88.

[16] Sandborn WJ, Fazio VW, Feagan BG, Hanauer SB. American Gastroenterological Association Clinical Practice Committee. AGA technical review on perianal Crohn's disease. *Gastroenterology.* 2003; 125:1508-1530.

In: Inflammatory Conditions of the Colon
Editor: Jia-ju Zheng

ISBN: 978-1-60692-240-8
© 2008 Nova Science Publishers, Inc.

Chapter XXXIII

Biological Therapy for Inflammatory Bowel Disease

Zhan-ju Liu
The Second Affiliated Hospital, Zheng-zhou University,
He-nan Province, P.R. China

Background of Biological Therapy

Idiopathic inflammatory bowel disease (IBD), including Crohn's disease (CD) and ulcerative colitis (UC), are chronic inflammatory disorders of the gastrointestinal tract which lead to an unpredictable clinical course with a succession of exacerbations and remissions of variable intensity. The etiology and pathogenesis of human IBD remain elusive. Dysfunction of the immune system, altered luminal flora, a defective mucosal barrier, and genetically predisposing factors as well as environmental factors have been implicated in the development of IBD [1-3]. Both diseases are characterized by chronic intestinal inflammation, accompanied by a number of extraintestinal manifestations (affecting eyes, joints, liver, skin). However, in the majority of cases, CD can be distinguished from UC. CD manifests primarily a transmural inflammation involving the full thickness of the bowel wall and frequently leading to bowel obstruction, fistulas, and abscess formation. Both diseases also differ with regard to their distribution in the bowel. CD can be found at any place in the gastrointestinal tract but with a predilection for the terminal ileum and ascending colon. It is discontinuous, with areas of inflammation alternating with normal areas. In contrast, UC is limited to the colon and usually begins in the rectal and sigmoid areas and progresses upward in a continuous manner. Additionally, 10-15% of cases have no characteristic diagnostic features and hence are called indeterminate colitis.

Histologial analysis has revealed that both CD and UC are characterized by an influx of activated leukocyte infiltrates in inflamed mucosa of IBD, e.g., $CD25^+$ $CD69^+$ $CD40L^+$ T cells, $CD40^+$ $CD80^+$ $CD86^+$ $CD54^+$ B cells, Mϕ and DC, and $CD25^+$ $CD56^+$ NK cells [1-3]. In CD, there is a dense accumulation of activated T cells and macrophages, which in some cases are organized into typical granulomas. The earliest microscopic lesions consist of epithelial patchy necrosis, mucosal microulcerations, aphthous ulcers, a naked surface of the dome, villous abnormalities, and damage of small capillaries. In UC mainly diffuse epithelial necrosis is seen. The cellular infiltrates are more changeable and acute inflammatory events are prominent. Lymphocytes and macrophages, but not granulomas, are present.

Both innate and adoptive immune responses are found to be involved in the pathogenesis of IBD [3-5]. Commensal bacteria and pathogens in gut lumen produce large amount of disease-related substances, namely pathogen-associated molecule patterns (PAMP), which are recognized by pattern recognition receptors (PPR) expressing on immune cells and intestinal epithelial cells. Toll-like receptor (TLR) and nucleotide-binding oligomerization domain (Nod) are major types of PPR. TLR is usually associated with cell membranes, whereas Nod (including Nod1, Nod2 or named as CARD4, CARD15) is present in the cytosol of intestinal epithelial cells, Paneth cells and immune cells. TLR1-9, Nod1 and Nod2 expressed on intestinal epithelial cells and Paneth cells indicate that they sense luminal bacterial infection and play an essential role in the initiation of the immune responses by detecting conserved microbial macromolecules. Alterations of the innate immune response contribute to disease development, as evidenced by the mutations in the Nod2 gene, which is considered as a susceptible gene in some CD patients (figure 33-1). Microbial recognition by TLR and Nod is essential for the induction of inflammation and plays an instructive role in the development of the adaptive immune response, particularly in IBD.

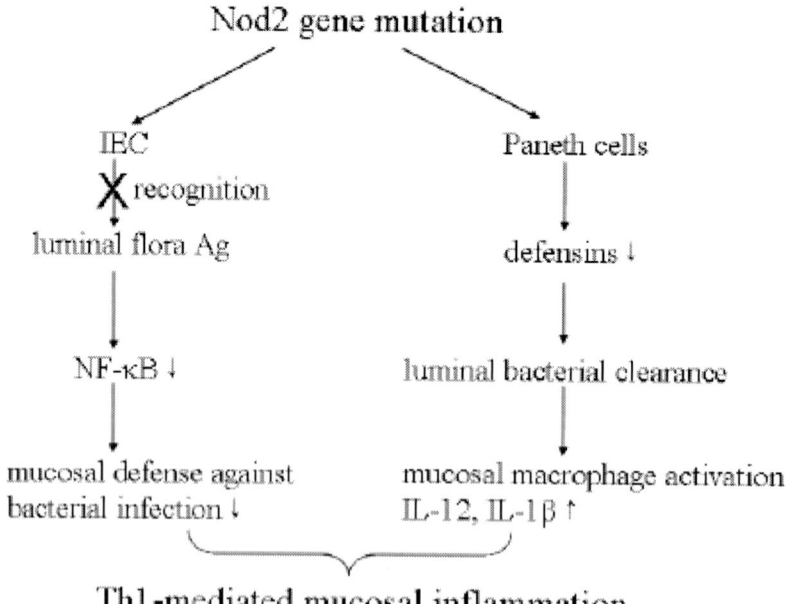

Figure 33-1. Association of Nod gene mutation with CD.

Several lines of evidences have pointed out that ongoing activation of lamina propria T cells and macrophages in inflamed mucosa is a central event in triggering the immunopathology in IBD. They function as effector cells in the intestine and secrete proinflammatory cytokines that cause and/or facilitate tissue damage. IBD lamina propria T cells from inflame mucosa exhibit a comparable or even higher proliferation than peripheral blood T cells in response to an antigen stimulation. These leukocytes as well as intestinal stromal cells express high levels of adhesion molecules (e.g., CD54、CD62L、CD106). Moreover, under inflammatory conditions, these immune cells are activated and express cytokine receptors, chemokine receptors (e.g., CCR5、CCR6、CCR7、CCR9) and integrins (e.g., LFA-1 or α2β2, α4β1, α4β7 integrins, MAdCAM-1). Importantly, endothelial cells of intestinal mucosal capillaries and fibroblasts express high levels of chemokines, selectins (e.g., P-selectin, E-selectin) and CD54 (ICAM-1). The interactions between these molecules induce circulatory leukocytes to immigrate and home into intestinal mucosa, leading to inflammatory damage in gut mucosa. Isolated lamina propria CD4$^+$ T cells from inflamed areas of CD patients, when stimulated in vitro, produce high levels of Th1-dominated proinflammatory cytokines such as TNF, IL-2 and IFN-γ. Recent years, several Th1-associated proinflammatory cytokines (e.g., IL-12、IL-15、IL-18) as well as IL-23 have also been detected in inflamed mucosa of CD patients. In contrast, mucosal CD4$^+$ T and NK-T cells from UC patients secrete high levels of Th2-like cytokines (e.g., IL-4, IL-13), when stimulated in vitro (figure 33-2).

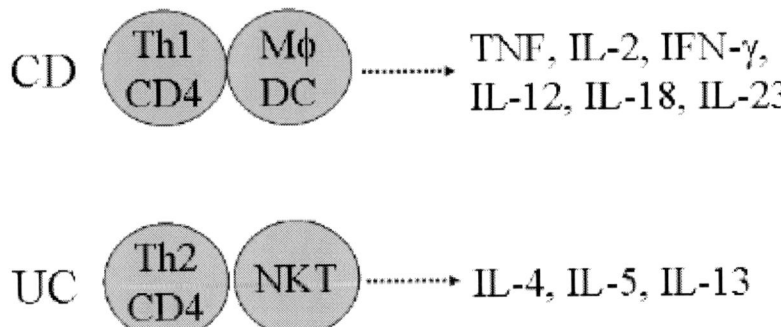

Figure 33-2. Cytokine profiles in lamina propria T cells in IBD.

New subset of T helper cells, namely Th17 cells, has recently been detected in inflamed mucosa of IBD [6,7]. These populations of Th17 cells play an important role in the induction of IL-22 and IL-23 secretion, and are involved in mucosal inflammatory response in CD patients (figure 33-3). In addition, some regulatory T cells (e.g., Treg. Th3, Tr1) with increased expression of FoxP3, CTLA-4 and GITR genes are also found in intestinal mucosa, and produce high levels of regulatory cytokines (e.g., TGF-β, IL-10). These cells play a critical role in the maintenance of intestinal mucosal immune tolerance. Evidences have proven that these regulatory T cells could prevent experimental colitis in mice, indicating that dysfunction of regulatory T cells may be associated with the development of IBD.

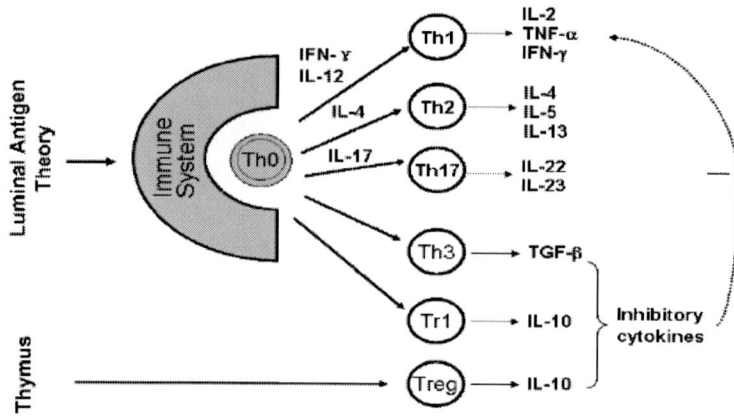
Figure 33-3. Intestinal mucosal T differentiation.

Over the past several years, understanding on intestinal mucosal immunology has promoted us to develop novel approaches in the treatment of IBD. Numerous biological agents have been generated and utilized in colitic models in animals and shown an encouraging result. Clinical trails in patients with IBD have also demonstrated to be statistical significance, and these biological agents have shed some light on the treatment of IBD. Biological therapies consist of monoclonal antibodies directed against proinflammatory cytokines, integrins and activation molecules, recombinant proteins and antisense oligonucleotides [8-10]. These agents are classified according to the mechanisms of action, mainly including TNF inhibitors, inhibitors of T-lymphocyte trafficking, inhibitors of T-lymphocyte polarization, inhibitors of T-cell activation, agents promoting epithelial repair, immune stimulators and others.

Inhibitors of TNF

TNF is mainly produced by activated T cells, macrophage and dendritic cells, and is a proinflammatory cytokine that induces inflammatory cell migration from circulation to local sites of inflammation [11]. It also induces edema, activates coagulation, and plays a role in the formation of granulomas. Granulomatous lesions may be found in up to 50% of CD cases. Currently, there are several biological agents directed against TNF in the treatment of CD and UC, such as Infliximab, CDP-571, CDP-870, Adlimumab, Thalidomide, Onercept and Etanercept [12]. Importantly, Infliximab and Adlimumab have shown to be effective in clinical trials, and will be described extensively in next Chapter.

Inhibitors of Lymphocyte Trafficking

Selective adhesion molecules (SAM) not only regulate the influx of leukocytes in normal and inflamed gut, but also involve intestinal lymphocyte stimulation and antigen presentation in gut mucosa (figure 33- 4). Increased expression of SAM (e.g., α4, β7, ICAM, MAdCAM-

1, VCAM-1) has been found in inflamed areas of IBD, and therapeutic compounds directed against trafficking of leukocytes have been designed as a novel class of drugs in the treatment of CD patients. Currently, biological agents directed against SAM in the treatment of IBD include Natalizumab, MLN-02 and Alicaforsen (figure 33-5) [13, 14].

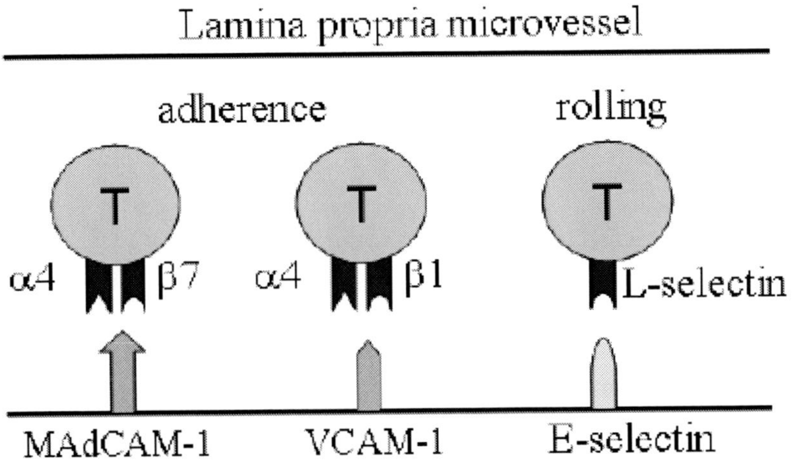

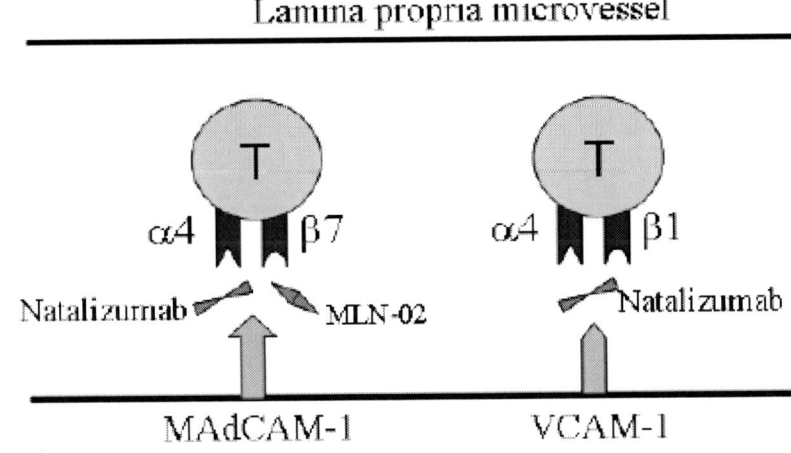

Figure 33-4. Gut T cell immigration and homing into lamina propria of intestinal mucosa, governed by the interaction between α4β7 or α4β1 and MAdCAM-1 or VCAM-1.

Figure 33-5. Target therapies directed against adhesion molecules, which govern T cell homing into gut mucosa.

α4β1 integrin (also named as very late antigen, VLA-4) is expressed on majority of leukocytes and affords to bind to VCAM-1 on endothelial cells and DC. However, α4β7 integrin is expressed on subsets of lymphocytes, NK cells and monocytes, and selectively binds MAdCAM-1 (figure 33-4). Accumulating evidences have demonstrated that α4 integrins are important in the recruitment and activation of cells in IBD. In IBD, anti-integrin molecule therapy has focused on two pathways: the α4-integrin/MAdCAM-1 and the β2-integrin/ICAM-1 interaction (figure 33-5). Natalizumab is a humanized anti-α4 integrin IgG4 Ab, which inhibits the interaction of α4β7–MAdCAM-1 as well as α4β1–VCAM-1. Clinical trial has demonstrated that natalizumab (300 mg or 3 to 4 mg/kg, i.v.) could efficaciously achieve remission in CD patients 2 weeks after administration [13]. A more specific humanized α4β7-integrin MLN-02 could block the α4β7–MAdCAM-1 interaction [14]. Preliminary clinical data have shown evidence of efficacy in UC and CD. Although anti-ICAM-1 mAb has demonstrated to effectively prevent experimental colitis in mice, several placebo-controlled with an ICAM antisense oligonucleotide (ISIS-2302, Alicaforsen) have been performed in active steroid-treated CD but have produced conflicting results [15]. Trials with ISIS-2302 in steroid refractory CD have provided conflicting efficacy data, while the efficacy in the control of active UC has been observed.

Inhibitors of T Cell Activation

For optimal T cell priming, T cells require the simultaneous recognition of Ag by the TCR and the engagement with costimulatory molecules (e.g., CD40, CD80) expressed on APC (figure 33-6). Evidence has shown that in situ expression of CD40 and CD40L is increased in inflamed mucosa of IBD, and that CD40 signaling could induce lamina propria T cell activation and production of TNF-α and IFN-γ. Blockage of CD40 signaling could prevent the development of experimental colitis in murine colitis model. Currently, target therapies directed against T cell activation include anti-human CD40 mAb (ch5D12) and anti-CD3 mAb (visilizumab). Phase II study using ch5D12 has performed in 18 patients with moderate to severe CD, and its overall response and remission rates were 72 and 22%, respectively [16]. Treatment with ch5D12 reduced microscopic disease activity and intensity of the lamina propria cell infiltrates, but did not alter percentages of circulating T and B cells. The side-effects included pyrexia, arthralgias, myalgias and headache. These preliminary data suggest that blockage of CD154-CD40 interactions with ch5D12 is a promising therapeutic approach for remission induction in CD. Visilizumab, a humanized anti-CD3 mAb, has been recently evaluated in patients with severe steroid-resistant UC [17]. The results showed that it could improve clinical disease and promote the healing of ulcers. Some patients had nausea, chills and arthralgias.

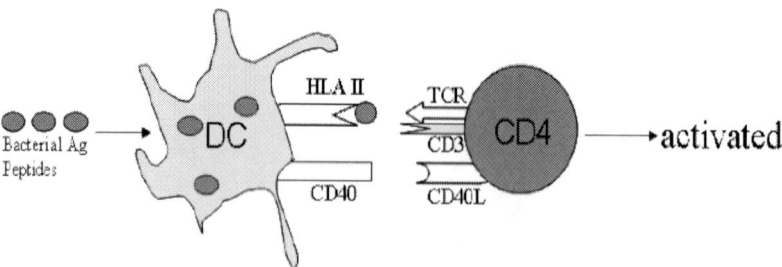

Figure 33-6. Two-signaling model for CD4$^+$ T cell activation.

Inhibitors of T Cell Polarization

These biological compounds include anti-IL-12, anti-IL-2R, anti-IFN-γ mAb, as well as IL-10 and IL-11. IL-12 regulates the differentiation and activation of Th cells and is the major factor promoting the Th1 immune response. Since IL-12 is increased expression in inflamed mucosa of CD patients, anti-IL-12 (ABT-874; 1 or 3 mg/kg, s.c., once weekly) has been evaluated in patients with active CD and demonstrated to markedly improve intestinal mucosal inflammation [18]. Moreover, it could decrease lamina propria mononuclear cells to secrete IFN-γ, IL-12 and TNF-α. The side-effects included local reaction at the injection site, hyperuricemia, hypoglycemia, hyperphosphatemia and hyperamylasemia. IL-2 plays an important role in inducting T cell activation and immune responses. Anti-IL-2R mAb (Basiliximab, 40 mg, i.v.; or Daclizumab, 1 mg/kg, i.v.) has been evaluated in patients with steroid-resistant UC, and shown to be effective at inducing remission, indicating anti-IL-2R mAb shows a promise moderate steroid-resistant UC [19]. Anti-IFN-γ mAb has been underwent clinical trials and the conflicting results enforce to stop further trials in the clinic.

IL-10 is potent anti-inflammatory activity and inhibits expression of HLA class II and B7 molecules as well as proinflammatory cytokine production (e.g., IL-1, IL-6, TNF-α). IL-10 KO mice develop spontaneous colitis resembling some of the features of human IBD in both macroscopic and histologic appearance. Therefore, IL-10 is considered as a potential therapy for Th1-drived inflammatory diseases. Previous reports have shown that patients with mild to moderately active CD had clinical improvement after receiving a dose of 5 or 10 μg/kg subcutaneously, down-regulated the activation of NF-κB in inflamed mucosa and proinflammatory cytokine secretion. However, multicentre trials have been performed in patients with mild/moderate or therapy refractory CD and indicated that IL-10 therapy did not lead to significantly higher remission rates or clinical improvement compared with placebo treatment. Adverse events include transient lymphopenia, headache, fever, back pain, decrease in hemoglobin concentration, dizziness and thrombocytytopenia. Recent report showed that oral administration of Lactococcus lactis, genetically expressing IL-10, was effective in the treatment of CD patients and avoided systemic side effects [20]. Further studies are needed to evaluate its clinical significance in the management of CD. IL-11 is a cytokine demonstrating anti-inflammatory, hematopoietic and mucosal-protective effects. The evaluation of IL-11 for use in mild to moderate CD was performed and showed that weekly subcutaneous injection with rhIL-11 (15 μ/kg) is safe and effective in inducing remission. While another study reported that subcutaneous injection with rhIL-11 (1 mg/kg once weekly) demonstrated to be significantly inferior when compared to prednisolone in short-term remission induction in active CD patients.

Biological Agents Promoting Epithelial Repair and Protection

These agents include human growth hormone (HGF), keratinocyte growth factor-2 (KGF) and epidermal growth factor (EGF) [8,9]. HGF is a regulatory peptide, decreases intestinal permeability, stimulates collagen synthesis through induction of expression of insulin-growth factor, and increases uptake of amino acids and electrolytes by the intestine. It has been evaluated in patients with moderate-to-severe active CD via subcutaneous injection at a dose of 5 mg/day for a week followed by a maintenance dose of 1.5 mg/day for 16 weeks. The results showed that HGF could significantly improve disease. KGF-2 (Repifermin) has been administrated i.v. in active UC patients and data showed that no clinical remission was seen 4 weeks after treatment. EGF stimulates cell proliferation within the gut. Patients with mild-to-moderate UC were treated with EGF enemas at a dose of 5 mg in 100 ml of an inert carrier, and the results demonstrated the EGF enemas are an effective treatment for active UC.

Immune Stimulators

These agents are IFN-α, IFN-β, granulocyte colony-stimulatory factor (G-CSF) and granulocyte-macrophage colony-stimulatory factory (GM-CSF). Previous study has shown that IFN-α is not effective in the treatment of active UC. Clinical trial using GM-CSF or G-CSF has been done in moderate-to-severe CD cases and shown that they are effective and safe in treating the disease.

Other Compounds Targeted Against Cytokines

Other compounds for biological therapies in IBD include anti-IL-6R mAb and rationally designed peptide (RDP-58). Increased expression of IL-6 has been found in patients with active CD. A humanized mAb against IL-6R was utilized in active CD patients and showed that it could improve the disease [21]. RDP-58 is found to inhibit production of TNF-α, IFN-α, IL-2 and IL-12 by interrupting cell-signaling events. Preliminary results have shown that it is effective in some active IBD patients.

Potential Therapeutic Approach Targeted Against Innate Immunity

TLR-4, TLR-5 and Nod molecules recognize commensal bacterial antigens, and the gene mutation and abnormal expression may lead to abundant luminal bacterial antigen absorption and induce intestinal mucosal inflammation. Blockage of TLR4 signaling has demonstrated to prevent experimental colitis in mice. Target therapy directed against TLR or Nod molecules may have a therapeutic approach in the treatment of IBD.

Leukocytapheresis

Leukocytapheresis selectively absorbs granulocytes, monocytes/macrophages and some lymphocytes in circulation. It has recently been used to induce remission in patients with active CD and UC who fail to respond to corticosteroids, and also decreases the concentration of serum IL-1Rα and IL-10. The side-effects are found to be relatively low [22].

References

[1] Podolsky DK. Inflammatory bowel disease. *N. Eng. J. Med.* 2002,347(6):417.
[2] Strober W, Fuss I, Mannon P. The fundamental basis of inflammatory bowel disease. *J. Clin. Invest.* 2007; 117: 514-21.
[3] Sartor RB. Mechanisms of disease: pathogenesis of Crohn's disease and ulcerative colitis. *Nat. Clin. Pract. Gastroenterol. Hepatol.* 2006; 3:390-407.
[4] Sartor RB. Microbial influences in inflammatory bowel disease. *Gastroenterology.* 2008;134: 577–94.
[5] Cobrin GM, Abreu MT. Defects in mucosal immunity leading to Crohn's disease. *Immunol. Rev.* 2005; 206:277-95.
[6] Schmechel S, Konrad A, Diegelmann J, et al. Linking genetic susceptibility to Crohn's disease with Th17 cell function: IL-22 serum levels are increased in Crohn's disease and correlate with disease activity and IL-23R genotype status. *Inflamm. Bowel. Dis.* 2008; 14:204-12.
[7] Liu Z, Jiu J, Zhang H. IL-23 is highly expressed inflammatory bowel disease and induces T cell proinflammatory cytokine secretion. *Gastroenterology.* 2008; 134(suppl 1):A645.
[8] Ardizzone S, Bianchi Porro G.. Biological therapy for inflammatory bowel disease. *Drugs.* 2005; 66:2253-86.
[9] Sandborn WJ, Faubion WA. Biologics in inflammatory bowel disease: how much progress have we made? *Gut.* 2004; 53:1366-73.
[10] Pizarro TT, Cominelli F. Cytokine therapy for Crohn's disease: advances in translational research. *Annu. Rev. Med.* 2007; 58:433-44.
[11] Aggarwal BB. Signaling pathways of the TNF superfamily: a double-edged sword. *Nat. Rev. Immunol.* 2003, 3: 745-56.
[12] Rutgeerts P, Van Assche G, Vermeire S. Optimizing anti-TNF treatment in inflammatory bowel disease. *Gastroenterology.* 2004, 126: 1593-610.
[13] Targan SR, Feagan BG, Fedorak RN, et al. Natalizumab for the treatment of active Crohn's disease: results of the ENCORE trial. *Gastroenterology.* 2007; 132:1672-83.
[14] Lanzarotto F, Carpani M, Chaudhary R, et al. Novel treatment options for inflammatory bowel disease. Targeting α4 integrin. *Drugs.* 2006; 66:1179-89.
[15] Yacyshyn B, Chey WY, Wedel MK, et al. A randomized, double-masked, placebo-controlled study of alicaforsen, an antisense inhibitor of intercellular adhesion molecule

1, for the treatment of subjects with active Crohn's disease. *Clin. Gastroenterol. Hepatol.* 2007; 5:215-20.

[16] Kasran A, Boon L, Wortel CH, et al. Safety and tolerability of antagonist anti-human CD0 Mab cd5D12 in patients with moderate to severe Crohn's disease. *Aliment Pharmacol. Ther.* 2005, 22(2): 111-22.

[17] Plevy S, Salzberg B, Van Assche G, et al. A phase I study of visilizumab, a humanized anti-CD3 monoclonal antibody, in severe steroid-refractory ulcerative colitis. *Gastroenterology.* 2007; 133:1414-22.

[18] Mannon PJ, Fuss IJ, Mayer L, et al. Anti-interleukin-12 antibody for acute Crohn's disease. *N. Eng. J. Med.* 2004, 351(20):2069-79.

[19] Creed TJ, Probert CS, Norman M, et al. Basiliximab for the treatment of steroid-resistant ulcerative colitis: further experience in moderate and severe disease. *Aliment Pharmacol. Ther.* 2006; 23:1435-42.

[20] Braat H, Rottiers P, Hommes DW, et al. A phase I trial with transgenic bacteria expressing interleukin-10 in Crohn's disease. Clin Gatroenterol Hepatol 2006; 4:754-9.

[21] Ito H. Treatment of Crohn's disease with anti-IL-6 receptor antibody. *J. Gastroenterol.* 2005; 40(suppl 16):32-34.

[22] Abreu MT, Plevy S, Sands BE, et al. Selective leukocyte apheresis for the treatment of inflammatory bowel disease. *J. Clin. Gastroenterol.* 2007; 41:874-88.

In: Inflammatory Conditions of the Colon
Editor: Jia-ju Zheng

ISBN: 978-1-60692-240-8
© 2008 Nova Science Publishers, Inc.

Chapter XXXIV

Anti-Tumor Necrosis Factor Therapy in Inflammatory Bowel Disease

Zhan-ju Liu
The Second Affiliated Hospital, Zheng-zhou University,
He-nan Province, P.R. China

Introduction

Inflammatory bowel disease (IBD), which includes Crohn's disease (CD) and ulcerative colitis (UC), is a relapsing and remitting condition characterized by chronic inflammation at various sites in the GI tract, which results in diarrhea and abdominal pain. The precise etiology is unknown, but evidence suggests that the normal intestinal flora trigger an immune reaction in patients with a multi-factorial genetic predisposition (perhaps involving abnormal epithelial barriers and mucosal immune defenses) [1-3]. Although no specific environmental, dietary, or infectious causes have been identified, the immune reaction involves the release of inflammatory mediators. Accumulating data have demonstrated that increased expression of pro-inflammatory cytokines is present in inflamed areas of IBD. The immune pathogenesis of CD is associated with increased Th1-mediated cytokines (e.g., TNF, IFN-γ, IL-12, IL-18) by lamina propria mononuclear cells in inflamed mucosa, whereas UC is associated with excess Th2-like cytokine production (e.g., IL-4, IL-13). The imbalance of mucosal immune responses (i.e., Th1/Th2) is considered to be involved in intestinal mucosal inflammation. Recent years, emerging therapies for IBD are focusing on major effector cytokines such as TNF and IL-12. Importantly, target therapy directed against TNF has shed some light in the control of the disease in the gut [1-3].

Tumor Necrosis Factor in Signaling Transduction

TNF is an important proinflammatory cytokine, which is mainly secreted by activated macrophages and T cells, and considered as a critical mediator against tumor and infection [4]. TNF is first produced as a 26-kD transmembrane protein with an intracellular tail, which is cleaved by the metalloproteinase TNF converting enzyme to be secreted as a 17-kD soluble protein. TNF functions through two receptors, namely TNFR1 (P^{55} subunit) and TNFR2 (P^{75} subunit), TNFR1 is a receptor for a soluble ligand, and TNFR2 mediates the signaling of the membrane-bound ligand. However, some work indicates that TNFR1 mediates apoptosis and TNFR2 mediates cell proliferation. It seems that the two TNFRs transfer their signals cooperatively (figure 34-1). TNF activates NF-κB through the degradation of IκBα and plays an important role in immune response. TNF represents a double-edged sword. It is an important cytokine and required for normal responses under physical conditions, whereas inappropriate expression is harmful. Therefore, TNF has both beneficial and harmful activities. In addition to its beneficial side such as anticancer potential, regulation of the immune response and protection against microbial infection, it shows to be harmful as a result of inappropriate activation of NF-κB, leading to cancer, autoimmunity and some chronic diseases.

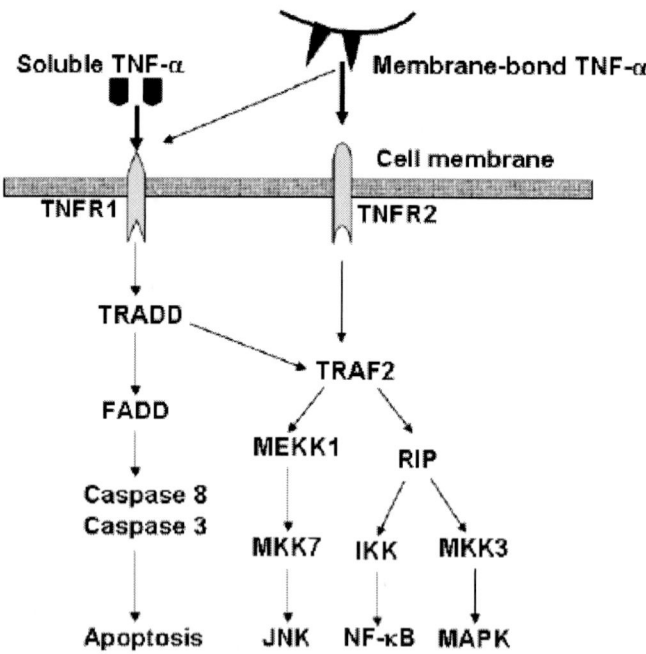

Figure 34-1. Signaling transduction by TNF.

Evidences have demonstrated that TNF is involved in many inflammatory diseases and is a key molecule in the cascade of inflammation of IBD. TNF is found to be significantly increased in inflamed areas of IBD, induces intestinal mucosal lymphocytes activation and pro-inflammatory cytokine secretion, triggers CD62E, CD54 and CD58 expression on endothelial cells, and induces leukocyte migration from circulation to local sites of inflammation. In addition, TNF also induces edema, activates coagulation, and plays a role in the formation of granulomas.

New approaches in the management of IBD have focused on the development of biologic agents (eg, mAb, recombinant proteins or peptides, antisense oligonucleotides) targeted at neutralizing specific proinflammatory proteins. Specifically, mAbs targeting TNF have proven to be highly effective in the treatment of IBD [5-7]. The anti-TNF agents, ranging from the introduction of infliximab, a chimeric mAb against TNF a decade ago to the fully human IgG1 anti-TNF mAb adalimumab, approved in early 2007, to the just approved certolizumab pegol, a humanized anti-TNF Fab' monoclonal antibody fragment linked to polyethylene glycol, have demonstrated the efficacy for induction and maintenance of remission in patients with moderate-to-severe CD [8,9]. These agents have reset the level for what is considered an acceptable symptomatic response to therapy in CD, paving the way for clinicians to look ahead to the possibility of modifying the natural history of the disease.

Up to date, several biological agents directed against TNF have been generated in the treatment of CD and UC, such as infliximab, CDP-571, CDP-870, adlimumab, thalidomide, onercept and etanercept (figure 34-2). Interestingly, some have shown to be effective in clinical trails. Both infliximab and adalimumab are approved by the US Food and Drug Administration (FDA) for the treatment of CD. Certolizumab pegol is a humanized anti-TNF Fab' monoclonal antibody fragment linked to polyethylene glycol; it is currently approved in Switzerland for the treatment of Crohn's disease and is undergoing review by the FDA in the United States.

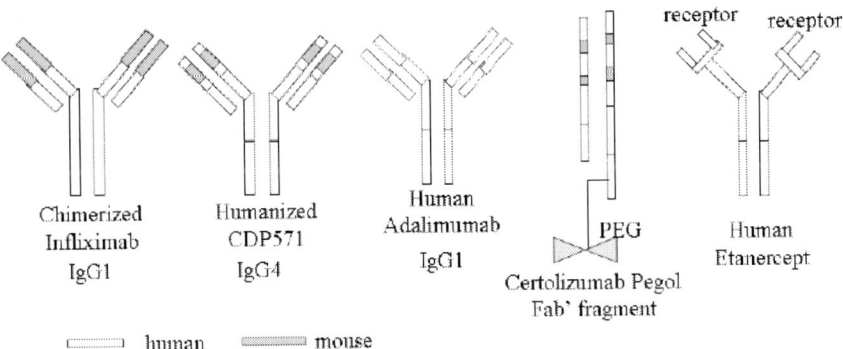

Figure 34-2. Biological agents directed against TNF-α in the treatment of IBD.

Infliximab

Infliximab is a chimeric, mouse anti-human, IgG1 mAb directed against anti-TNF which consists of human constant and murine variable regions. Currently, it is commercially available for rheumatoid arthritis, ankylosing spondylitis, psoriasis, and psoriatic arthritis, and is FDA approved for reducing signs and symptoms and inducing and maintaining clinical remission in adult and pediatric patients with moderately to severely active luminal and fistulizing CD who have had an inadequate response to conventional therapy [10]. In 2006, it was also approved for reducing signs and symptoms and inducing and maintaining clinical remission in adult patients with moderately to severely active UC who have had an inadequate response to conventional therapy [11].

Currently this compound has set the standard for future development of IBD therapies. In these patients, a series of three infusions of 5 mg/kg of infliximab at weeks 0, 2 and 6 results in a good response with mucosal healing and complete cessation of drainage. The optimal strategy is systematic maintenance treatment with 5 mg/kg intravenous (i.v) every 8 weeks. Long-term maintenance therapy with infliximab results in a reduction of the rate of complications, hospitalizations and surgeries associated with CD. This effect of infliximab is probably achieved by elimination of inflammatory cells expressing TNF on their membranes mainly by induction of apoptosis of T cells and monocytes.

In addition, infliximab has a proven efficacy in some patients with moderately to severely active UC, and reduces the colectomy rate in patients with acutely exacerbated steroid-refractory disease [12]. Results from two international active ulcerative colitis trials, ACT1 and ACT2, have shown that patients received placebo or infliximab at two different dosages (5, 10 mg/kg) at weeks 0, 2 and 6 followed by maintenance treatment every 8 weeks. Clinical response was observed in 66.9% (infliximab 5 mg/kg), 65.3% (infliximab 10 mg/kg) and 33.2% (placebo) at week 8. It reached in 49.6%, 55.4% and 27.9% respectively at week 30. Moreover, clinical response was found in 45.5%, 44.3% and 19.8% respectively 54 weeks after extended treatment.

Infliximab is effective corticosteroid-sparing agent in patients with CD. Infliximab alone or in combination with azathioprine can be an effective induction and maintenance therapy for patients who are steroid-dependent or steroid-naive. It demonstrates to be effective for the partial or complete healing of fistulas, the induction of mucosal healing, and improvement of the health-related quality of life (HRQL) in patients with CD.

Since the anti-TNF antibodies have been used longer in rheumatology, most of the safety data with these drugs have been extrapolated from this literature. Evidences have shown that the long-term use of this drug increases the immunogeneicity and the risk for infectious complications [13]. Treatment with infliximab may result in the development of antibodies to infliximab (ATI). Patients treated episodically with infliximab developed ATI more frequently (30–61%) than those with maintenance treatment (7–10%). Patients with ATI had a 2-fold-increased incidence of infusion reactions (16–30%) compared to those individuals without ATI (8–16%). Other studies demonstrated that the development of ATI was associated with a 12% absolute increase in infusion reactions, characterized by symptoms of headache, dizziness, nausea, injection-site irritation, flushing, chest pain, dyspnea or pruritus. Infliximab administration can also result in the development of double stranded DNA (dsDNA, 23.3%-34%), antinuclear antibody (ANA, 46%-56%), drug-induced reactions without major organ involvement (0.2%), infection involved in upper respiratory tract and urinary tract (30%-34%), opportunistic infection (e.g., nocardiosis, cytomegalovirus, histoplasmosis, invasive pulmonary aspergillosis), active tuberculosis, lymphoma, optic neuritis, multifocal motor neuropathy and drug-induced lupus.

CDP-571

CDP-571 (Certolizuman or Humicade), an approximately 95% humanized mAb to TNF, was created by linking the complement-determining region of a murine-derived TNF mAb to human IgG4 [14]. CDP-571 seeks out and binds TNF. Unlike infliximab, CDP-571 does not fix complement or lead to antibody-dependent lysis of the cells producing TNF. Additionally, since CDP-571 is only about 5% chimeric, it may produce fewer adverse effects than infliximab. Patients with moderate to severe CD were randomly treated with CDP-571 (10 mg/kg) or placebo every 8 weeks to week 24 and had significant clinical response with a decrease in the Crohn's disease activity index (CDAI) score $\geqslant 100$ points 2 weeks after administration (34.2% vs 21.2%, $P = 0.011$) [15]. Therefore, CDP-571 is modestly effective for short but not long-term treatment of CD patients.

Clinical trial has also done in patients with corticosteroid-dependent CD had prednisolone (15-40 mg/day) or budesonide (9 mg/day) for at least 8 weeks. These patients were treated with intravenous CDP-571 (20 mg/kg at week 0 and 10 mg/kg at week 8) and corticosteroid therapy was decreased following a predefined schedule. The results demonstrated that CDP-571 was effective and well-tolerated at week 16 in patients with corticosteroid-dependent CD. However, another report demonstrated that patients with corticosteroid-dependent CD received intravenous CDP-571 (10 mg/kg) every 8-weekly through to week 32. The results showed that CDP-571 is ineffective for sparing steroids in these patients at week 36. Ab to CDP-571 developed in 2.6%-10.9% of patients treated with active drug. Infusion reactions were also observed in 10.5%–12% patients. Anti-dsDNA Ab, ANA, upper-respiratory-tract infections were also occasionally seen in patients treated with CDP-571.

CDP-870

CDP-870 (Certolizumab pegol) is a polyethylene glycol (PEG) ylated anti-TNF mAb fragment modified to obtain a prolonged plasma half-life (approximately 14 days) [16]. Randomized placebo controlled trials have been done in patients with moderate-to-severe CD, who were administered intravenously at a single dose (1.25, 5, 20 mg/kg) or subcutaneously (100, 200, 300 mg). The results appeared to be good clinical response, particularly in patients with high levels of serum C-reaction protein. The most common side effects by intravenous administration included headache (38%), exacerbation of disease (7.6%), urinary tract infection (7.6%), abdominal pain (4.3%), fever (4.3%) and nausea (4.3%). However, the most frequent adverse events by subcutaneous injection were headache (13.2%), aggravation of disease (11.9%), nausea (11.4%) and nasopharyngitis (9.1%).

Adalimumab

Adalimumab (D2E7 or Humira), a fully human IgG1 anti-TNF mAb that has been commercially available in the United States for rheumatoid arthritis, ankylosing spondylitis, and psoriatic arthritis, was FDA approved in early 2007 for reducing signs and symptoms and inducing and maintaining clinical remission in adult patients with moderately to severely active CD [8,9]. A randomized, double-blind, placebo-controlled trail was performed to evaluate the efficacy of adalimumab induction therapy in patients with moderate to severe CD. The data pointed out that adalimumab was effective in the induction of remission of active disease, and the optimal induction dosing regimen was 160 mg at week 0 followed by 80 mg at week 2 via subcutaneous injection. Adalimumab was well tolerated and the frequencies of adverse events were low, e.g., injection-site reaction, infection, and aggravation of CD. Moreover, adalimumab is also safe and effective in patients with CD who have previously allergic or intolerant to infliximab.

Recent work has reported on the efficacy of adalimumab in patients with moderately to severely active CD after infliximab failure [17,18]. The clinical trials have demonstrated that adalimumab was significantly more effective than placebo in inducing remission in patients previously exposed to infliximab. In this 1-year follow-up to that study, they found that remission was preserved in 40% of patients and that 66% of patients maintained response.

Thalidomide

Thalidomide inhibits TNF production in certain inflammatory cells [19]. In the multicenter trial, patients with refractory CD received treatment of thalidomide (200 mg/day), 14 of the 22 patients responded well and CDAI was decreased at 12 weeks. This preliminary data suggest that thalidomide is useful for treatment of CD in patients who are steroid refractory or who have refractory fistulizing disease.

CNI-1493

CNI-1493 (Semapimod) is a small molecule, which blocks TNF gene expression by inhibiting mitogen-activated protein kinase (MAPKs) [20]. Previous study has reported that 12 patients with severe CD were randomly treated i.v. either 8 or 25 mg/m^2 daily for 12 weeks and shown that 8 patients were well tolerated and had remission. Further analysis presented that CNI-1493 could down-regulate MAPK signaling and cytokine production by macrophages. Phospho-MEK was also significantly decreased in patients with a good clinical response to CNI-1493. The side-effects were elevation of liver enzymes and phlebitis. The agents in the treatment of CD need further investigation.

Onercept

Onercept, a recombinant, soluble human P^{55} receptor to TNF, is a human protein with a possible mechanism of action through neutralization of soluble TNF [21]. Previous study showed that 12 patients with active CD were randomized to receive onercept at either 11.7 or 50 mg three times weekly for 2 weeks. The results demonstrated that 7 patients had clinical improvement with decreased CDAI scores 6 months after the end of treatment. Further clinical trial was performed and showed that patients with moderate-to-severe acute or chronic active CD were randomized to receive subcutaneous onercept (10, 25, 35, or 50 mg) or placebo 3 times weekly for 8 weeks. The results demonstrate that onercept was well tolerated but was not effective at the doses studied in patients with active CD. The most common adverse events include headache, prutitus, arthralgia, fatigue and influenza-like syndrome. Therefore, the utility of onercept in CD patients has questioned the efficacy of this compound, which has been quitted in clinical trial.

Etanercept

Etanercept is a recombinant product consisting of 2 chains of soluble TNF receptor P^{75} fused to human IgG1. This agent has been approved by the US FDA and used for treatment of rheumatoid arthritis, ankylosing spondylitis and psoriatic arthritis. A subsequent trail in patients with CD has also been done and shown that is safe and well tolerated but not effective for patients with mild-to-moderate CD [22].

Since the slight increased risk of infection and lymphomas is present at anti-TNF therapy, not all CD patients will need or warrant treatment with a biologic. Ideally, clinicians must be able to identify those patients who might benefit the most from early intervention with an anti-TNF agent before they develop complications. Treatment with infliximab, adalimumab, and certolizumab is effective for the induction and maintenance of remission in patients with moderate-to-severe CD. Infliximab and adalimumab have demonstrated efficacy in achieving steroid-free remission. The use of infliximab in lieu of corticosteroids has demonstrated benefit in the steroid-naive patient, serving as a bridge to azathioprine maintenance therapy. This approach does, however, raise concern for future lack of response to the agent. Infliximab and adalimumab have also demonstrated efficacy in the partial and complete closure of fistulas. Infliximab is associated with higher rates of mucosal healing and reduced rates of surgery. Therapy with infliximab and adalimumab is also associated with lower hospitalization rates. All 3 TNF antagonists–infliximab, adalimumab, and certolizumab–are associated with improvements in HRQL. Future long-term prospective studies may document that medical therapy is finally changing the natural history of this disease, allowing more patients to live a healthy and full life.

References

[1] Sartor RB. Mechanisms of disease: pathogenesis of Crohn's disease and ulcerative colitis. *Nat. Clin. Pract. Gastroenterol. Hepatol.* 2006; 3:390407.

[2] Xavier RJ, Podolsky DK. Unravelling the pathogenesis of inflammatory bowel disease. *Nature.* 2007; 448:42734.

[3] Sartor RB. Microbial influences in inflammatory bowel disease. *Gastroenterology.* 2008; 134:57794.

[4] Aggarwal BB. Signaling pathways of the TNF superfamily: a double-edged sword. *Nat. Rev. Immunol.* 2003; 3:745-56.

[5] Rutgeerts P, Van Assche G, Vermeire S. Optimizing anti-TNF treatment in inflammatory bowel disease. *Gastroenterology.* 2004; 126:1593-610.

[6] Pizarro TT, Cominelli F. Cytokine therapy for Crohn's disease: advances in translational research. *Annu. Rev. Med.* 2007; 58:433-44.

[7] Thkral C, Cheifetz A, Peppercorn MA. Anti-tumour necrosis factor therapy for ulcerative colitis. Evidence to date. *Drugs.* 2006; 66:2059-65.

[8] Sandborn WJ, Hanauer SB, Rutgeerts P, et al. Adalimumab for maintenance treatment of Crohn's disease: results of the CLASSIC II trial. *Gut.* 2007; 56:1232-9.

[9] Ho GT, Smith L, Aitken S, et al. The use of adalimumab in the management of refractory Crohn's disease. *Aliment. Pharmacol. Ther.* 2008; 27:308-15.

[10] Osteman MT, Lichtenstein GR. Infliximab in fistulizing Crohn's disease. *Gastroenterol. Clin. North Am.* 2006; 35:795-820.

[11] Thukral C, Cheifetz A, Peppercorn MA. Anti-tumour necrosis factor therapy for ulcerative colitis. *Drugs.* 2006; 66:2059-2065.

[12] Rutgeerts P, Sandborn WJ, Feagan BG, et al. Infliximab for induction and maintenance therapy for ulcerative colitis. *N. Eng. J. Med.* 2005; 353:2462-76.

[13] Blonski W, Lichtenstein GR. Complications of biological therapy for inflammatory bowel disease. *Curr. Opin. Gastroenterol.* 2006; 22:30-43.

[14] CD571, a humanized monoclonal antibody to tomour necrosis factor α, for moderate to severe Crohn's disease: a randomized, double blindm pacebo controlled trial. *Gut.* 2004; 53:1485-93.

[15] Feagan BG, Sandborn WJ, Lichtenstein G, et al. CDP-51, a humanized monoclonal antibody to tomour necrosis factor-α, for steroid-dependent Crohn's disease: a randomized, double-blind, placebo-controlled trial. *Aliment. Pharmacol. Ther.* 2006; 23:617-28.

[16] Schreiber S, Rutgeerts P, Fedorak RN, et al. Aandomized,placebo-controlled trial of certolizumab pegel (CDP870) for treatment of Crohn's disease. *Gastroenterology.* 2005; 129:807-18.

[17] Panaccione R, Sandborn WJ, D'Haens G, et al. Adalimumab maintains long-term remission in moderate to severely active Crohn's disease after infliximab failure: 1-year follow-up of gain trial. *Gastroenterology.* 2008; 134(suppl 1):A133.

[18] panaccione R, Colombel JF, Sandborn WJ, et al. Adalimumab maintains long-term remission in moderately to severely active Crohn's disease through 2 years. *Gastroenterology.* 2008; 134(suppl 1):A134.

[19] Efficacy and safety of thalidomide in children and young adults with intractable inflammatory bowel disease: long-term results. *Aliment. Pharmacol. Ther.* 2007; 25:419-27.

[20] Hommes D, van den Blink B, Plasse T, et al. Inhibition of stress-activated MAP kinases induces clinical improvement in moderate to severe Crohn's disease. *Gastroenterology.* 2002; 122:7-14.

[21] Rutgeerts P, Lemmens L, van Assche G, et al. Treatment of active Crohn's disease with onercept (recombinant human soluble p55 tumour necrosis factor receptor): results of a randomized, open-label, pilot study. *Aliment. Pharmacol. Ther.* 2003; 17:185-92.

[22] Chang JT, Lichtenstein GR. Drug insight: antagonists of tumor-necrosis factor-a in the treatment of inflammatory bowel disease. *Nat. Clin. Pract. Gastroenterol. Hepatol.* 2006; 3:220-8.

Section Six: Disorders That Simulate Idiopathic Colitis: Non-Infections Colitis

In: Inflammatory Conditions of the Colon
Editor: Jia-ju Zheng

ISBN: 978-1-60692-240-8
© 2008 Nova Science Publishers, Inc.

Chapter XXXV

Collagenous and Lymphocytic Colitis

Ping Zheng
The First People's Hospital of Shang-hai Jiao-tong University,
Shang-hai, P.R. China

Collagenous colitis and lymphocytic colitis (collectively known as microscopic colitis) are characterized by chronic diarrhea, normal endoscopic and radiologic findings, and typical findings on histologic examination of colonic tissue [1,2]. The etiology of microscopic colitis is uncertain. Most patients with microscopic colitis are middleaged or older, and there is a distinct female predominance [2,3]. The classic presentation is chronic or intermittent watery diarrhea with or without abdominal pain, weight loss, and other symptoms [1]. Pathologically, microscopic colitis is subdivided into collagenous colitis (characterized by an increase in intraepithelial lymphocytes with a thickened subepithelial collagen band) and lymphocytic colitis (characterized by a marked increase in intraepithelial lymphocytes without a thickened subepithelial collagen band) [1,2]. Population-based studies have reported an annual incidence of collagenous colitis ranging from 1.1 to 5.2 per 100,000 population and of lymphocytic colitis ranging from 3.1 to 4.4 per 100,000 population [1,2-4].

Collagenous Colitis

Collagenous colitis is a clinicopathologic syndrome characterized by: (1) chronic watery diarrhea and crampy abdominal pain, and (2) distinctive colorectal histopathology that includes a subepithelial collagen band, prominent chronic inflammation in the lamina propria, and increased intraepithelial lymphocytes [3-5].

This disease is found mainly in "Western" countries in Europe, Australia, and North America, but cases have been reported from around the world, including Africa [2]. The cause of collagenous colitis is unknown [1,2]. Hypotheses for the etiology of collagenous colitis include: (1) immune dysregulation, (2) abnormalities in pericryptal fibroblasts, (3) intraluminal bacterial agents or toxins, and (4) drug-induced damage.

Collagenous colitis is a disease primarily of women with a female to male ratio of 9:1 in recent Swedish studies [2,3-5]. This disorder is seen primarily in middle-aged patients in their 50s and 60s. Chronic watery diarrhea is the main symptom and in most patients have been present months to years [3-5]. Nocturnal diarrhea is not uncommon. The patients often also have crampy diffuse abdominal pain, symptoms which cause misdiagnosis with irritable bowel syndrome. Enteropathic arthritis is seen in approximately 7% of collagenous colitis patients, with the arthritis being seronegative for rheumatoid factor and nondestructive. A variety of other immunologic disorders have been noted in this patient population, with of patients having coexistent autoimmune illnesses. Routine laboratory studies are usually normal. However, antineutrophilic cytoplasmic antibodies have been described. Importantly, gastrointestinal radiographic and endoscopic examinations usually show normal mucosa. Thus, it is essential for clinicians to biopsy grossly normal mucosa to establish this diagnosis.

As the name implies, there are two main histologic components to collagenous colitis: (1) increased collagen deposition and (2) colitis. In normal colon, a delicate basement membrane is visible just beneath the lumenal epithelium, measuring less than 3 um in thickness [3-5]. In collagenous colitis, there is abnormal deposition of collagen immediately beneath the basement membrane. By immunohistochemical staining, this band contains collagens type I, III, and VI as well as tenascin.

Lymphocytic Colitis

Lymphocytic colitis has similar clinical features to collagenous colitis [1,5,6]. Watery diarrhea is the main symptom with most individual also noting a mild, intermittent, crampy abdominal pain [1,2]. Most patients are middle-aged, but in contrast to collagenous colitis, there is less of a gender gap, with a female:male ratio of 2.4:1 [2,6]. The incidence of lymphocytic colitis is reported as 5.7/100,00 individuals, in Sweden from 1996 to 1998 [1,2]. Routine hematologic tests are usually normal. Some patients have increased titers of antinuclear antibodies, antiparietal cell antibodies, and antimicrosomal antibodies. Lymphocytic colitis patients have an increased frequency of HLA A1 and of a diminished frequency of HLA A3 compared with controls [2,4-6].

The main histologic feature of lymphocytic colitis is increased intraepithelial lymphocytes [1,6]. In a normal colon, the number of intraepithelial lymphocytes (IELs) is approximately 5 per 100 epithelial cells, whereas in lymphocytic colitis, the median number of IELs is 30 lymphocytes per 100 epithelial cells (range 10 to 50).

References

[1]   Olesen M, Eriksson S, Bohr J, et al. Lymphocytic colitis: a retrospective clinical study of 199 Swedish patients. *Gut.* 2004; 53:536-541.

[2] Fernandez-Banares F, Salas A, Forne M, et al. Incidence of collagenous and lymphocytic colitis: a 5-year population-based study. *Am. J. Gastroenterol.* 1999; 92:418-4 23.

[3] Agnarsdottir M, Gunnlaugsson O, Orvar KB, et al. Collagenous and lymphocytic colitis in Iceland. *Dig. Dis. Sci.* 2002; 47:1122-1128.

[4] Lazenby AJ. Collagenous and lymphocytic colitis. *Semin. Diagn. Pathol.* 2005 22:295-300

[5] Nilesh C, David K D, Richard P E R. Collagenous colitis and lymphocytic colitis: Patient characteristics and clinical presentation. *Scand. J. Gastroenterol.* 2005; 40: 343-347

[6] Pardi DS, Ramnath VR, Loftus EV, et al. Sandborn WJ. Lymphocytic colitis: clinical features, treatment, and outcomes. *Am. J. Gastroenterol.* 2002; 97:2829-2833.

In: Inflammatory Conditions of the Colon
Editor: Jia-ju Zheng

ISBN: 978-1-60692-240-8
© 2008 Nova Science Publishers, Inc.

Chapter XXXVI

Colonic Ischemia

Long-dian Chen
Department of Digestive Disease, Drum Tower Hospital, affiliated with
Nan-jing University Medical School, Jiang-su Province,
P.R. China

Introduction

Mesenteric ischemia is caused by a reduction in intestinal blood flow, which most commonly arises from occlusion, vasospasm, and/or hypoperfusion of the mesenteric vasculature.

Ischemic colitis (IC) is the most frequent form of mesenteric ischemia, affecting mostly the elderly [1].

The majority of patients (85 percent) develop non-gangrenous ischemia, which is usually transient and resolves without sequelae [2]. Only a minority of these patients develop long-term complications, which include persistent segmental colitis and the development of a stricture. On the other hand, approximately 15 percent of patients with colonic ischemia develop gangrene, the consequences of which are life-threatening.

Nonocclusive colonic ischemia. It is most commonly affects the "watershed" areas of the colon that have limited collateralization, such as the splenic flexure and rectosigmoid junction [3,4].

A study of more than 1000 patients with IC demonstrated that the left colon was involved in approximately 75 persent of patients, with about one-quarter of lesions affecting the splenic flexure [5]. The rectum was involved in only 5 percent of patients.

Situations associated with IC include (table 36-1): Aortoiliac surgery, Cardiopulmonary bypass, Myocardial infarction, Hemodialysis, Mesenteric vein thrombosis and Cardiac embolism.

Several drugs have been implicated in the development of colonic ischemia. alosetron, a synthetic 5-HT3 antagonist association with ischemic colitis. Tegaserod, a 5-HT4 partial agonist has also been associated with a few cases of ischemic colitis.

Table 36-1. Causes of colonic ischemia

Classification	Causes
1. non-inflammation associated cardiovascular disorders	inferior mesenteric artery thrombosis
	arterial embolus
	cholesterol emboli
	cardiac failure or arrhythmias
	shock
	pheochromocytoma
	volvulus
	strangulated hernia
	amyloidosis
	pancreatitis
2. vasculitis	systemic lupus erythematosus
	polyarteritis nodosa
	rheumatoid vasculitis
	buerger's disease
	takayasu's arthritis
	kawasaki's disease
3. hematologic disorders and coagulopathies	sickel cell disease
	polycythemia vera
	parocysmal nocturnal hemoglobinuria
	protein C and S deficiency
	antithrombin deficiency
	activated protein C resistance
	prothronbin 20210A mutation
4. infections	parasites (angiostrogylus costaricensis)
	bacteria (escherichia coli O157;H7)
	viruses (hepatitis B, cytomegalovirus)
5. iatrogenic causes	a. surgical
	aneurysmectomy
	aortoiliac reconstruction
	gynecological operations
	exchange transfusions
	colon bypass
	lumbar aortography
	colectomy with inferior mesenteric artery
	colonoscopy and barium enema examination
	b. medications and drugs
	digitalis
	estrogens
	progestins
	danazol
	vasopressin
	pseudoephedrine
	phenylephrine
	sumatriptan
	methamphetamine
	ergot
	gold
	psychotropic drugs
	nonsteroidal anti-inflammatory drugs

Classification	causes
	oral saline laxatives
	golytely
	glycerin enema
	interferon-α
	flutamine
	penicillin
	immunosuppressive agents
	alosetron
	pit viper toxin
	cocain
6. allergy (some seefood)	
7. trauma, blunt or penetrating	
8. raptured ectopic pregnancy	
9. competitive long-distance running	

Extreme exercise (as occurs in marathon running or triathlon competition) has been associated with intestinal ischemia.

Acquired and hereditary thrombotic conditions also are possible that specific types of thrombophilic disorders may predispose to particular forms of colonic ischemia such as chronic ischemic colitis and stricture formation. Younger patients and those with recurrent colonic ischemia may be reasonable candidates.

Park et al. performed a study of a total of 467 patients who underwent sigmoidoscopy or colonoscopy because of lower abdominal discomforts with or without blood in stool were consecutively enrolled; 147 patients were diagnosed endoscopically and histologically as having ischemic colitis; they found that old age, hemodialysis, hypertension, diabetes mellitus, hypoalbuminemia, and constipation-inducing medications are clinically important risk factors for ischemic colitis in patients experiencing lower abdominal discomfort with or without bloody stool [6]. In any personal experiences of the 84 cases of ischemic colitis in recent two years, I also found that most of these cases were associated with basic diseases including hypertension, cardiovascular disorders, diabetes mellitus and hematological diseases as well as a history of abdominal operation. These data are well consistent with a number of clinical analysis in Chinese populations [7-9].

Clinical Features

Patients with acute colonic ischemia usually present with rapid onset of mild abdominal pain and tenderness over the affected bowel, most often involving the left side. Mild to moderate amounts of rectal bleeding or bloody diarrhea usually develops within 24 hours of the onset of abdominal pain. Several features distinguish colonic ischemia from acute mesenteric ischemia involving the small bowel. In particular, the pain that accompanies colonic ischemia usually is not as severe, is felt laterally rather than periumbilically, and often is associated with hematochezia. three progressive clinical stages have been described. Hyperactive phase: Soon after occlusion or hypoperfusion, severe pain dominates with frequent passage of bloody, loose stools. Blood loss is usually mild without the need for transfusion. More than 80 percent of all patients with colonic ischemia show only mucosal and submucosal injury, symptoms resolved with conservative measures, and no long-term sequelae. Paralytic phase: The pain usually diminishes, becomes more continuous, and diffuses. The abdomen becomes more tender and distended without bowel sounds. Shock phase: Massive fluid, protein, and electrolytes start to leak through a damaged, gangrenous mucosa. Severe dehydration with shock and metabolic acidosis may develop, requiring rapid surgical intervention. Fortunately, this most severe form affects only 10 to 20 percent of patients.

Diagnosis

The diagnosis is usually established based upon the clinical setting, physical examination, and radiological and/or endoscopic studies. Invasive studies such as angiography or laparoscopy are rarely needed but may be valuable when the diagnosis is unclear or as a means to follow patients after surgery for ischemia. Magnetic resonance angiography and Duplex sonography are more recently introduced vascular studies to assess patients with suspected proximal arterial mesenteric vessel or mesenteric venous disease, but are hardly ever required in the evaluation of suspected colonic ischemia. The differential diagnosis includes infectious colitis, inflammatory bowel disease, diverticulitis, radiation enteritis, solitary rectal ulcer syndrome, and colon carcinoma. Clostridium difficile infection produces marked thickening of the colon on CT scan as well as very high total white blood counts which resemble the findings of ischemic colitis. However, bloody stools are quite rare in C difficile infection.

There are no specific laboratory markers for ischemia, although an increased serum lactate, LDH, CPK, or amylase may indicate advanced tissue damage. White blood count above 20,000 µL and metabolic acidosis in a patient with signs and symptoms of acute colitis are highly suggestive of intestinal ischemia with infarction.

A plain abdominal x-ray is frequently non-specific. Distension or pneumatosisare typically seen only in advanced ischemia. In one series of 23 cases, specific signs such as thumbprinting (indicating submucosal edema) and hemorrhage could be identified in only 30 percent of patients with mesenteric infarction [10]. Typical findings of CT scan are thickening of the bowel wall in a segmental pattern. Pneumatosis and gas in the mesenteric veins may be seen in the more advanced stages. CT findings are generally nonspecific and scans may initially be norma.

Endoscopic and Histologic Features

Colonoscopy can be considered and there is no clinical or radiologic evidence of peritonitis or perforation. Over distention and associated high intraluminal colonic pressures should be avoided during colonoscopy since they may worsen ischemic damage. Colonoscopic findings in the acute setting frequently include pale mucosa with petechial bleeding. Bluish hemorrhagic nodules may be seen representing submucosal bleeding; these are the equivalent to "thumbprints" detected on radiological studies. More severe disease is marked by cyanotic mucosa and hemorrhagic ulcerations. Segmental distribution, abrupt transition between injured and non-injured mucosa, rectal sparing, and rapid resolution on serial endoscopy favor ischemia rather than inflammatory bowel disease (figure 36-1a and b). A single linear ulcer running along the longitudinal axis of the colon (the "single-stripe sign") may also favor an ischemic cause of colitis [11]. Biopsies taken from affected areas may show non-specific changes such as hemorrhage, crypt destruction, capillary thrombosis, granulation tissue with crypt abscesses, and pseudopolyps, which may mimic Crohn's disease [12]. In the chronic phase of ischemic colitis, mucosal atrophy and areas of granulation tissue may be found. Biopsy of a post-ischemic stricture is marked by extensive transmural fibrosis and mucosal atrophy.

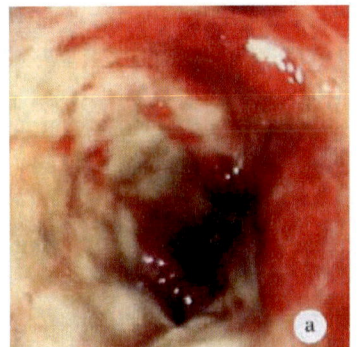 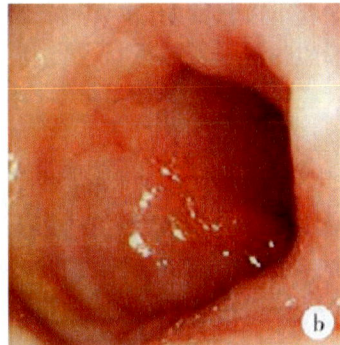

Figure 36-1. Endoscopic features of ischemic colitis: a. diffused inflammation in active stage, which can be easily confused with ulcerative colitis; b. inflammation in resolving; luminal stricture is indicated.

Treatment

Nonocclusive ischemia — Supportive care is appropriate in the absence of colonic gangrene or perforation. Intravenous fluids should be given to ensure adequate colonic perfusion, and patients should be placed on bowel rest. Empiric broad spectrum antibiotics are recommended in moderate to severe cases. A nasogastric tube should be inserted if an ileus is present. Any medications that can promote ischemia should be withheld promptly. Cardiac function and oxygenation should be optimized. Careful monitoring for persistent fever, leukocytosis, peritoneal irritation, protracted diarrhea, and bleeding is imperative. If clinical deterioration is evident despite conservative therapy, laparotomy and segmental resection are indicated.

Colonic infarction — Colonic infarction develops as a consequence of severe hypoperfusion leading to transmural necrosis of the bowel wall, which can progress to sepsis, peritonitis, free intraabdominal air, or extensive gangrene. Such patients require urgent surgical intervention. As a general rule, the bowel should not be cleansed in preparation for surgery, because bowel preparations can precipitate perforation or toxic dilatation of the colon.

Mesenteric vein thrombosis —treatment should include evaluation for hypercoagulability and may include anticoagulant therapy. and do not have a contraindication to anticoagulation should be anticoagulated with warfarin for three to six months or for life if there is a hypercoagulable state or cardiac source. Thrombectomy and thrombolysis have been described in the acute setting, but experience is limited.

Most patients with nonocclusive ischemia improve within one or two days, and have complete clinical and radiological resolution within one to two weeks. More severe ischemia causes ulceration and inflammation, which may develop into segmental ulcerating colitis or strictures. These lesions may be asymptomatic, but they should be followed to document healing or the development of persistent colitis or stricture. The prognosis may be worse in patients who have peripheral vascular disease or right colonic involvement [13].

As a general rule, non-gangrenous colonic ischemia is associated with a low mortality (approximately 6 percent), in contrast to gangrenous ischemia, which is associated with a mortality as high as 50 to 75 percent with surgical resection and is almost always fatal if treated conservatively.

It has been reported that, in comparison with control rats, intravenous administration of sodium ferulate (an active component of traditional Chinese Medicine with enhancing bleed circulation effect) given 40-80 mg·kg^{-1} significantly ameliorates ischemic colitis injury in rats, which is associated with inhibition of endothlin-1 and malonyl dialdehyde generation tumor necrosis factor-α and intercellular adhesion moleche-1 expression in colonic mucosa [14].

References

[1] Higgins, PD, Davis, KJ, Laine, L. Systematic review: the epidemiology of ischaemic colitis. *Aliment. Pharmacol. Ther.* 2004; 19:729.
[2] Greenwald, DA, Brandt, LJ. Colonic ischemia. *J. Clin. Gastroenterol.* 1998; 27:122.
[3] Gandhi, SK, Hanson, MM, Vernava, AM, et al. Ischemic colitis. *Dis. Colon. Rectum.* 1996; 39:88.
[4] Greenwald, DA, Brandt, LJ, Reinus, JF. Ischemic bowel disease in the elderly. *Gastroenterol. Clin. North Am.* 2001; 30:445.
[5] Reeders, JW, Tytgat, GN, Rosenbusch, G, et al. Ischaemic colitis. Martinus Nijhoff, The Hague 1984. p.17.
[6] Park CJ, Jang MK, Shin WG, et al. Can we predict the development of ischemic colitis among patients with lower abdominal pain? *Dis. Colon Rectum.* February 1, 2007; 50(2): 232-8.
[7] Chao G-q, Lü B, Fan Y-h. Clinical analysis of ischemic colitis in 36 patients. *Chin. J. Gastroenterol.* 2007; 12(10):585-588 (Chinese).
[8] Yang X-s, Lü Y-m, Yu C-f, et al. Clinical features, endoscopic findings and outcome of ischemic colitis. *Chin. J. Dig. Dis.* 2002; 22(5):282-284 (Chinese).
[9] Ou X-l, Shun W-h, Cao D-z, et al. Ischemic colitis: an analysis of 52 cases. *Chin. J. Dig. Endosc.* 2008; 25(3):155-156 (Chinese).

[10] Smerud, MJ, Johnson, CD, Stephens, DH. Diagnosis of bowel infarction: A comparison of plain films and CT scans in 23 cases. *AJR. Am. J. Roentgenol.* 1990; 154:99.

[11] Zuckerman, GR, Prakash, C, Merriman, RB, et al. The colon single-stripe sign and its relationship to ischemic colitis. *Am. J. Gastroenterol.* 2003;98:2018.

[12] Mitsudo, S, Brandt, LJ. Pathology of intestinal ischemia. *Surg. Clin. North Am.* 1992; 72:43.

[13] Medina, C, Vilaseca, J, Videla, S, et al. Outcome of patients with ischemic colitis: review of fifty-three cases. *Dis. Colon Rectum.* 2004; 47:180.

[14] Liu Y, Wu B-y, Guo Y, et al. Effect of sodium ferulate on ischemic colitis in rats. *Chin. J. New Drugs.* 2007;16(24):2024-2026 (Chinese).

Chapter XXXVII

Eosinophilic Colitis

Ming Zhang
Drum Tower Hospital Affiliated, Nan-jing University Medical School,
Jiang-su Province, P.R. China

Definition and Etiology

Eosinophilic colitis (EC) is a relatively uncommon and benign entity of eosinophilic gastroenteritis, and was first described by Kaijser in 1937 [1]. There are no precise data on the incidence or prevalence of it and no predominance between the two genders. It is most often occurred during adolescence or early adulthood, and the typical symptoms are diarrhea, abdominal distension, periumbilical pain, anorexia, vomiting, and weight loss [2].

Eosinophilic colitis, with unknown etiology, may be idiopathic or due to allergies to foods (in allergic proctitis, most common in children, usually is due to allergy to cow's milk, soy protein or boty), drugs (5-ASA, Clozapine, carbamazepine), parasites (dog hookworm, herring worm, whipworm) or hypereosinophilic syndrome, leukemia, or systemic vasculitis [3]. Recently, evidence supports the idea that EC develops as a result of an interaction between genetic and environmental factors. Approximately 10% of patients with EC have a close family member who suffers from the same disorder and approximately 50% of patients have an atopic disease [4]. And it has been reported EC associated with rheumatoid arthritis and connective tissue diseases including scleroderma and dermatomyositis [5].

Histologica and Endoscopic Features

In contrast to the normal colon, which contains only a few eosinophils, the colon of patients with EC is defined by pure or dominamt eosinophilic infiltrates, usually without crypt destruction. In addition to the mucosal and submucosal areas, the eosinophilic infiltration can be deep, affecting the muscularis propria or even the serosa [6]. The distinction between EC and other colitis is somewhat arbitrary and there is no exact cutoff point proposed in the literature, but the predominance of eosinophils over other inflammatory cells maybe helpful in the differentiation of EC from other causes of eosinophilic infiltration.

Endoscopic appearances vary from normal to nonspecific inflammatory changes. On endoscope a nodular pattern or patchy distribution of the disease along the mucosa is seen. Typically, mucosal granularity, friability, nodularity, patchy erythema, and mucosal ulcerations are observed in only a minority of patients. For this reason, diagnosis can be missed and panendoscopic examination and multiple biopsies are suggested. The intervening mucosa was endoscopically normal. Crypt abscesses were not present, but sporadic cryptitis was seen. In patients with chronic idiopathic inflammatory bowel disease (IBD) experiencing a clinical flare of disease, prominent eosinophilic infiltrates in otherwise mildly active or inactive colitis should raise the possibility of an allergic reaction to therapeutic drugs.

Clinical Manifestations

Almost very part of the colon could be affected, and the cecum and ascending colon are the most common sites of involvement in the large bowel. The clinical manifestations of EC are similar to those found in most colon diseases, which including: abdominal pain (acute or chronic), altered bowel evacuation habit (diarrhea, constipation or both), nausea, vomiting, weight loss, palpable mass, bleeding, abdominal distention, ascites, ileus, perforation or severe perianal disease. As for individual the major manifestations are related to the location, extension and depth of eosinophilic infiltration of the bowel wall. Extra-colonic symptoms, such as iron-deficiency anemia, pruritic erythematous papules and urticaria, also can be seen in some EC patients and those symptoms can occur concurrently or subsequently with the colonic symptoms. In some rare cases it can be asymptomatic.

Diagnosis and Treatment

Even though diagnostic reliability has been improved, EC are also often misdiagnosed because of its rarity, the nonspecific clinical manifestations and lab data and difficult radiologic interpretations. In some cases it can be misdiagnosed as colon cancer, inflammatory bowel disease, acute appendicitis, allergy or colon, small-bowel obstruction, cecal volvulus and so on [7,8].

Tissue eosinophilia, without granuloma and subtotal villous atrophy, is a universal feature of EC. While eosinophils are a recognized feature in numerous gastrointestinal conditions, such as benign and malignant tumors, inflammatory bowel diseases, peptic ulcer diseases, granulomatous polyps, amoebiasis and other enteroinvasive parasites, milk protein induced colitis and the systemic hypereosinophilic syndromes. Histologically, the whole thickness of the bowel could be involved, which mimic the histological feature of Crohn's disease. It was reported that some UC maybe misdiagnosed as EC at the early stage of the disease because of the mass eosinophilic infiltration in the colon mucosa [9], the degree of which has been suggested as a possible differentiating factor between EC and IBD.

Colonoscopy will probably turn out to be one of the most useful tools in diagnosing EC and, in turn, monitoring its follow-up.

Peripheral eosinophilia may be of value in diagnosis, but this is not universal. It was reported that about 25 percent of cases had a normal eosinophil count and the initial eosinophil count did not appear to indicate either the severity of the disease or the prognosis. Thus peripheral eosinophilia is not a satisfactory diagnostic tool. In some cases the level of IgE in serum and ascitic may provide some diagnostic clues.

No radiologic appearance is specific enough for precise diagnosis. Typically, the radiologic findings are: strictures, thickening of the bowel wall and mucosal folds, a rigid ileocecal valve open to reflux, and ulcerative and polypoidal lesions. The rigidity of the ileocecal valve has also been suggested as a differentiating factor between EC and Crohn's disease.

Steroids could lead to prompt clinical improvement rapidly and have been proposed as the best form of treatment once the diagnosis has been established; however steroid resistance has been reported in some cases. "Diagnostic treatment" by steroid is not recommended in suspected cases, for some other diseases (such as malignant tumors) could be misdiagnosed as EC.

Ketotifen is a benzocycloheptathiophene derivative which has been used in the place of sodium cromoglycate for the treatment of severe asthma. In a patient with severe osteoporosis, it was reported that ketotifen maybe effective. And even discontinue using of ketotifen one year later the patient free of the initial symptoms [10,11]. Other choices for the treatment of EC included hydroxyurea, cyclosporine, etoposide, vincristine, cyclophosphamide, metronidazole and IFN-a. Dietary elimination of provocative foodstuffs has been tried in some cases but is ineffective.

References

[1] Kaijser R. Zur kennt nis der allergischen affektionen des verdauungskanals yore standpunkt des chirurgen aus. *Arch. Klin. Chir.* 1937; 188:36-74.

[2] Khan S. Eosinophilic gastroenteritis. *Best Pract. Res. Clin. Gastroenterol.* 2005; 19(2): 177–98.

[3] Wang L-j Zhu F, Qian J-m. Eosinophic gastroenteritis and hypereosiniphilic syndrome. *Chin. J. Dig. Dis.* 2003; 23(8):455-7 (Chinese).

[4] Gonsalves N. Food allergies and eosinophilic gastrointestinal illness. *Gastroenterol. Clin. North Am.* 2007; 36(1):75-91.

[5] Khan S, Orenstein SR. Eosinophilic gastroenteritis: epidemiology, diagnosis and management. *Paediatr. Drugs.* 2002; 4(9):563-70.

[6] Carpenter HA, Talley NJ. The importance of clinicopathological correlation in the diagnosis of inflammatory conditions of the colon: histological patterns with clinical implications. *Am. J. Gastroenterol.* 2000; 95 (4):878-96.

[7] Lim K, Black R. Eosinophilic colitis masquerading as colonic cancer. *Aust. N.Z. J. Surg.* 2000; 70: 682–4.

[8] Velchuru VR, Khan MA, Hellquist HB, et al. Eosinophilic colitis. *J. Gastrointest. Surg.* 2007;11(10):1373-5.

[9] Uzunismail H, Hatemi I, Doğusoy G, et al. Dense eosinophilic infiltration of the mucosa preceding ulcerative colitis and mimicking eosinophilic colitis: Report of two cases. *Turk J. Gastroenterol.* 2006;17(1):53-7

[10] Katsinelos P, Pilpilidis I, Xiarchos P, et al. Oral administration of ketotifen in a patient with eosinophilic colitis and severe osteoporosis. *Am. J. Gastroenterol.* 2002; 97(4):1072-4.

[11] Moore D, Lichtman S, Lentz J, et al. Eosinophilic gastroenteritis presenting in an adolescent with isolated colonic involvement. *Gut.* 1986; 27(10):1219-22.

In: Inflammatory Conditions of the Colon
Editor: Jia-ju Zheng

ISBN: 978-1-60692-240-8
© 2008 Nova Science Publishers, Inc.

Chapter XXXVIII

Behcet's Disease and Tangier Disease

Fu-xing Xu
Hua-dong Hospital, Fu-dan University, Shang-hai, P.R. China

Behcet's Disease

The disease, a chronic and multisystemic vasculitis that may involve the small bowel with pathology closely resembling Crohn's disease (CD), is associated with oral ulcers, iridocyclitis, arthritis, erythema nodosum, and thrombophlebitis [1]. In Behcet's disease, however, ocular symptoms and painful ulcerations of the mouth and genitalia usually dominate the clinical picture, whereas bowel complaints are less prominent [1-2].

Whenever systemic vasculitis is considered in a differential diagnosis of ileitis, it is important to remember that idiopathic (primary) inflammatory bowel disease (ulcerative colitis or Crohn's colitis) may give rise to a secondary vasculitis, and the clinical histories generally indicate that the bowel disease was pre-existing [1].

Involvement of the esophagus includes ulcer, varices, and perforation. The intestinal ulcers are predominantly ileocecal and often involve the colon segmentally.

The rate of postoperative recurrence of these ulcers is high [1].Intestinal ulcerations may perforate and bleed. In endoscopic appearance, it can be strikingly similar to CD. Although some lesions respond to corticosteroid therapy, the effects are often transient and inconsistent [1].

Tangier Disease

The disease is an autosomal-recessive disorder characterized by accumulation of cholesterol esters in macrophages in tonsils, thymus, lymph nodes, marrow, liver and the gut [3]. .

They have very low levels of plasma cholesterol and high density lipoproteins (HDLs), owing to a lack of apolipoprotein A I and A II. The striking clinical findings include yellow-orange and enlarged tonsil in 80% of cases, hepatosplenomegaly, and peripheral neuropathy. Patients may have diarrhea without steatorrhea.

Colonoscopy reveals orange-brown mucosal "spots" throughout the colon and rectum, and laparoscopy reveals similar yellow patches on the surface of the liver due to cholesterol esters in hepatic reticuloendothelial cells [3].

References

[1] Kanabata H, Miyata M, Kanaguchi Y et al. Intestinal Behcet's disease with an esophageal ulcer. *Gastrointestin. Edosc.* 2003; 58:151-154

[2] Morita H, Kawai S , Kobori O et al. Incomplete form of Behcet's colitis in Japan ,is it a distinct entity?(letter) *Am. J. Gastroenteral.* 1995; 90:523

[3] Frosini G, Marini M, Gaglgan P et al. Tangier disease: an unusual diagnosis for the endoscopist, *Endoscopy.* 1994; 26:373

Chapter XXXIX

Radiation Colitis

Ping Xiang
Hua-dong Hospital, Fu-dan University, Shang-hai, P.R. China

Definition

Injury of rectal and distal colon due to radiotherapy of intrapelvic, intraperitioneal and retroperitoeal tumors is termed radiation colitis, whereas the proximal colon and small bowel are rarely injured [1].

Clinical and Endoscopic Feature

Acute radiation colitis occurs a few days after radiotherapy, most patients complain of transient diarrhea and tenesmus, but bloody diarrhea is uncommon at this time point [2]. The endoscopic picture is similar to that of ulcerative colitis, with mucosal edema, fragility, hemorrhage, and some erosions or ulcers (figure 39-1). The clinical manifestation of chronic radiation colitis usually occurs 1-2 years after radiation. Pale mucosa with telangiectasia and rarefaction of mucosal vessels is typical in the mild forms endoscopically. In severe radiation colitis, excessive hemorrhage, necrosis, and ulcerations occur, lead to extensive bleeding, perforation fistula formation and stenosis of colon lumen (figure 39-1).

Endoscopic Classification

Sherman classification of endoscope [2,3]: Degree I: limited or extensive hyperemia of mucosa, telangiectasia, frailty of tissue, bleeding tendency, with erosion but no ulceration. Degree II: ulcer formation, round or irregular in shape, grey-whitish mossy crust or necrosis in the surface, flat in margin. Degree III: former variations plus stenosis of colon lumen.

Degree IV: complicated with fistula, usually vaginarectal fistula, and perforation occasionally.

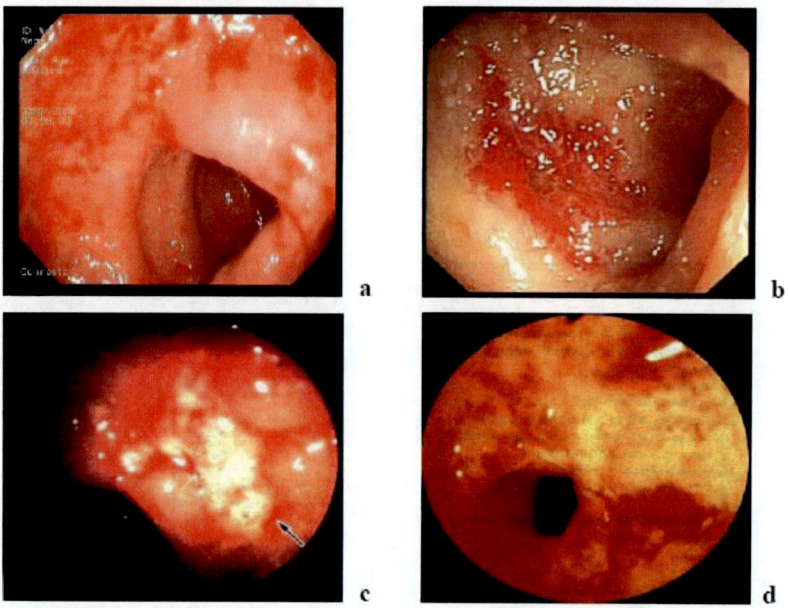

Figure 39-1. Radiation colitis showing mucosal edema (a), erosion (b), ulceration (c), and stenosis (d).

References

[1] LeupinN, Curschmann J, Kranzbuhler H et al. Acute radiation colitis in patients treated with short-term preoperative radiotherapy for rectal cancer. *Am. J. Surg. Pathol.* 2002;26(4): 498-504

[2] Jahraus CD, Bettenhausen D, Malid U et al. Prevention of acute radiation-induced proctosigmoiditis by balsalazide: a randomized, double-blind, placebo controlled trial in prostate cancer patients. *Int. J. Radiat. Oncol. Biol. Phys.* 2005 1; 63(5): 1483-1487

[3] Fajardo LF. The pathology of ionzing radiation as defined by morphologic patterns. *Acta Oncol.* 2005; 44(1): 13-22

[4] Nagar AB. Isolated colonic ulcers: diagnosis and management. *Curr. Gastroenterol. Rep.* 2007 Oct;9(5):422-8.

In: Inflammatory Conditions of the Colon
Editor: Jia-ju Zheng

ISBN: 978-1-60692-240-8
© 2008 Nova Science Publishers, Inc.

Chapter XL

Portal Hypertensive Colopathy

Ping Xiang
Hua-dong Hospital, Fu-dan University, Shang-hai, P.R. China

Definition

Portal hypertensive colopathy (PHC) is defined as colitis-like abnormalities and/or vascular lesions [1].

Endoscopic Features

PHC has a characteristic endoscopic appearance of edema, erythemas, cherry red spots, diffuse hyperemia, spider angiomas, telangiectasia, angiodysplasia and anorectal varices [2,3]. Telangiectasia is defined as hyperemia, engorgement and tortuosity and of small vessels in the mucosal area of the colon [4]. Angiodysplasia, usually locates on colonic mucosa, has a fur-ball appearance and a diameter approximately 1cm with a feeding vessel. Cherry red spots are sparse, clear red hyperemia spots on mucosa surrounded with normal mucosa. Anorectal varices appear bluish or gray distended, tortuous, extending into the rectum. Prominent vessels lose their normal pattern. Vascular ectasia is classified into two types: type1, solitary vascular ectasia; and type 2, diffuse vascular ectasia.

PHC is classified into three levels [2,3]: Degree I: erythemas and telangiectasias; Degree II: erythemas, telangiectasias, and angiodysplasias; and Degree III: erythemas telangiectasias, angiodysplasias, cherry red spots, and rectal varices.

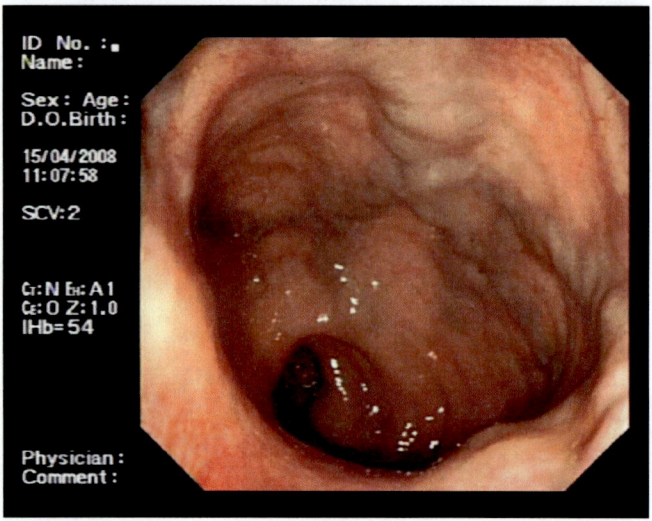

Figure 40-1. Portal hypertension.

References

[1] Ito K, Shiraki K, Sakai T et al. Portal hypertensive colopathy in patients with liver cirr,hosis. *World J. Gastroenterol.* 2005 28; 11(20): 3127-3130
[2] Misra SP, Dwivedi M, Misra V et al. Colonic changes in patients with cirrhosis and in patients with extrahepatic portal vein obstruction. *Endoscopy.* 2005; 37(5): 454-459
[3] Justo CR, Brandt CT, Lucena MT et al. Effect of splenectomy and ligature of the left gastric vein on portal hypertensive colopathy in carriers of surgical hepatosplenic schistosomiasis mansoni. *Acta Cir. Bras.* 2005; 20(1): 9-14
[4] Miranda MA, Domingues AL, Dias HS et al. Hypertensive portal colopathy in schistosomiasis mensoni-proposal for a classification. *Men Inst. Oswaldo Cruz.* 2004; 99(5 Suppl 1): 67-71
[5] Bresci G, Parisi G, Capria A. Clinical relevance of colonic lesions in cirrhotic patients with portal hypertension. *Endoscopy.* 2006; 38(8): 830-835

Chapter XLI

Solitary Rectal Ulcer Syndrome

Ping Xiang
Hua-dong Hospital, Fu-dan University, Shang-hai, P.R. China

Definition

Solitary Rectal Ulcer syndrome (SRUS) is rare disorder; the pathogenesis is likely to vary in different patients [1]. SURS is a rectal inflammatory disorder, which is characterized by a combination of symptoms including rectal bleeding, disordered defecation and anal pain, endoscopic evidence of benign rectal lesion that has a characteristic histological appearance, and in patients that are often less than 50 years of age. It has been noted recently that the term "solitary rectal ulcer" is a misnomer because only one fourth of the patients with SRUS have true rectal ulcer.

Endoscopic Features

The lesion may appear endoscopically as erythema, single ulcer, multiple ulcers or polypoid lesion [2,3]. Ulcers usually locate on the anterior rectal wall approximately 6 to 10 cm from the anal verge (68%-95% of cases), but also locate on the other places, such as posterior rectal wall. Some ulcer may extend around rectum very quickly to cause a circumferential stricture. In some cases, only rectal polypoid lesions are present. It was reported that prevalence of ulceration was 57%-64.3%, of polypoid lesions 25-32.1% and of patches of hyperaemic mucosa in 18% of patients. In addition, rectal lesion may not be consistent with clinical feature of SRUS.

Diagnosis and Treatment

The diagnosis is confirmed by colonscopy and histological examination, which demonstrates fibrosis of the lamina propria and distortion and hypertrophy of the muscular mucosa [4]. The colonic crypts are decreased in number, and may show architectural distortion [5]. A neutrophilic infiltration is present. In clinical practice, the lesions are often confused with adenomas, but no dysplastic tissue is present. Medical treatment is the mainstay of management [6-8]. Intake of high dietary fiber food and regulation of bowel movement may ameliorate symptoms and prevent frequent onset of symptoms. Metronidazole is effective if infection exists. Ulcer can be relapsed after surgery.

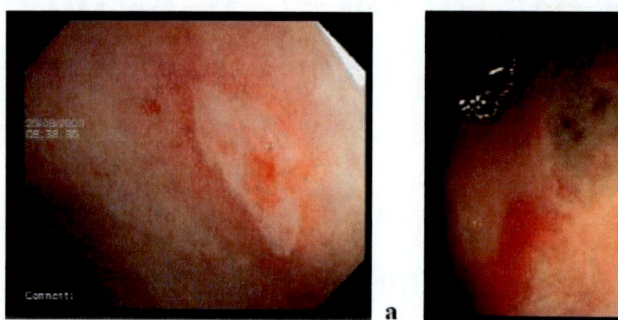

Figure 41-1. Rndoscopic images of solitary rectal ulcer syndrome before (a) and after (b) treatment.

References

[1] Perrakis E, Vezakis A, Velimezis G et al. Solitary rectal ulcer mimicking a malignant stricture. A Case Report. *Rom. J. Gastroenterol.* 2005; 14(3): 289-291

[2] Chong VH, Jalihal A. Solitary rectal ulcer syndrome: characteristics, outcomes and predictive profiles for persisitent bleeding per rectum. *Singapore Med. J.* 2006;47(12): 1063-1068

[3] Uza N, Nakase H, Nishimura k et al. Solitary ulcer syndrome associated with ulcerative colitis. *Gastrointest. Endosc.* 2006;63(2):335-356

[4] Shaara AL, Azar C, Amr SS et al. Solitary rectal ulcer syndrome endoscopic septum and review of the literature. *Gastrointest. Endosc.* 2005 Nov;62(5): 755-762

[5] Singh B, Mortensen MJ, Warren BF. Histopathological mimicry in mucosal prolapsed. *Histopathology.* 2007; 50(1): 97-102

[6] Torres C, Khaikin M, Bracho J et al. Solitary rectal ulcer syndrome: clinical findings, surgical treatment, and outcomes. *Int. J. Colorectal Dis.* 2007 Nov; 22(11):1389-93.

[7] Keshtgar AS. Solitary rectal ulcer syndrome in children. *Eur. J. Gastroenterol. Hepatol.* 2008 Feb;20(2):89-92.

[8] Li N, Gao K, Ma Q-z, et al. Solitary rectal ulcer syndrome: one case study. *Chin. J. Dig. Endosc.* 2008;25(2):109-110 (Chinese).

Chapter XLII

Diverticula-Associated Colitis

Fu-xing Xu
Hua-dong Hospital, Fu-dan University, Shang-hai, P.R. China

Introduction

Ulcerative colitis (UC) rarely is confused with diverticulitis because UC patients usually present with persistent rectal bleeding and have a typical endoscopic appearance [1]. Overlap between UC and diverticular disease rarely is reported [1,2].

Clinically and radiographically, however, diverticulitis can be confused with Crohn's disease (CD); both diseases can share similar features of fever, abdominal pain, tender abdominal mass, leukocytosis, elevated sedimentation rate, partial obstruction, and fistula complications [1]. Furthermore, both may respond to bowel rest and antibiotic therapy.

A history of constipation is more likely in diverticulitis, and diarrhea usually precedes a diagnosis of CD. As a rule, blood in the stools is more likely in CD than in diverticulitis.

Endoscopic Features

Endoscopically, significant mucosal abnormalities are more likely in CD than in diverticulitis. Mucosal changes in diverticulitis tend to be milder, consisting of erythema or edema, whereas in CD, the mucosa tends to be friable and ulcerated, with aphthae or "cobblestoning" around islands of edematous mucosa [1,2].

Diverticular-associated chronic colitis usually appears in elderly patients with painless, chronic hematochezia and, in more severe cases, large bowel obstruction.

Edoscopically, mucosal abnormalities are limited to the sigmoid and descending colon with rectal sparing. A diffuse mononuclear expansion of the lamina propria with crypt abscesses can be identified histologically [1,2].

Principles of Management

These patients may respond to antibiotics, 5-aminosalicylic acid (5-ASA), and immunosuppressive therapy but tent to require surgery more frequently than patients with diverticular disease alone [1].

References

[1] Tamura S, Yokoyama Y, Ockavauchi K et al. Colonic Diverticulitis. *Gastrointestin, Endosc,* 2003;158(1):96-97

[2] Simmand CL, Shires GT. Diverticular disease of the colon, In: Feldman M, Scharsschmidt BF, Sleisenger MH. (eds). Sleisenger and Fordtran's Gastrointestinal and Liver Disease. 6th ed. Printed in China Harcourt Asia W.B. Saunders Company. 1998; P.1989

Chapter XLIII

Drug-Induced Proctitis and Colitis

Jia-ju Zheng
Su-zhou Institute for Digestive Disease and Nutrition,
Su-zhou Municipal Hospital, Nan-jing Medical University,
Su-zhou, Jiang-su Province, P.R. China

Introduction

A variety of drugs given either topically or systemically can cause colitis or proctitis [1]. Overlook or neglect of medication as an etiology of colitis in practice is not uncommon.

A drug history must be taken in the investigation of patients with diarrhea. Non steroids anti-inflammatory drugs (NSAIDs), gold, sulfasalazine, methyldopa and penicillamine have all been indicated as the cause of a mild diffuse colitis [1-3].

Ingestion of laxatives remains a relatively common cause of diarrhea [1]. Anthraquinone ingestion as manifested by pseudomelanosis coli also remains relatively common [1-3]. Both enemas and laxatives can cause mucin depletion. In rat cathartic colon, the stimulant laxatives rhubarb containing anthraquinone cause abnormal expression of enteric nerve growth factor (NGF) and its receptor P75, and lead to cellular apoptosis of enteric nervous system and related pathologic changes of intestinal nerve plexus, and then lower colonic motility [4]. The long term abuse of stimulant laxatives is considered the cause of the cathartic colon.

NSAIDS- and Salicylates-Associated Colitis

NSAIDs may cause neutrophils aggregation to the terminal ileum, presumably causing acute inflammation in this location. NSAIDs can cause a similar spectrum of diseases in the large bowel [1,2]. The fenemates (mefenamic acid in particular) are associated with bloody diarrhea and an endoscopic appearance mimicking ulcerative colitis (UC), although histologically only a mild colitis has been reported.

NSAIDs can cause exacerbations of established UC and Crohn's disease and induce perforation, bleeding, and fistula formation in other pre-existing diseases, such as diverticulitis [1,2,4].

NASIDs have also been associated with their own de novo nonspecific colitis, and are considered to relate to prostaglandin inhibition and increased permeability [5]. Symptoms include hematochezia, diarrhea, ulcerations, perforations, abdominal pain, and iron deficiency anemia. The diagnosis is depending on a history in combination with endoscopic evidence of submucosal fibrosis and focal inflammatory lesions [5].

Salicylates may rarely cause a colitis [6]. These patients may be misdiagnosed as UC, and continuously treated with drugs containing 5-amina salicylic acid (5-ASA). This treatment invariably makes them worse.

Recently, the concept of apoptotic bodies as an indication of drug-associated disease has been reported, other than for cytotoxic drugs [1]. In normal conditions apoptotic bodies seldom were seen and the mean apoptotic count was less than 1.0 [1]. In untreated inflammatory bowel disease the mean apoptotic count was marginally increased, but during a partial response to drug treatment, the apoptotic count rose to 13.1. In colonic lesions directly attributable to drugs, the apoptotic count always was increased, reaching its highest level with 5-fluorouracil.

References

[1] Riddell RH. Pathology of idiopathic inflammatory bowel disease. In: Kirsner JB (ed.) Inflammatory Bowel Disease. 5th ed. Philadelphia: W.B. Saunders Company. 2000; P.427-448.

[2] Zheng J-j Medical treatment of chronic constipation. *Chin. J. Dig. Dis.* 2004; 24(1):45-46 (Chinese).

[3] Gu T-j, Xiang P, Zhang W. Drug associated colopathy. In: Xiang P and Bao Z-j (eds). Progress of diagnosis and treatment in large intestinal disease. 1st ed. Shang-hai, Shanghai Press of Scientific and Technological Literatures 2005; P.236-246 (Chinese).

[4] Lü B, Wang M, Fang Y-h, et al. The study on expression of nerve growth factor and its receptor in the rat cathartic colon. *Chin. J. Dig.* 2004;24(11):684-687 (Chinese).

[5] Krok KL, Lichtenstein GR. Inflammatory bowel disease. In: Ginsberg GG, Kochman ML, Norton I. Gostout CJ (eds.). Clinical Gastrointestinal Endoscopy. Printed in China. Elsevier Saunders 2005; P.325.

[6] Jewell DP. Ulcerative colitis. In: Feldman M, Scharschidt BF, Sleisenger MH (eds). Sleisenger and Fordtran's Gastrointestinal and Liver Disease. 6th ed. Philadelphia: Saunders 1998; 1735-1761.

Chapter XLIV

Iatrogenic Lesions

Jia-ju Zheng
Su-zhou Institute for Digestive Disease and Nutrition,
Su-zhou Municipal Hospital, Nan-jing Medical University,
Su-zhou, Jiang-su Province, P.R. China

Preparation-Related Lesions

Any toxic or caustic materials, if introduced therapeutically or incidentically into the rectum by enema or suppository, can cause colitis with variable degree of severity. Phosphosoda enemas cause endoscopic abnormalities, such as loss of the normal vascular pattern, granularity, and friability in the distal colon, and are therefore usually avoided as preparative agents in patients with clinically suspected inflammatory bowel disease (IBD) [1].

Mucosal abnormalities recently have been reported following the use of oral sodium phosphate for colonic preparation prior to colonoscopy. The lesions consist of multiple tiny (2 to 3 mm) "red ring" lesion (small aphthoid-like erosions) in the distal sigmoid and rectum that endoscopically may resemble, and must be differentiated from aphthous ulcers in Crohn's disease (CD) [1-3]. The lesion probably is activated lymphoid follicles [3].

These lesions generally are not friable, and their pathologic appearances are not typical of idiopathic IBD and are easily differentiated. Nonetheless, grossly, they may be misinterpreted as characteristic IBD lesions, particularly in a patient for whom the indication for colonoscopy is diarrhea [1,3].

Disinfectant Colitis

Hydrogen peroxide and glutaraldehyde solutions are routinely used to disinfect endoscopes, and both have been associated with colonic mucosal damage [1].

Glutaraldehyde reportedly directly injures crypt epithelium, and hydrogen peroxide causes compromise of the mucosal stroma, resulting in white plaque-like lesions, a form of colitis known as "pseudolipomatosis" and sometimes referred to as the "Snow White" sign [1,2]. Both agents may result in tissue necrosis, and fever, and cramps, etc. Bloody diarrhea have occasionally, been reported in patients within 24 hours after colonoscopy when exposed to these agents. Appropriate rinsing of the colonoscpe after disinfecting circumvents these rare complications [1].

Diversion Colitis

The problem is the sequela of surgical operation [1]. It is the inflammation that occurs in segments of colon excluded from the fecal stream by surgeries (an ileostomy or a colostomy). Diversion colitis can be found endoscopically in the excluded colonic segments in over 90% of patients within approximately 3 months following any diversion procedure, and the tissue reaction resolves when bowel continuity is re-established (reanastomosis).

Lymphoid follicular hyperplasia is a major pathologic change [1,2]. Other changes diagnostic of ulcerative colitis (UC) are present, including surface epithelial degeneration and ulceration, mucosal inflammation with crypt abscesses, and crypt branching.

Re-establishment of luminal continuity is the treatment of choice when medically feasible [4]. Corticosteroid enemas or orally produced variable results. Although initial hopes were high that this was a deficiency disease curable by rectal administration of short-chain fatty acids (SCFA), subsequent reports have been less enthusiastic [1,3]. However, treatment with SCFA enemas is still reasonable; potentially providing relief for patients in whom re-establishment of fecal flow to the excluded segment is not possible.

The SCFA enema solution consists of three SCFAs: 1. sodium acetate (60 mmol), 2. sodium propionate (30 mmol), and 3. sodium n-butyrate (40 mmol) to yield an osmolarity of 280 to 290 mOsm/L, with the pH adjusted to 7.0 by titration with 1 normal sodium hydroxide [4]. The solution can be kept stable at 4^0 for 4 months. A dose of 60 ml should be instilled into the rectum twice daily for 2 to 4 weeks. Possibly, symptoms can be controlled by less frequent treatment thereafter.

References

[1] Krok KL, Lichtenstein GR. Inflammatory bowel disease. In: Ginsberg GG, Kochman ML, Norton I. Gastout CJ (eds.). Printed in China Clinical Gastrointestinal Endoscopy. Elsevier Saunders 2005; P.311-332.

[2] Riddell RH. Pathology of idiopathlogic inflammatory bowel disease. In: Kirsner JB (ed) Inflammatory Bowel Disease. 5th ed. Philadelphia: W.B. Saunders Company.2000; P.427-450.

[3] ChutKan RK, Waye JD. Endoscopy in inflammatory bowel disease. In: Kirsner JB (ed.) Inflammatory Bowel Disease. 5th ed. Philadelphia: W.B. Saunders Company.2000; P.453-477.

[4] Davila AD and Willenbucher RF. Other disease of the colon and rectum. In: Feldman M, Scharschidt BF, Sleisenger MH (eds). Sleisenger and Fordtran's Gastrointestinal and liver disease. 6th ed. Philadwlphia: Saunders 1998; P.1997-1998.

In: Inflammatory Conditions of the Colon
Editor: Jia-ju Zheng

ISBN: 978-1-60692-240-8
© 2008 Nova Science Publishers, Inc.

Chapter XLV

Endoscopic and Pathologic Features and Treatment in Colonic Graft-versus-Host Disease

Wei-chang Chen
The First Affiliated Hospital of Soo-chow University,
Jiang-su Province, P.R. China

Introduction

Graft-versus-host disease (GVHD) is one of the frequent complications after allogeneic hematopoietic stem cell transplantation (Allo-HSCT) [1].There are more organ systems involved in GVHD, but skin, liver and gastrointestinal tract are prominent. Skin rash, jaundice and diarrhea are seen in clinical manifestations. The colonic GVHD happens frequently and severely and can lead to many complications which aggravate GVHD. The effects of Allo-HSCT are influenced by colonic GVHD. So, the prognosis and appropriate treatments depend on early diagnosis of colonic GVHD.

GVHD is often divided into two types: acute GVHD and chronic GVHD. The acute form can be observed beyond 100 days. Chronic GVHD has been defined as onset after the first 100 days [1]. The development of GVHD is closely related with "cytokine storm" [1,2].

Symptoms and Severity Evaluation

About 62% gastrointestinal complaints in acute GVHD and chronic GVHD are attributable to colonic GVHD [3].The common symptoms in acute colonic GVHD are diarrhea with abdominal cramps, nausea and vomiting. The whole gut can be involved in severe cases. The incidence of moderate to severe bleeding in acute GVHD has been reported to be as high as 31 to 35%.Although a decrease in frequency of GI bleeding and death decline, GI bleeding remains associated with an overall poor prognosis. T he differentiation between intestinal thrombotic microangiopathy and colonic GVHD is difficult[4].Chronic GVHD patients commonly have GI complaints, with 74% complaining for diarrhea;45% for abdominal pain; and 33% for nausea/vomiting[5].If GI symptoms are the only clinical manifestations of GVHD, we should rule out transplantation preconditioning(the symptoms often disappear two weeks later) and enteric infection(especially cytomegalovirus colitis).Stool routine test and stool culture can make a definitive diagnosis of infectious colitis. Infectious giant cell found in mucous biopsies by HE dying is the diagnostic golden standard.

The volume of diarrhea is used in assigning gastrointestinal GVHD grades [6]. Grade I indicates diarrhea (stool volume 500-1000 ml/d) or persistent nausea and vomiting; Grades II indicates diarrhea (stool volume 1000-1500 ml/d), biopsy confirms GVHD; Grades III indicates diarrhea (stool volume 1500-2000 ml/d); GradesIV indicates diarrhea (stool volume > 2000 mL/d) with obstruction and severe abdominal pain. Accurate gastrointestinal grading is good for proper treatment.

Diagnostic Significance of Endoscopy and Biopsy

Endoscopy and biopsies play significant role in diagnosing colonic GVHD. The endoscopic appearance in GVHD varied from normal to necrotic erosion and bleeding. The colonoscopic appearance of acute colonic GVHD presented with diffuse and continus mucosal edema, erosion, hemorrhage and necrosis. These endoscopic patterns were similar to ulcerative colitis. Ileum also presented with scattered hemorrhagic spots. He et al [7] reported the tortoiseshell-patter mucosa in GI-GVHD and deep ulcer in CMV colitis are characteristic lesions after 50 times colonoscopies on 47 Allo-HSCT patients. But endoscopic findings are usually reported lack of specificity and having no correlation with histologic or clinical grading of GVHD severity. Endoscopically normal examinations are reported in 18% of GI GVHD patients.

Histopathology has played a major role in understanding the pathophysiology and aiding in the diagnosis and management of acute and chronic GVHD. The histologic diagnostic threshold ranged from rare isolated apoptotic enterocytes to extensive lymphocytic infiltration with glandular or crypt destruction and crypt abscesses filled with apoptotic debris. Apoptosis is not specific for GVHD.Some entities as preconditioning regimen or CMV colitis can also demonstrate apoptosis, but its absence makes the diagnosis unwarranted[8].

We performed colonoscopy on a chronic colonic GVHD patient five months later after Allo-HSCT and found that diffuse and continues erosions and bleeding [9] (figure 45-1). Another young male patient diagnosed with CML 3 months after Allo-HSCT showed diffuse ulcers and bleeding (figure 45-2).Biopsy specimen has inflammatory cells infiltration, crypt loss and numerous apoptotic changes (figure 45-3).

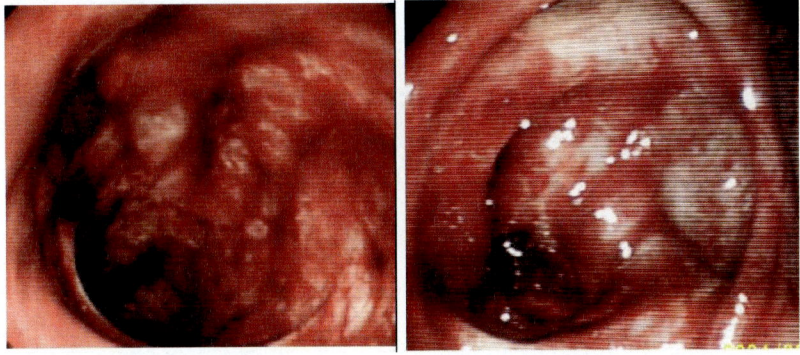

Figure 45-1. A 23-year-old male patient presented with diffuse erosions and bleeding at coloscopy 180 days later after Allo-HSCT.

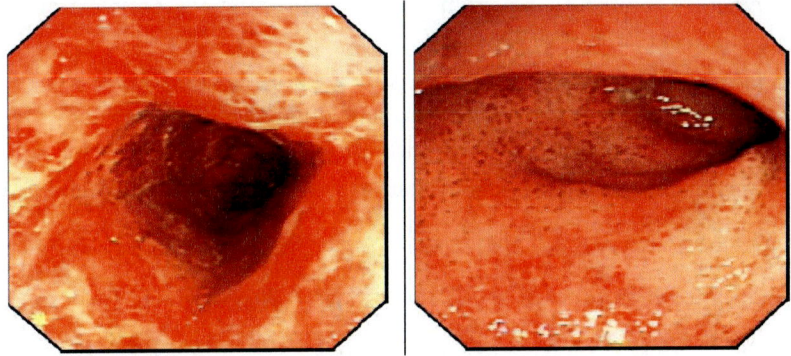

Figure 45-2. A young male patient diagnosed with CML 3 months after Allo-HSCT showed diffuse ulcers and bleeding.

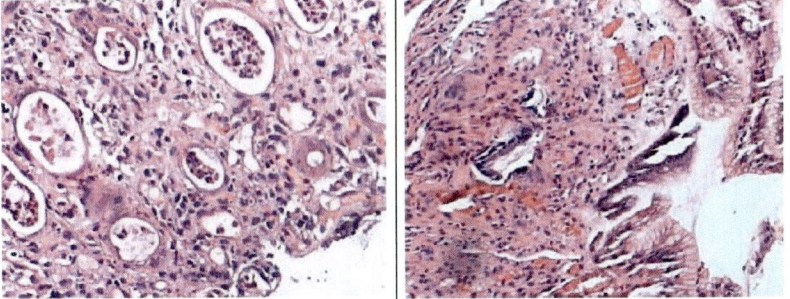

Figure 45-3. Biopsy sample show inflammatory cells infiltration, crypt loss and numerous apoptotic changes.

The segment of gut to target for diagnostic biopsy is a topic of debate. The most severely affected areas may not be sampled, particularly in the lower gastrointestinal tract. Some reporters believe that small bowel biopsies are more fruitful. Our practice is more biopsies on different spots in gut. More biopsies are good for evaluation of GVHD.

Performing endoscopy and mucosal biopsies in the post-HSCT is procedural risk. Endoscopic procedural mortality in HSCT patients has been reported as high as 1.8%. Patients with thrombocytopenia and neutropenia have the risk of bleeding and infection. Some centers do not prefer biopsies until platelet counts are more than 5×10^9/L.

Prophylaxis and Management

The prophylaxis of GVHD included protecting target organs, immunosuppressive agents and T cell depletion [10]. Reduction in doses of chemotherapy and total body irradiation used for preconditioning and retaining the anti-tumor potential can reduce GVHD and prevent from injury of host tissues. Use of antibiotics can eradicate or reduce the load of gram-negative bacteria and LPS in the GI tract. Commonly used immunosuppressive agents contained cyclosporin, tacrolimus, corticosteroids, methotrexate and anti-thymus globulin. Immunosuppressive agents should be used together and play roles in different phases to achieve good prophylactic effect. T cell depletion means to use monoclonal antibody, chemic or physical methods to deplete T cells. Although T-cell depletion is effective in the prevention of GVHD, he survival of T-cell depletion is less than expected due to delayed recovery of immunity, increased rejection rate and leukemia relapse. immunosuppressive agents also used to treat GVHD.

Cytokine plays an important role in the pathogenesis of GVHD. So use of protective cytokines and monoclonal antibody of anti-inflammation cytokines including IL-11, KGF, HGF, monoclonal antibody of TNF-α and infliximab have been important ways to treat GVHD. Blocking agents of co-stimulants can stop T cells activation and treat GVHD effectively.

The main symptom of colonic GVHD is diarrhea. Sousing drugs to control diarrhea is very important. Some drugs as SASP,5-ASA and topical glucocorticoid (budesonide) to treat ulcerative colitis are effective. For symptom relief, octreotide is reported to control diarrhea in post-irradiation and post-chemotherapy, especially at the onset of diarrhea.

The mechanisms of GVHD is complicated and GVHD remains difficult to treat. Colonic GVHD is a lethal complication of HSCT. To prevent and treat colonic GVHD effectively and appropriately can reduce the incidence and grades of GVHD so as to increase the successful rate of transplantation.

References

[1] Ross WA, Couriel D. Colonic graft-versus-host disease. *Curr. Opin. Gastroenterol.* 2005; 21:64-69.

[2] Vogeisang GB, Lee L, Bensen-kennedy DM. Pathogenesis and treatment of graft-versus-host disease after bone marrow transplant. *Annu. Rev. Med.* 2004; 54:29-52.

[3] Schwartz JM, Wolford JL, Thornquist MD, et al. Severe gastrointestinal bleeding after hemopoietic cell transplantation, 1987-97 :incidence, causes and outcome. *Am. J. Gastroenterol.* 2001; 96:385-393.

[4] Nevo S, Swam V, Enger C, et al. Acute bleeding after bone marrow transplantation-incidence and effect on survival: a quantitative analysis in 1402 patients. *Blood.* 1998; 91:1469-1477.

[5] Akpek G, Valladares JL, et al. Gastrointestinal involvement in chronic graft-versus-host disease: a clinicopathologic study. *Biol. Blood Marrow Transplat.* 2003; 9:46-51.

[6] Przepiorka D, Weisdorf D, Martin P, et al. Consensus conference on acute GVHD grading. *Bone Marrow Transplant.* 1995; 15:825-828.

[7] He J-d, Liu Y-l, Wang Z-f, et al. The role of colonoscopy in diagnosis of gastrointestinal graft-versus-host disease and cytomegalovirus colitis after allergenic hematopoietic stem cell transplantation. *Chin. J. Dig. Endosc.* 2006; 23:421-425 (Chinese).

[8] Shidham VB, Chang C-C, Shidham G, et al. Colon biopsies for evaluation of acute graft-versus-host disease in allogenic bone marrow tranplant patients. *BMC Gastroenterl.* 2003; 3:5.

[9] Xu C-f, Zhu L-xi, Xu X-m, et al. Endoscopic diagnosis of gastrointestinal graft-versus-host disease. *Chin. J. Dig. Endosc.* 2004; 21:297-300 (Chinese).

[10] Bolaños-Meade J. Update on the management of acute graft-versus-host disease. *Curr. Opin. Oncol.* 2006; 18:120125 .

Chapter XLVI

Cap Polyposis

Ming Zhang
Drum Tower Hospital Affiliated, Nan-jing University Medical School,
Jiang-su Province, P.R. China

Definition

Cap polyposis,which was first reported in 1985 by Williams et al. [1], is a rare but distinct disorder with characteristic endoscopic and histological features [2]. This disorder could be found at any age and no obvious difference was found between the two genders.

Symptoms and Signs

Patients of cap polyposis present with abdominal pain, acute diarrhea associated with blood or mucus and tenesmus [2,3-6]. Some patients manifested protein-losing enteropathy. Habitual straining at defecation and chronic constipation existed in most patients. Digital rectal examination may revealed polypoidal masses in some patients and could be misdiagnosed as rectal carcinoma or solitary rectal ulcer syndrome. The most common sites involved are the rectum and sigmoid colon. The number of polyps ranged immensely (from 1 to more than 100).

Endoscopic and Histologic Features

Typical endoscopic features are small, red and sessile polyps dotted along the colon (figure 46-1). For this reason it is sometimes misdiagnosed as pseudopolyps present in ulcerative colitis. However, cap polyps tend to be situated commonly on the apices of transverse mucosa folds and the intervening mucosa are normal, which are distinct from ulcerative colitis. Surfaces of the polyps are often covered with fibrinopurulent exudates [7].

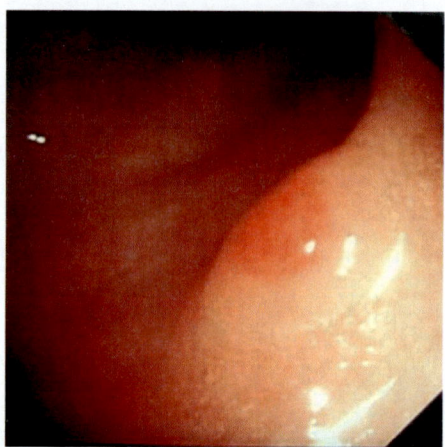 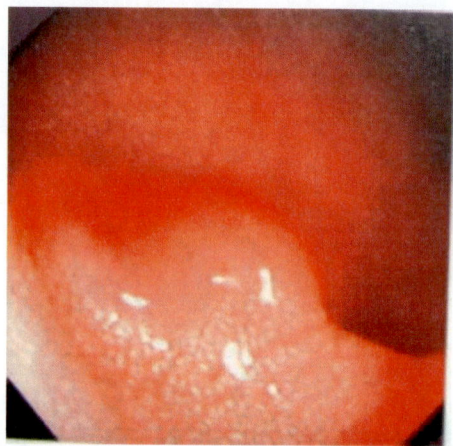

Figure 46-1. Typical endoscopic views of cap polyposis: small, red and sessile polyps, which are commonly situated on the apices of transverse mucosal folds and the intervening mucosa are normal.

There are three major histologic features of cap polyposis [7]: firstly, the polyps consist of elongated, distended, tortuous, and hyperplastic crypts that become attenuated toward the mucosal surface; secondly, these polyps contain large amount of inflammatory cells; and thirdly, the surface of these sessile polyps are ulcerated and covered by a thick layer of fibrinopurulent exudates.

Mucus secreted by these distorted polyps is different from that of normal colon: abnormal ultrastructure of the mucus in the goblet cells, predominance of non-sulphated mucins, and abnormal expression of the *MUC3*, *MUC4* and *MUC5AC* genes [8]. *MUC3* indicated very weak signal through the epithelium on the cap polyps, whereas it strong expressed in the upper part of the normal crypts. *MUC4* was strong expressed in all epithelial cells on the cap polyps, however in normal colon it only moderately expressed. As for *MUC5AC*, it weakly expressed in the surface of some epithelial cells, but not detected in normal colonic mucosa. This abnormal mucus was considered involved in the protection of trauma.

Mechanisms

The exact pathogenesis of cap polys is still unknown. The clinical and histological appearances are similar to those observed in mucosal prolapse syndrome (MPS); therefore, abnormal colonic motility causing mucosal prolapse has been proposed as a possible cause of this disorder [1]. This can be supported by the findings that most cap polyposis patients exist habitual straining at defecation and chronic constipation. Resection of the lesion colon could relief the symptoms also support the causation. Infection has also been postulated as a possible cause of cap polyposis, even though no infective organisms have been identified, and treatment of cap polyposis with antibiotics had been shown to be ineffective. Even though metronidazole was effective in some cases, it was considered its anti-inflammatory effects rather than its antibiotic action [9]. Inflammation was postulated as another etiology of cap polyposis [10,11]. Infection of *Helicobacter pylori (HP)* in the stomach, meanwhile no infection sign was found in colon, was also proposed as the possible pathogenesis of cap polyposis, which was confirmed by the fact that once *HP* was eradicated cap polyposis could be cured [12-14].

Treatment

Until now there is no accepted curative treatment for cap polyposis. Avoid straining and constipation is not only the primary management but also the first step to prevent recurrence. Drug therapies usually used for other inflammatory bowel disease, such as 5-ASA and immunosuppressives, are often ineffective, and surgery resection has generally been the treatment choice [2,4-6]. But before surgery each patient should be treated medically, and only after medical management failed could surgery be considered. If the number of the cap polyps is no more than 10 endoscopic polypectomy should be preferentially considered. Rapid recurrence is described after a limited surgical resection [4,15], and this often necessitates repeat surgery. Some cap polyposis patients, meanwhile infected with *HP*, *HP* eradication therapy could be try.

Infliximab may be an effective treatment for cap polyposis and avoid the requirement for surgery [5]. The dramatic and sustained response after infliximab therapy suggests tumor necrosis factor (TNF)- α play a pivotal role in the causation of this disorder. However, another researcher documented that cap polyposis could be spontaneous regression [16] and the effect of Infliximab on cap polyposis may be a coincidence. Also there was report that infliximab failures in cap polyposis [4], all the controversial issues suggest that the effects of Inflixmab on cap polyposis should be explored in the future.

References

[1] Williams GT, Bussey HJR, Morson BC. Inflammatory 'cap' polyps of the large intestine. *Br. J. Surg.* 1985; 72(S):S133.

[2] Campbell AP, Cobb CA, Chapman RWG, et al. Cap polyposis-an unusual cause of diarrhoea. *Gut.* 1993;34:562-564.

[3] Williams GT, Bussey HJR, Morson BC. Inflammatory "cap" polyps of the large intestine. *BR. J. Surg.* 1985; 72(Suppl):S133.

[4] Mounoury V, Breisse M, Desreumoury P, et al. Infliximab failures in cap polyposis. *Gut.* 2005; 54(2):313-314.

[5] Bookman I, Redston M, Greenberg GR. Successful treatment of cap-polyposis with infliximab: a case report. *Gastroeanlerot.* 2004;126:1868-1871

[6] Busine MP, Colombel J-F, Lecomte-Houche M, et al. Abnormal mucus in cap polyposis. *Gut.* 1998;42:135-138

[7] Ng KH, Mathur P, Kumarasinghe MP, et al. Cap polyposis: further experience and review. *Dis. Colon Rectum.* 2004; 47(7):1208-15.

[8] Buisine MP, Colombel JF, Lecomte-Houcke M, et al. Abnormal mucus in cap polyposis. *Gut.* 1998; 42(1):135-8.

[9] Shimizu K, Koga H, Iida M, et al. Does metronidazole cure cap polyposis by its ntiinflammatory actions instead of by its antibiotic action? A case study. *Dig. Dis. Sci.* 2002; 47:1465–8.

[10] Konishi T, Watanabe T, Takei Y, et al. Confined progression of cap polyposis along the anastomotic line, implicating the role of inflammatory responses in the pathogenesis. *Gastrointest. Endosc.* 2005; 62(3):446-7.

[11] Konishi T, Watanabe T, Takei Y, et al. Cap polyposis: an inflammatory disorder or a spectrum of mucosal prolapse syndrome? *Gut.* 2005; 54(9):1342-3.

[12] Akamatsu T, Nakamura N, Kawamura Y, ea al. Possible relationship between Helicobacter pylori infection and cap polyposis of the colon. *Helicobacter.* 2004;9(6):651-6.

[13] Oiya H, Okawa K, Aoki T, et al. Cap polyposis cured by Helicobacter pylori eradication therapy. *J Gastroenterol.* 2002; 37(6):463-6.

[14] Liu Z-l, Zhang P-f, Yin Q. Cap polyposis: one case report. *Chin. J. Dig. Endosc.* 2007; 24(4):265.

[15] Gehenot M, Colombel JF, Wolschies E, et al. Cap polyposis occurring in the postoperative course of pelvic surgery. *Gut.* 1994;35:1670-1672.

[16] Ohkawara T, Kato M, Nakagawa S, et al. Spontaneous resolution of cap polyposis: case report. *Gastrointest. Endosc.* 2003; 57(4):599-602.

In: Inflammatory Conditions of the Colon
Editor: Jia-ju Zheng

ISBN: 978-1-60692-240-8
© 2008 Nova Science Publishers, Inc.

Chapter XLVII

Watermelon Colon

Ming Zhang
Drum Tower Hospital Affiliated, Nan-jing University Medical School,
Jiang-su Province, P.R. China

Clinical and Endoscopic Characteristics of GAVE

Watermelon stomach was coined by Jabbari et al. in 1984 [1]. It is a term used to describe the endoscopic appearance of gastric antral vascular ectasia (GAVE). [1] The typical picture of watermelon stomach is an array of reddish stripes radiating from the pylorus. There are rare reports of "watermelon" lesions besides stomach in GI tract. As far as we know, only 11 cases of watermelon colon were reported [2-4].

GAVE is an uncommon but important cause of GI blood loss and iron deficiency anemia [1]. Clinical manifestations included abdominal pain, fever, hematochezia, rectal fullness, generalized edema and diarrhea. Associated conditions have included eosinophilia, chronic anemia, protein-losing enteropathy, systemic sclerosis, watermelon stomach, alcohol and mitral valve disease with supraventricular tachycardia.

Clinical, Endoscopic and Histologic Features

The colonic lesions resembled typical watermelon stomach but sites of involvement varied: 7 rectal, 2 cecum, and 2 entire colon except for cecum. Anemia is frequently the first clinical manifestation of watermelon stomach, but only 6 of the 11 patients with watermelon colon were anemic [1,2].

The distinctive histologic features of watermelon stomach are mucosal capillary ectasia with thrombosis and fibromuscular hyperplasia [1]. In most cases, endoscopic biopsy specimens are sufficient for histopathologic diagnosis. However, in several cases, no histopathologic findings or only nonspecific inflammation were noted [1]. Lymphatic ectasias in the submucosa and hemosiderin-laden macrophages in the muscularis mucosa and submucosa were found.

Dilated capillaries with thrombi were found in one reported case [1,2], and vascular ectasia is common in other GI lesions known to be associated with trauma and mucosal prolapse. Prolapse of antral mucosa throughout the pylorus has been proposed as a possible etiology of GAVE [1].

Interestingly, in most of the cases of watermelon colon, either the cecum or rectum was involved, sites also frequently affected by disorders with a traumatic etiology such as intussusception, solitary rectal ulcer syndrome, and rectal prolapse [1].

Because the relation between this entity and GI blood loss remains uncertain, the use of endoscopic hemostatic methods and other local treatment should be individualized.

References

[1] Tan S-l, Huang W-s, Lin J-w. Watermelon colon: case report and review. *Gastrointest. Endosc.* 2003; 58(1):160-161.

[2] Altintas E, Sezgin O, Cinel L. Watermelon colon: is there an association with alcohol? *Med. Sci. Monit.* 2007; 13(11):CS137-140.

[3] Chen SC, Liangpunsakul S, Rex DK. Watermelon colon treated by argon plasma coagulation. *Gastrointest. Endosc.* 2005; 61(4):631-633.

[4] Fu K, Ikematsu H, Hurlstone DP, et al. "Watermelon rectum" associated with multiple vascular ectasia in the colon. *Gastrointest. Endosc.* 2007; 66(3):601-602.

Section Seven: Disorders That Simulate Idiopathic Colitis – Specific Infections

Ulcerative colitis (UC) and Crohn's disease (CD) account for only a small proportion of the number of patients with inflammatory colitis in the world; the majority of colitides are due to infectious causes [1]. This is probably more prominent in the developing countries where account for the most portion of population of the world.

Infections involving a healthy colon, once sought, usually are readily diagnosed and antimicrobials generally are effective [1,2]. However, it can mimic the clinical presentation of UC or CD [1-3]. Colonic infections may be due to either specific or general (viral, bacterial, protozoal, or fungal etc.) in origin.

Chapter XLVIII

Intestinal Tuberculosis

Long-dian Chen
Department of Digestive Disease, Drum Tower Hospital affiliated to
Nan-jing University Medical School, Jiang-su Province, P.R. China

Pathogenesis

Mycobacterium tuberculosis is the pathogen responsible for most cases of intestinal tuberculosis (intestinal TB), although in some parts of the world cases caused by M. bovis, an organism found in dairy products, are still reported [1].

The pathogenesis of TB enteritis has been attributed to four mechanisms: 1. swallowing of infected sputum; 2. hematogenous spread from active pulmonary or miliary TB; 3. ingestion of contaminated milk or food, a rarity in the Western world; 4. contiguous spread from adjacent organs. Multiple areas (any regions) of the gastrointestinal tract can be involved with TB, but the ileocecal region is clearly the most frequent. Both sides of the ileocecal valve are usually involved (deformity), leading to incompetence of the valve, a point that distinguishes tuberculosis from Crohn's disease (CD).

Clinical Features

The most common complaint is chronic abdominal pain, which is nonspecific and is reported in 80% to 90% of individuals. Weight loss, fever, diarrhea or constipation, and blood in the stool may be present. An abdominal mass, usually in the right lower quadrant of the abdomen, can be appreciated. Intractable hematochezia as a unusual manifestation of intestinal TB was reported [2].

Diagnosis

The diagnosis is made most directly by colonoscopy with biopsy and culture [3]. The definitive diagnosis of intestinal TB is made by the identification of the organism in tissue, either 1.by direct visualization with an acid-fast stain (Ziehl-Neelson stain) in the sections of the involved region in about one third of patients, 2.by culture of the excised tissue, or 3.by a PCR assay. Colonoscopic findings, although nonspecific, consist of superficial areas of ulceration and a nodular friable mucosa [3]. Colonoscopy may demonstrate diffuse nodules, linear ulcerations, and stricture. The ulcerations usually are bordered by edema and erythema and as in CD. They are frequently located in areas of otherwise normal-appearing mucosa. Mass lesions or tuberculomas can develop, and fistulization may occur between loops of bowel. Cobblestoning as a result of submucosal involvement has been reported, with thickening of the bowel wall and inflammatory pseudopolyps. The differentiation between CD and tuberculosis can be difficult because the two illnesses closely resemble each other. In contrast to CD, the superficial ulcers are seen in 60% of TB patients, and ulcers tend to be circumferential, with the long axis perpendicular to the lumen. Histologically, the distinguishing lesion is a granuloma. Caseating granuloma are seen in TB patients, which is found with regularity in regional lymph nodes, but not always seen in the mucosa in particular (the muscularis is usually spared). Small bowel obstruction has been reported. The presence of ascites may help to distinguish ileocecal TB from CD, since ascites is uncommon in the latter.

Standard antituberculosis treatment gives a high cure rate for intestinal tuberculosis. Four drug regimen using Isoniazid (INH, 300 mg/day), rifampin (600 mg/day), pyrazinamide (15 to 30 $mg \cdot kg^{-1} \cdot d^{-1}$),and either ethambutol (0.75/day) or streptomycin (0.75 /day) for 2 months (or for 9-12 months in China) .Surgery is usually reserved for patients who have developed complications, including free perforation, confined perforation with abscess or fistula, massive bleeding, complete obstruction, or obstruction not responding to medical management

References

[1] Akgun Y. Intestinal and peritoneal tuberculosis. Changing trends over 10 years and review of 80 patients. *Can. J. Surg.* 2005;48:131-136

[2] Rabkin DG☐Caiat JM☐Allendorf JA, et al. Intractable hematochezia☐an unusual presentation of intestinal tuberculosis. *Surgery.* 2003;133:592-593

[3] Sato S, Yao K, Yao T et al. Colonoscopy in the diagnosis of intestinal tuberculosis in asymptomatic patients. *Gastrointest. Endosc.* 2004;59:362-368

Chapter XLIX

Pseudomembranous Colitis

Jia-ju Zheng
Su-zhou Institute for Digestive Disease and Nutrition, Su-zhou Municipal Hospital,
Nan-jing Medical University, Su-zhou, Jiang-su Province, P.R. China

Definition

Pseudomembranous colitis (PMC) is an acute mucosal injury characterized by punctate pseudomembrane formation on the colonic mucosa (figure 49-1) [1]. However, the term "pseudomembrane" is a common denominator, which indicates the presence of pseudomembranes on the intestinal mucosa, either in the small bowel (pseudomembranous enteritis), colon (PMC), or both (pseudomembranous enterocolitis)[2]. In early time, studies showed high rates of small bowel involvement. However, nearly all cases reported in the past two decades follow antibiotic use, and show changes restricted to the colon; rare cases with small bowel involvement are reported, both with and without antecedent antibiotic exposure [2]. The colitis without plaque formation, if it is believed to be associated with prior ingestion of antibiotics, is called antibiotic-associated colitis.

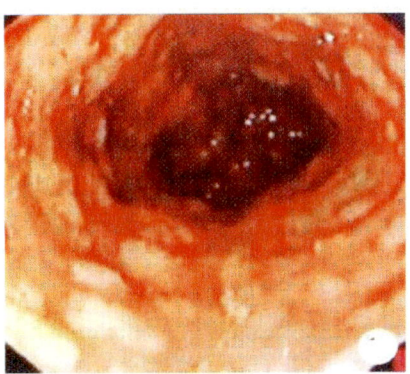

Figure 49-1. Pseudomembranous colitis. The characteristic colonoscopic feature: a pseudomembrane consisting of raised, yellow white adherent plaques that range from 2 mm to 8 mm in diameter.

Etiology

PMC usually refers to the lesion secondary to Clostridium difficile (C.difficile, a gram-positive anaerobic bacillus) infection, and is called clostridium difficile-associated disease (CDAD) [1,2]. Nosocomial infection is common. C. difficile infection may be the result of disruption of the normal colonic flora, usually following use of antibiotics or chemotherapeutic drugs, most commonly the cephalosporings, ampicillin, amoxicillin, and clindamycin. On the other hand, aminoglycosides such as gentamycin, some fluoroquinolones such as ciprofloxacin, and the antipseudomonal penicillin, ticarcillin, clavulanate, have little or no propensity to cause C. difficile infection, probably due to lack of effect on endogenous anaerobic gut flora.

Other toxin-producing bacteria (e.g., Verotoxin E. coli 0157) and early or mild ischemia of other causes may induce this pattern of colitis [2,3].

Symptoms

Disease is mediated by toxin production, and virulent strains are produced by toxin A (enterotoxin) and toxin B (cytotoxin). C. difficile infection causes a spectrum of conditions in susceptible patients, ranging from the asymptomatic carrier state to severe fulminate disease with toxic megacolon. Symptoms develop within a few days to 2 months after starting antibiotics, with up to 10 watery stools per day; blood streaks may be present, but gross bloody stools are uncommon except in patients with underlying inflammatory bowel disease (IBD) or colonic neoplasm. Crampy abdominal pain, tenesmus, nausea, vomiting, and anorexia are common [3-5]. Infection may be asymptomatic, particularly in healthy newborns; serologic studies show antibodies to toxin A and B in up to 50% of children by age 2. On physical examination, abdominal distention and tenderness may be present; peritoneal signs are rare.

Diagnosis

The diagnosis is confirmed by the identification of the C. difficile toxin in the stools, present in 95% of patients with pseudomembranous colitis and 30% of patients with antibiotic-associated colitis. Toxin detection by cytotoxicity testing is the gold standard and results usually are available in 24 hours. Toxin antigen techniques have been developed and allow detection in 2 to 4 hours, with specificity of 75% to 100% [4-7]. The C. difficile culture is widely useful for epidemiologic studies. Toxin assays and cultures will continue to be positive for days or weeks after symptoms resolve, and follow-up stool studies are not clinically useful in asymptomatic patients. Abdominal CT scan in patients with pseudomembranous colitis reveals pronounced thickening of the colonic wall that may involve the entire colon.

Endoscopic and Histologic Features

PMC has a readily identifiable endoscopic appearance: numerous, discrete, small (2-5 or 8 mm), elevated creamy and yellowish adherent plaques (punctate pseudomembranes) that stud the surface of a moderately inflamed mucosa (figure 49-1) [1,5,6]. The mucosa between plaques is not ulcerated but as with ulcerative colitis, it may be edematous and friable or hemorrhagic. In severe cases, the punctate pseudomembranes may coalesce, forming large segmental membranes endoscopically indistinguishable from those seen in well developed ischemic colitis. Although the rectum usually is involved, the distribution is not always uniform and may be confined to the right colon, or sigmoid area alone, or involved the entire colon. Importantly, C. difficile may not always produce inflammatory pseudomembranes, and, endoscopically, the mucosa resembles other infectious colitides. Colonoscopy should be avoid in patients with severe symptoms because of the risk of perforation.

Not only the endoscopic findings are typical but also histopathologic features of the pseudomembrane are characteristic. The pathological feature are usually a consequence of relatively weak bacterial toxins that damage the endothelium producing numerous minute foci of early superficial ischemic necrosis (in superficial crypt and surface epithelium) characterized by punctate inflammatory psendomembranes [6,7]. Ischemia rarely can produce a similar picture. Pathologically, diffuse pseudomembranous changes are more consistent with C. difficile and focal full-thickness necrosis is more consistent with ischemic disease [5,8]. Biopsy may demonstrates a typical "volcano" lesions: polymorphonuclear exudates (neutrophil-rich edema fluid) in the lamina propria bursts through tiny breeches in the surface epithelium, like a volcanic eruption, to from characteristic punctate inflammatory pseudomembranes [2].

In early stages of ischemia, the histological and endoscopic appearances may be identical, but diffusely distributed punctate pseudomembranes seen on endoscopy favor C. difficle. In the resolving phase, the histological changes may be subtle. Biopsy samples taken during the resolution phase may show only an occasional dilated crypt lined by elongated degenerating or regenerating epithelial cells and containing a few luminal neutrophils.

Treatment

Initial therapy for C. difficile colitis is to discontinue the offending antibiotic or chemotherapeutic drugs, which results in resolution of symptoms in about 15% of patients without other specific treatment [4-6]. Specific therapeutic options are oral metronidazole, 250 mg three times daily for 7 to 10 days, or oral vancomycin, 125 mg four time per day for 7 to 10 days with similar response rates with either agent in the range of 77% to 100%. Higher doses of vancomycin do not appear to be more effective. Vancomycin significantly shortens the duration of symptoms compared to metronidazole, with a mean duration of 3 days compared to 4.6 days. For patients who are unable to take oral therapy, intravenous vancomycin plus metronidazole should be given to ensure adequate concentrations in the gut. Relapse occur with both metronidazole and vancomycin in up to 24% of patients, although

DNA-typing studies show that at least half of so-called relapse actually are infections with different strains of C. difficile.

A recent retrospective cohort study conducted in a tertiary-care Canadian hospital showed that the efficacy of vancomycin was no more superior over metronidazole after the year of 2003. This was coincided with the emergence of hypervirulent stain (NAP1/027), which was demonstrated to be tolerate vancomycin treatment. Thus, exploring novel therapeutic approaches was needed [9].

Prevention of Relapse

Several strategies have been used to prevent relapse, including oral lactobacilli or sacchromyces boulardii [2,6]. Tapering the dose of vancomycin followed by pulse dose therapy has been used to kill vegetative spores, and combination oral vancomycin and rifampicin has been used in patients with multiple relapse. Cholestyramine can be initiated following antibiotics to bind residual toxin. Antibiotics use concurrently with cholestyramine should be avoided because of binding and inactivation of the antibiotic by the cholestyramine. Intravenous gamma globulin has been prescribed for relapsing C. difficile colitis, although the role of immunotherapy is unclear.

References

[1] Krok KL, Lichtenstein GR. Inflammatory bowel disease. In: Ginsberg GG, Kochman ML, Norton I, Gostout CJ (eds.). *Clinical Gastrointestinal Endoscopy.* Elsevier Saunders 2005; P.311-332.

[2] Barlett JG. Pseudomembranous enterocolitis and antibiotic-associated colitis. In: Feldman M, Scharschmidt BF, Sleisenger MH. (eds). Sleisenger and Fordtran's Gastrointestinal and Liver Disease. 6th ed. Printed in China Harcourt Asia W.B. Saunders Company. 2001; P.1633-1647.

[3] Li P, Yand Z-j, Song H-m, et al. Early diagnosis and treatment of severe pseudomembranous colitis. *Mord Dig. Intervent.* 2005;10(3):167 (Chinese).

[4] Wen Z-f, Cheng X-l, Zheng F-p, et al. Clinical analysis of pseudomembranous colitis. *Mord Dig. Intervent.* 2005;10(5):156 (Chinese).

[5] Zheng J-j, Zhou C-l. Colonoscopic and histopathologic features and treatment of pseudomembranous colitis. *Chin. J. Dig. Dis.*8 (1):35-41.

[6] Chutkan RK, Waye JD. Endoscopy in inflammatory bowel disease. In: Kirsner JB (ed.).5th ed. Inflammatory Bowel Disease. Philadelphia. New York. St. Louis. Syd. W.B.Saunders Company. 2000;P453-478.

[7] Përia AS, Heunissen SGH. Diagnosis of the first attack of colitis. *Res. Clin. Forum.* 1998;20(1);67-76.

[8] Cappel M.S. Intestinal vasculopathy II: ischemic colitis and chronic mesenteric ischemia. *Gastroenterol. Clin. Nor. Am.* 1998;27(4):827-860.

[9] Pépin J, Valiquette L, Gagnon S, et al. Outcomes of Clostridium difficile-associated disease treated with metronidaole or vancomycin before and after the emergence of NAP1/027. *Am. J. Gastroenterol.* 2007; 102:2781-2788.

Section Eight: Disorders That Simulate Idiopathic Colitis-Other Forms of Acute Infectious Colitis and Acute Self-Limited Colitis

In: Inflammatory Conditions of the Colon
Editor: Jia-ju Zheng

ISBN: 978-1-60692-240-8
© 2008 Nova Science Publishers, Inc.

Chapter L

Acute Infectious Colitis and Acute Self-Limited Colitis

Jia-ju Zheng

Su-zhou Institute for Digestive Disease and Nutrition, Su-zhou Municipal Hospital, Nan-jing Medical University, Su-zhou, Jiang-su Province, P.R. China

Acute Infectious Colitis

Infectious colitis (IC) may produce mucosal inflammation that resembles ulcerative colitis (UC), clinically or endoscopically and histologically [1-3]. For example, bacillary dysentery and gonococcal proctitis produce mucosal inflammation with a macroscopic distribution similar to that of UC (or proctitis). In addition, IC may affect deeper portion of the colon wall that mimics Crohn's disease (CD), such as the condition seen in Cytomegalovirus induced colitis [1-3].

The diagnosis of IC is usually established by [1,2]:

1. typical clinical picture;
2. occasionally, positive identification of specific infectious agents with standard microbiological studies of the stool or mucus. Special methods are necessary to Campylobacter or Yersinia. Salmonella infection has been reported in some patients with UC and CD, or exacerbations of UC occur as Clostridium difficile is infected;
3. identifying the organism in the biopsy;
4. demonstrating a rise in a specific serum antibody titer.

Acute Self-Limited Colitis

In some patients who have the acute onset of colitis with negative cultures and who subsequently achieve spontaneous remission in a few weeks, the presumptive diagnosis of "acute self-limited colitis" (ASLC) can be made [1,2].

Colonoscopy may play a significant role of diagnosis, and can be performed safely [3]. However, it is not done routinely because, in the emergency setting, uncontrollable hemorrhage, toxic megacolon, and bowel perforation remain indications for surgery, and the role of endoscopy in evaluating these situations is limited.

Table 50-1 and table 50-2 depict some endoscopic and histologic features useful for differentiating (IC) from idiopathic colitis (UC and Crohn's colitis), respectively [1-5]:

Table 50-1. Colonoscopic features of infectious and idiopathic colitis [1-7]

Mucosal changes	Acute IC	UC	CD
surface appearance	a patchy intensely[1] red-to-magenta	deeper red	deeper red
vascula pattern	may be normal	distorted or loss	segmental distorted, or loss
mucosal folds	preserved	loss	loss
haustral markings	preserved	loss	loss
erythema	present	continuous uniform involved	skip distributed
edema	present	diffuse	segmental
ulcers	superficial	superficial, with abnormal mucosa	linear or serpiginous, with normal mucosa
granularity	unusual	wet "sandpaper-like"	unusual
friability (contact bleeding)	unusual	frequent	unusual
cobblestoning from submucosal edema	no	no	frequent
fistulas	no	no	yes

[1] Patchy inflammation: consisting of multiple small areas of inflammation with intervening normal-appearing mucosa within the same colonic segment [3]. Patchy inflammation is one of the more characteristic endoscopic features of IC [5].

Table 50-2. Histologic features of infectious and idiopathic colitis [1-7]

Histologic features[1]	Acute IC	UC	CD
inflammatory cells			
neutrophils	predominate	persist	persist
monouclears	confined to upper lamina propria	predominate	predominate
focal	common	no	common
(basal lymphoid or plasma cell aggregates)	absent	yes	very common
mucin depletion	less	more	more
crypt	preserved	destroyed	destroyed
abscesses	less and superficial	prominently basal	prominently basal
branching and distortion	no	yes	yes

Histologic features	Acute IC	UC	CD
diffused mucosal atrophy	not frequent	yes	yes
Paneth cell metaplasia	no	yes	yes
granuloma			
epithelioid	no	no	yes
"micro"	unusual	no	yes

[1] an absence of crypt architecture distortion, increased number of plasma cells in the lamina propria, or Paneth cell metaplasia excludes idiopathic IBD in most cases [6].

References

[1] Riddell RH. Pathology of idiopathic inflammatory bowel disease. In: Kirsner JB (ed.) Inflammatory Bowel Disease. 5th ed. Philadelphia: W.B. Saunders Company. 2000; P;427-450.

[2] Haggitt RC. Pathology of bowel inflammatory. In: AGA Postgraduate course: idiopathic inflammatory bowel disease. New Orleans, Louisiana 1984;P.53-63.

[3] Chutkan RK, Waye JD. Endoscopy in inflammatory bowel disease. In: Kirsner JB (ed.). 5th ed. Inflammatory Bowel Disease Philadelphia. London. New York. St. Louis. Syd. W.B. Saunders Company.2000; P. 453-477.

[4] Carpenter HA, Talley NJ. The importance of clinicopathological correlation in the diagnosis of inflammatory conditions of the colon: histological patterns with clinical implications. *An. J. Gastroenterol.* 2000; 95(4):878-896.

[5] Krok KL, Lichtenstein GR. Inflammatory bowel disease. In: Ginsberg GG, Kochman ML, Norton I, Gastout CJ (eds). Clinical Gastrointestinal Endoscopy. Printed in China Elsevier Saunders 2005; P311-332.

[6] Lee SD, Cohen RD. Endoscopy in inflammatory bowel disease. *Gastroenterol. Clin. N. Am.* 2002; 31(1):119-132.

[7] Tremaine WJ. The other colitides. In: Kirsner JB (ed.). 5th ed. Inflammatory Bowel Disease. Philadelphia. London. New York. St. Louis. Syd. W.B. Saunders Company. 2000; P.410-423.

In: Inflammatory Conditions of the Colon
Editor: Jia-ju Zheng

ISBN: 978-1-60692-240-8
© 2008 Nova Science Publishers, Inc.

Chapter LI

Viral Colitis, Bacterial Colitis, Protozoal and Fungal Infections

Jia-ju Zheng

Su-zhou Institute for Digestive Disease and Nutrition, Su-zhou Municipal Hospital,
Nan-jing Medical University, Su-zhou, Jiang-su Province, P.R. China

Viral Colitis

It is most commonly seen in immunosuppressed patients, however, Cytomegalovirus (CMV) and herpes simplex virus (HSV) infection (HVS proctitis) also may occur in immunocompeteut individuals [1,2]. Table 51-1 shows the characteristics of common viral colitis.

In the later course of HIV infection, patient's immune function is markedly diminished, and diarrhea or/and colitis usually are due to a readily identifiable infection, often one of the following [2]:

1. A bacterial infection, particularly Mycobacterium avium complex, Salmonella, Shigella, or Campylobacter;
2. A parasitic infection with Cryptosporidium, Microsporidium, or Isospora;
3. A viral infection such as CMV, adenovirus, or herpes simplex. Using a comprehensive approach to diagnosis, a specific pathogen can be identified in 85 % of patients (table 51-2). The principle of management is to treat gastrointestinal infection and systemic supportive therapy.

There may be a relationship of HIV infection to the course of inflammatory bowel disease including UC, CD and indeterminate colitis [2]. With a progressive decline in the CD4 counts, IBD activity may improve or remit. The CD4 counts at which remission occurs may reflect severe immunodeficiency and the risk of AIDS-related infection, with symptoms due to the infection rather than to IBD. Active symptoms of IBD may occur in patients with HIV infection who have lesser degree of immunodeficiency

CMV infection was first reported in China in 2003 in a patient with diarrhea after surgery of rectal cancer [9]. Colonoscopy showed a tumorous lesion with gray-white color (figure 51-1, and intranuclear inclusions were identified in mucosal biopsies with hematoxylin) and eosin staining. The patient was successfully treated with acyclovir, and discharged 2 weeks thereafter.

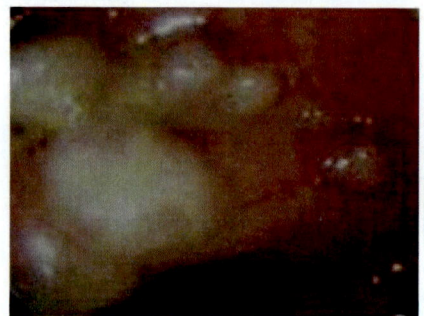 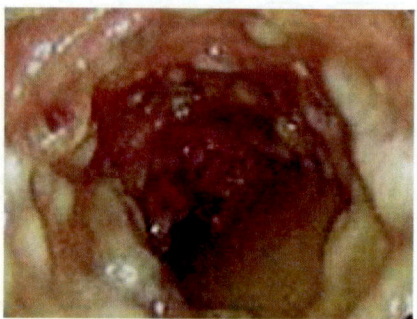

Figure 51-1. Colonoscopic view of CMV infection in a patient with 4-week diarrhea after rectal caner surgery: nodular lesions with gray color were shown. CMV antibody positive (Torch test), CMV-PCR (polymer chain reaction) positive, and the patient was cured with antiviral therapy.

Table 51-2. Evaluation of diarrhea in patients with AIDS [2]

Steps	Examinations	Contents
1	*stool examination* routine exams direct, concentrated, or both for	parasites using saline, trichrome, and acid-fast preparations
	routine cultures three times	bacterial pathogens including Salmonella, Shigella, Campylobacter)
	special exams	Clostridium difficile toxin assay
2.	*gastroduodenoscopy* duodenal fluid examination duodenal biopsies hematoxylin-eosin stain methenamine silver fite, Giemsa stain acid-fast stains	parasites cultures for CMV and Mycobacteria protozoa and viral inclusions Fungi; Mycobacteria
3.	*colonoscopy* mucosal biopsies hematoxyline -eosin methenamine silver Giemsa stain for fite, acid-fast stains	CMV, Adenovirus, Mycobacteria, and HSV Protozoa and viral inclusions Fungi Mycobacteria
4.	*electron microscopy* mucosal biopsies for	Microsporidia (duodenum) Adenovirus (colon)

Table 51-1. Characteristics of viral colitis [1,3-9]

Characteristics	Cytomegalovirus (CMV)	Human immunodeficiency virus (HIV)	Herpes simplex virus (HSV)	Adenovirus	Chlamydia trachomatis
DNA or RNA	DNA	DNA	DNA	DNA	DNA and RNA
inclusions	large intranuclear, and small cytoplasmic inclusions in epithelial cells	intranuclear inclusions	intranuclear inclusions in epithelial cells (or brain cells)	intranuclear inclusions in epithelial cells	cytoplasmic inclusions in epithelial cells
GI involvements	esophagus, colorectum (cecum) small intestine (terminal ileum)		oropharynx, esophagus, anorectum, perianal areas		rectal stenosis and fistula formation
symptoms	abdominal pain, bloody diarrhea, fever, weight loss	diarrhea, nausea, vomiting, anorexia,	anorectal pain, tenesmus, rectal discharge, constipation inguinal adenopathy, difficulty with urinary voiding lumbo sacral dysesthesias, importence, mucoid stools, but diarrhea is uncommon	watery diarrhea with weight loss	LGV proctitis [It is the etiologic agent for lymphogranuloma venereum (LGV)]
an opportunistic infection	yes		sexually transmitted direct contact with pts, or		
affects immunocom-promised patients (most commonly in patients with AIDS[1] or those on immunosuppressive therapy	yes		indirect contact with contaminated saliva or dinner ware		

Table 51-1. (Continued).

Characteristics	Cytomegalovirus (CMV)	Human immunodeficiency virus (HIV)	Herpes simplex virus (HSV)	Adenovirus	Chlamydia trachomatis
affects immunocompetent patients with UC	yes	yes	individuals who engage in receptive anal intercourse		sexually transmitted
CD4 count	< 100	IBD activity may improve or remit, with a progressive declined CD4 count	usually not affects the colon		NA[2]
Complications	ischemic necrosis, intestinal perforation	low-grade small bowel bacterial overgrowth fat malabsorption	ulcers in perianal area		rectal structure, fistula formation, may mimic CD
colonoscopic view	may mimic UC (with a granular or friable mucosa), or CD (focal hemorrhagic ulcers with normal intervening mucosa discrete, punched-out shallow, usually single, and vary in size from 2-6mm)	with a bacterial, a parasitic, or a viral	highly suggestive lesion: external perianal vesicles plus rectal mucosa lesion (erythmatous ulcer in the distal 10 cm of the rectum)	may be normal, or small (a few mm) erythematous raised lesions	rectum: discrete ulcers friable mucosa, may extend to the descending colon
Diagnosis	identification of intranuclear inclusions in mucosal cells, immunohistochemical studies, cultures of mucosal biopsies	small intestinal biopsies: partial villous atrophy (not correlated with the occurrence of diarrhea)	sigmoldoscopy with culture of biopsy or swab samples	identification of virus in biopsies of inflamed colonic mucosa by electron microscopy, immunohistochemistry, or culture of the virus on epithelial cells	cultures, serologic tests and/or specific identification with PCR technique

Characteristics	Cytomegalovirus (CMV)	Human immunodeficiency virus (HIV)	Herpes simplex virus (HSV)	Adenovirus	Chlamydia trachomatis
Treatment	1. ganciclovir, i.v. (5 mg/kg, Bid ×14 d) or 2. foscarnet, i.v. (90 mg/kg, Bid×3 wks)	treat GI infection, and systemic supportive therapy including vaccines and highly active antiviral agents antiretroviral therapy (HAAPT) with integrase inhibitor ?	Acyclovir, p.o. (200 mg five times daily×14 d), or i.v. (5 mg/kg t.i.d) Or long-term suppressive therapy (recurrent infection is common).		rifampicin, or other antibiotics such as tetracycline, chloramphenicol and sulfonamides

[1] AIDS: acquired immunodeficiency syndrome. [2] NA: no data available.

Bacterial Colitis

1. Campylobacter Jejuni

This is a curved or spiral gram-negative rod organism [2]. It is a part of the natural flora in many wild and domesticated animals, including household pets, and is one of the most commonly identified bacterial pathogen in cases of diarrhea in the some developed countries. It is spread by fecal-oral contamination, usually from eating unwashed food, and the incubation period is 2 to 5 days.

It typically causes self-limited infectious diarrhea [2,6]. Symptoms include severe bloody or watery diarrhea, fever, abdominal pain, malaise, and nausea. However, 20 % of infected patients remain asymptomatic. Extraintestinal manifestations, such as arthralgias, erythema nodosum, and hepatosplenomegaly, may be present [6]. Bacteremia may occur in elderly or immurocompromised patients. The mortality rate is 2.4 per 1000 infections. Infection is associated with Guillain-Barré syndrome in 20 to 40% of cases. Twenty percent of patients may relapse or have a prolonged illness that may mimic IBD [7]. Persistent infection may occur in patients with AIDS.

Endoscopic features: Campylobacter colitis, typically, produces mucosal erythema and friability in the early stages, and diffuse exudates over the mucosa that may mimic the endoscopic appearance of severe UC. Campylobacter infection can cause a relapse of established UC. Colonic mucosal biopsies also can be confused with either UC or CD [6]. Less commonly, the colonoscopic appearance resembles Crohn's disease with hyperemia, friability, edema, and scattered small ulcers.

The rectum is usually involved and the right colon is rarely affected; up to 50% of patients may present with rectal bleeding and tenesmus similar to UC [2,8].

Diagnosis is made by stool culture [2]; dark-field or phase-control examination of fresh stool may be otherwise diagnostic [6].

Treatment: the disease is self-limited, and the role of antibiotics is controversial [2]. In patients with severe symptoms in whom the diagnosis is confirmed, erythromycin 250 to 500 mg four times daily for 7 days or ciprofloxacin 500 mg twice daily can be prescribed; antidiarrheal drugs should be avoided.

2. Escherichia Coli (E. Coli)

This gram-negative rod is an abundant portion of the normal flora of the colon. There are five categories of pathogenic E. coli, including three that cause colitis: enterohemorrhagic E coli (EHEC), enteroinvasive E.coli (EIEC), and enteroaggregative E coli (EaggEC).

Both EIEC and EaggEC occur primarily in the tropics. EIEC is rarely encountered in industrialized countries. It causes an illness similar to Shigella infection, with direct invasion of the distal ileal and colonic mucosa. EaggEC (primarily in children) form a stacked brick aggregate appearance on epithelial cells and cause injury both by adherence to epithelial cells and by toxin elaboration.

EHEC produces a hemorrhagic colitis, and also lead to a hemolytic uremic syndrome and thrombocytopenic purpura [2,6].

Major food outbreaks have been reported from consumption of contaminated undercooked beef products like hamburger, unpasteurized milk, or drinking water and contact with swimming pool water or cow manure [2,6].

Lesions are present in the terminal ileum and colon; the mucosa appears edematous, hyperemia, and friable, mimicking CD [2]; and on biopsy can be confused with ischemic injury. Although EHEC and EIEC can complicate IBD, these virulent strains with adherence factors were no more common in control patients than among those with symptomatic or asymptomatic UC or CD of the colon [2].

Diagnosis is made by stool culture. Treatment is supportive; antibiotics are not effective.

3. Neisseria Gonorrhoeae

This bacteria, like other sexually transmitted disease such as HSV and LGV (see Table 51-1), produces a proctitis [6]. Anal intercourse is the largest risk factor for developing this proctitis.

A creamy rectal discharge or rectal bleeding, rectal friability, and erythema are usually present. Culture are required to distinguish this from UC [6,11].

Treatment: antibiotics including Quinolones or Cephalosporins are all effective, with a cure rate of 98% to 100% [9]. One of the following oral agents or injections can be selected individually: ofloxacin (0.4 - 0.6 once daily); or Norfloxacin (0.8 - 1.0 once daily); or Ciprofloxacin (0.5 once daily); or Ceftriaxone (250 mg i.m. once daily); Cefotaxime (1.0 i.m. once daily) [11].

4. Salmonella Infection

These gram-negative rods are now part of the normal flora of cattle and poultry and infections occur via contaminated food or water.

The organism primarily invades the epithelium of the small bowel such as the ileum; the infection spares the rectum and only affects the colon sporadically [6]. In the early stage, there is edema, hyperemia, and granularity of the mucosa that then progresses to petechial hemorrhages and mucosal friability [2].

For typhoid fever cases, multiple ulcers in the ileum can be observed in 90% of patients (usually between two to three weeks after onset of the disease) [12]. However, ulcerative lesions also can be seen in the area between ileo-cecum to right colon. The positive rates for Widal reaction, blood culture and bone marrow culture are 79%, 72% and 88%, respectively.

Symptoms include nausea and vomiting followed by watery or bloody diarrhea and fever. A distinctive acute systemic febrile infection caused by Salmonella typhosa is called typhoid fever, which is the result of heat-labile enterotoxin that on invasion of the intestinal mucosa causes an influx of water and electrolytes into the lumen of the bond [2,12].

The illness is self-limited and usually resolves over 2 to 5 days (at most, lasts less than 2 months [2,6]. Less than 1% of infected patients become asymptomatic carriers.

5. Shigella Dysenteriae

This gram-negative bacterium causes bacillary dysentery or Shigellosis [2]. The pathogen produces toxins (both Shiga and Shiga-like) that inhibit protein synthesis and are associated with the development of hemolytic uremic syndrome.

Symptoms begin with watery diarrhea, abdominal pain, and fever followed by rectal tenesmus and by the passage of blood and mucus per rectum.

Although patchy in appearance, the endoscopic appearance often resembles UC because there are multiple ulcers with considerable exudates [6]. The mucosa often appears magenta colored because of the intense erythema.

Diagnosis is made by stool culture, which only positive in 50% of cases [6].

Infection usually is self-limited, but for severe symptoms ciprofloxacin 500 mg twice daily for 3 to 5 days is effective.

6. Yersinia Enterocolitica

This gram-negative coccobacillus, including several variant species, is found primarily in the cooler regions of Europe and North America [2]. Infection results from eating contaminated foods, particularly pork.

The organism causes injury by invasion of the epithelium overlying Peyer's patches and also produces an enterotoxin, although injury from this toxin has not been documented.

Endoscopy: the bacteria may cause enterocolitis, and affects primarily the terminal ileum and causes aphthous ulcers adjacent to normal mucosa, and thickening of the ileal wall resembling CD [2, 6]. Infection also may cause diffuse erythema, friability, and edema throughout the entire colon mimicking UC.

Symptoms include diarrhea, fever, and abdominal pain that usually resolve over 14 to 17 days, although in some patients, symptoms are more persistent (may last for months) [2, 6].

Arthritis occurs in about 2% of patients, more commonly in those with HLA-B27 phenotypes. Other extraintestinal symptoms include polyarthritis, erythema nodosum, and erythema multiforme.

Diagnosis is made by stool culture on selective media.

Infection usually is self-limited, but antibiotics may be indicated in patients with severe symptoms. Effective agents include ciprofloxacin, co-trimoxazole, or tetracycline.

Protozoa Infection

Protozoa parasites may cause acute self-limited illness in immunocompetent patients or chronic debilitation diarrhea in immunosuppressed patients, particularly those with AIDS

1. Balantidium Coli

It is a ciliate protozoan that infects the colon rarely, and transmitted by pigs [2, 6]. The infection causes varying degrees of ulceration in the rectosigmoid that initially may resemble CD or amebiasis. The inflammation varies from scattered and superficial ulcers to multiple and deep lesions. The characteristic trophozoites may be found in scrapings from the rectal ulcers or in tissue samples.

2. Cryptosporidium

These tiny (2 to 6 μm) coccidial organisms are attached to the gut and biliary epithelium. Infection occurs via contaminated water supplies.

The diarrhea is large in volume and watery, with associated cramping, abdominal discomfort, and weight loss.

Diagnosis is made by identification of organism in the stool or in jejunal aspirates using a modified acid-fast stain.

There is no proved effective therapy, although there are anecdotal reports of efficacy using spiramycin, paromomycin, and azithromycin.

3. Entamieba Histolytica

Ten percent of the world's population is infected with Entamoeba histolytica or a related species, and these infections will result in about 50 million cases of invasive amebiasis and up to 100,000 total deaths [2]. It is one of the most common causes of infectious diarrhea in developing countries [5].

Infection usually is a result of ingestion of contaminated food or water, but it also can be sexually transmitted among male homosexuals through anal intercourse, and following colonic irrigation with unsterilized equipment.

GI involvement: amebiasis primarily affects the large bowel [1], however, trophozoites develop from cysts in the small intestine that adhere to the colonic mucosa with invasion of the epithelium by proteolytic action.

Symptoms: vary from none (up to 90% of Entamoeba infections are asymptomatic) to a fulminate illness with explosive bloody diarrhea, abdominal cramps, tenesmus and fever. Frequent loose stools containing blood and mucus, and tenderness on abdominal examination are seen in acute phase patients.

Colonoscopic examination shows focal punctate hemorrhagic ulcers with normal intervening mucosa in the cecum (in 80% to 90% of patients) or right colon segments in chronic phase [1, 2, 6]. The ulcers may be covered with a yellowish-white exudates and may resemble CD [3]. In acute amebic colitis, there may by diffuse granularity and friability with an appearance similar to UC [2, 6, 13].

The diagnosis of amebic colitis is made by colonoscopic biopsy from a ulcer edge with identification of amebic cysts or trophozoites (with a 60% to 90% positive rates) [1, 6]. A diarrhetic patient who recently traveled to developing countries should be considered amebic infection [6].

Serum antibodies to amoeba are detected in up to 95% of patients with invasive colitis or liver abscess, but antibodies persist for years after acute infection so that a definitive diagnosis of current infection cannot be based on serologic tests alone.

Treatment of invasive colitis is metronidazole, 750 mg orally three times daily, or 500 mg intravenously every 6 hours for 10 days.

Less severe colitis responds to tetracycline, 500 mg four times daily for 14 days and dehydroemetine, 0.5 to 0.75 mg/kg (maximum of 90 mg/day) IM twice daily for 5 days.

Amebiasis is an uncommon cause of exacerbation of UC, but identification is important, particularly for patients treated with corticosteroids.

4. Isospora Belli

Cysts of this organism invade epithelium and develop into trophozoites.

It is an uncommon cause of traveler's diarrhea among otherwise healthy hosts and causes an acute self –limited diarrhea with fever and abdominal pain. Isospora infection occurs in less than 3% of AIDS patients in the United States and cause chronic profuse watery diarrhea, weight loss, and abdominal cramping pain.

Diagnosis is made by identification of oocysts using acid-fast stains of a stool sample or duodenal aspirate.

Treatment is with trimethoprim-sulfamethoxazole, but recurrences are common, and ongoing prophylaxis often is necessary.

5. Microsporidium

These organisms are among the smallest of the eukaryotes and are obligate intracellular parasites.

Infection occurs almost exclusively among HIV-1 infected individuals and causes chronic watery diarrhea and weigh loss.

One of the microsporidia, Enterocytozoon bieneus, can be identified by light microscopy examination of stool stained with Giemsa or modified trichrome.

Treatment with albendazole, 400 to 800 mg twice daily, appears promising, but there are no controlled trials.

6. Schistosoma Japonica

Schistosoma japonica is a parasite that may be difficult to diagnose because it is not commonly seen in the hospital; The encysted schistosomes are found in biopsies.

Schistosomiasis produces a severely inflamed colon. Often the rectum and sigmoid colon are involved and may mimic UC; in the cases, there are shallow ulcerations with hyperemia, friability, and edema of the mucosa (figure 51-2).

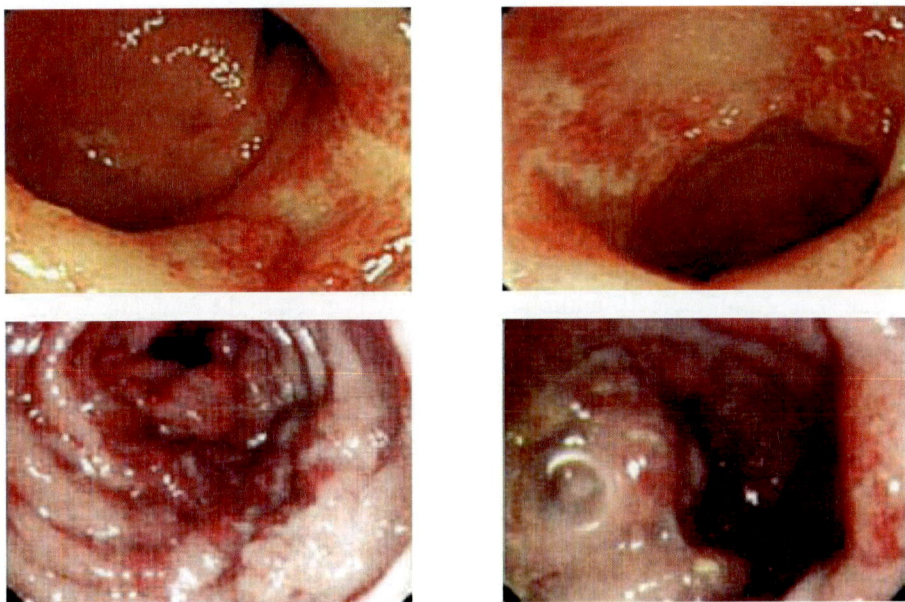

Figure 51-2. Colitis in active schistosma japonica showing edema, hyperemia and ulcers (A and B); and hypertrophic lesions including scar and polypoid changes in chronic stage of the infection (C and D).

In chronic cases, ova were calcified and deposited (figure 51-3) with numerous lymphocytes, plasma cells infiltration and submucosal fibrosis [14].

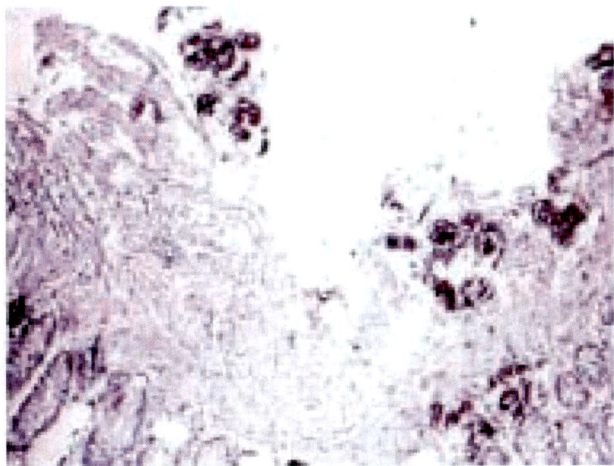

Figure 51-3. Colonoscopy biopsy specimen showing calcified ova deposited in the mucosa with submucosal fibrosis.

Fungal Infection

1. Actinomycosis

Actinomycosis israelii: this is an anaerobic gram-positive bacterium, and is found in the mouth, lungs, and GI tract.

GI tract involvement: the most common site is the ileocecal region, and it can produce a suppurative, granulomatous infection with a propensity for fistula formation and a release of "sulfur granules."

Symptoms include weight loss, night sweats, draining fistulas, and abdominal masses.
The diagnosis is confirmed by culture and histopathologic evaluation.
Treatment: Penicilline G is highly effective, and a high dose is choice of better efficacy. In general, a dose of 2-million to 10-million units per day is given in the beginning according to patient condition, and the dose is tapered when the condition is stabilized. Treatment should be maintained 1 to 3 months, or until the lesion is resolved [15].

2. Candida And Aspergillus

In severely immunocompromised patients, including those with AIDS or patients receiving chemotherapy for malignancy, Candida or Aspergillus infections can be identified in the submucosa.

These infections have a high mortality rate despite specific therapy probably because of underlying debility of the hosts.

3. Histoplasmosis

It is a mycotic infection that rarely infects the colon. Involvement of the ileocecal area usually occurs in the setting of acute disseminated histoplasmosis in severely immunocompromised patients. Common findings are fever, hepatosplenomegaly, lymphadenopathy, and jaundice.

The transmural inflammatory changes in the bowel can mimic the appearance of CD, although the intestinal symptoms usually are minimal. When it is present, there are usually mucosal hyperemia, friability, ulcerations, and pseudopolyps in the ileocecal region. However, the overall clinical picture with systemic involvement, including the lungs, usually is easily distinguishable from CD, friability, ulcerations, lymph node hypertrophy, and pseufopolyps in the ileocecal region. Rarely, the infection can be misdiagnosed as Kala azar (figure 51-4) [16].

This mimics CD in the predominantly right-sided distribution and its noncontiguous nature.

The diagnosis should be considered in immunocompromised hosts and traverlers from endemic area. The organism is identified by serology, culture or by DNA probe.

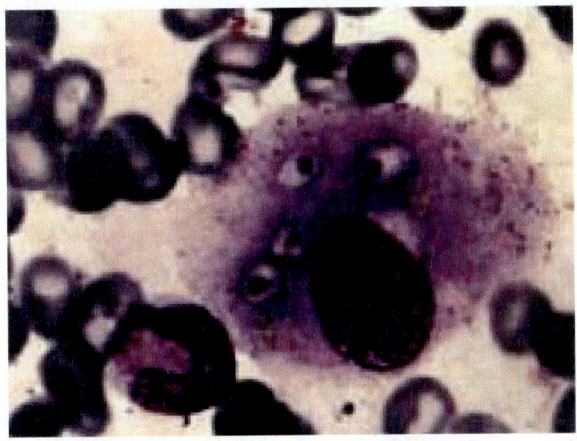

Figure 51-4. The organism of histoplasmosis was identified within a macropage in the bone marrow smear specimen (Giemsa stain).

Treatment: Amphtericin B (initial dose is 2.5 mg once daily or every other day, and the dose is increased gradually to 50 mg to 60 mg once daily; each dose should not be greater than 1.0 mg/kg once daily; and a total dose of 0.8 to 1.0 gram) is given intravenously for ten weeks [2,17]. The dose may be doubled for disseminated type of disease. Other antifungal agents such as ketoconazole, and clotrimazole also may be used, and itraconazole can be used for mild cases.

Treponema Infection

Treponema Pallidum

It causes primary or secondary syphilis, and is another sexually transmitted infection that leads to a nonspecific proctitis.

Anal or anorectal lesions may be accompanied by symptoms or asymptomatic; it can resemble both CD and UC [2, 6, 18].

Penicillin is an effective agent to relief the symptoms or to cure the infection [18]

References

[1] Chutkan RK, Waye JD. Endoscopy in inflammatory bowel disease. In: Kirsner JB (ed.). 5th ed. Inflammatory Bowel Disease Philadelphia. London. New York. St. Louis. Syd. W.B. Saunders Company. 2000; P.453-477.

[2] Tremaine WJ. The other colitides. In: Kirsner JB (ed.). 5th ed. Inflammatory Bowel Disease. Philadelphia. London. New York. St. Louis. Syd. W.B. Saunders Company. 2000; P.410-423.

[3] Riddell RH. Pathology of idiopathic inflammatory bowel disease. In: Kirsner JB (ed.) Inflammatory Bowel Disease. 5th ed. Philadelphia. London. New York. St. Louis. Syd.: W.B. Saunders Company. 2000; P; 427-450.

[4] Haggitt RC. Pathology of bowel inflammatory. In: AGA Postgraduate course: idiopathic inflammatory bowel disease. New Orleans, Louisiana 1984; P.53-63.

[5] Carpenter HA, Talley NJ. The importance of clinicopathological correlation in the diagnosis of inflammatory conditions of the colon: histological patterns with clinical implications. *An. J. Gastroenterol.* 2000; 95(4):878-896.

[6] Krok KL, Lichtenstein GR. Inflammatory bowel disease. In: Ginsberg GG, Kochman ML, Norton I, Gastout CJ (eds). Clinical Gastrointestinal Endoscopy. Printed in Beijing Elsevier Saunders 2005; P311-332.

[7] Lee SD, Cohen RD. Endoscopy in inflammatory bowel disease. *Gastroenterol. Clin. N. Am.* 2002; 31(1):119-132.

[8] Zheng J-j. Inflammatory conditions of the colon: the importance of clinicopathological correlation in the diagnosis. *Chin. J. Dig.* 2002;22(2):36-37 (Chinese).

[9] Marion JF, Rubin PH, Present DH. Differential diagnosis of Chronic ulcerative colitis and Crohn's disease. In: Kirsner JB (ed.). Inflammatory Bowel Disease.5th ed. Philadelphia. London. New York. St. Louis. Syd. W.B. Saunders Company. 2000; P.315-325.

[10] Liu H-j, Wang A, Yang Y-m. Cytomegalovirus infection: one case report. *Chin. J. Dig. Endosc.* 2003; 20(1). (Chinese).

[11] Xu Y-c, Li F, Wen Q-s, et al. Colonoscopic diagnosis of gonorrheal proctocolitis. *Chin. J. Dig. Endosc.* 2002; 19(1):13-14. (Chinese).

[12] Huang X-f, Zhou J-p, Yang Z-s, et al. Colonoscopy in the diagnosis of intestinal typhoid fever. 2002; 19 (1):40. (Chinese).

[13] Wang Y-z, Lu X-p, Yang J. Entamoeba infection in ulcerative colitis. *Chin. J. Dig. Dis.* 2006; 26(3):146. (Chinese).

[14] Guo J, Shen L, Shen Z-x, et al. Endoscopic and histologic characteristics of the intestinal schistosomiasis. *Chin. J. Dig. Dis.* 2006; 23(2):90-93. (Chinese).

[15] Zhao B-f, Xu Y-h. Primary actinomycosis of the bowel: one case study. *Chin. J. Gener. Surg.* 2000; 15(10):637.

[16] Li J-h. Report on a histoplasmosis patient misdiagnosed as kala azar. *Chin. Trop. Med.* 2005; 2:1.

[17] Xu S-p, Yi S-q, Cheng W-x. Fever, diarrhea, and emaciation: clinical case conference.. *Chin. J. Dig. Dis.* 2004; 24(7):445-446 (Chinese).

[18] Liu J. Syphilitic ulcer in the rectum: one case report. *Chin. J. Dig. Endosc.* 2002; 19 (6):380 (Chinese).

Acknowledgments

The editor is grateful to my professional colleagues in the Section of Gastroenterology of Su-zhou Municipal Hospital for their warm academic help and support. The editor is also grateful to the many contributing authors whose experience and scholarship fill the pages of the book. The editor also wishes to express his deep gratitude to Mrs. Xia-shuang Zhu for her expert secretarial support and assistance in processing book manuscripts. It would have been impossible to accomplish this work in such a short period of time without her hard work. I am grateful to Mr. Frank Columbus, President and Editor-in-Chief, Nova Science Publishers, Inc. for his warm invitation to publish this book; to Mr. Michael Nespler for his expert editorial assistance; and for their guidance through the process of publication. I am grateful for the understanding of my wife.

Index

A

abdomen, 31, 315, 364
abdominal, 31, 55, 71, 76, 126, 147, 148, 149, 151, 153, 158, 160, 168, 239, 249, 251, 260, 273, 277, 293, 299, 307, 308, 309, 314, 315, 318, 321, 322, 339, 342, 350, 355, 359, 363, 368, 382, 387, 390, 391, 392, 395
abdominal cramps, 350, 392
abnormalities, 19, 25, 55, 79, 128, 133, 152, 160, 163, 164, 220, 280, 308, 333, 339, 340, 345
abortion, 266
absorption, 7, 89, 91, 92, 96, 198, 204, 206, 209, 214, 218, 221, 234, 235, 236, 240, 247, 256, 265, 289
academic, 399
access, 60
accounting, 206
accuracy, 90, 94, 95, 106, 107, 108, 114, 116, 127, 180, 182
acetate, 347
acetylation, 206
acid, 135, 136, 138, 165, 173, 174, 197, 198, 200, 205, 210, 211, 228, 237, 243, 252, 254, 255, 256, 273, 340, 342, 364, 380, 381, 391, 393
acoustic, 60
acquired immunodeficiency syndrome, 386
ACTH, 215, 219
actinomycosis, 398
activation, 203, 213, 214, 254, 281, 283, 285, 286, 287, 294, 295, 353
acupuncture, 251
acute, 11, 13, 15, 39, 44, 55, 112, 134, 140, 172, 179, 211, 224, 228, 232, 234, 241, 259, 266, 272, 280, 291, 301, 314, 315, 316, 317, 322, 323, 330, 342, 349, 350, 351, 354, 355, 367, 376, 389, 391, 392, 395
acute infection, 39, 392
adalimumab, 295, 296, 299, 300, 301, 302
adenocarcinoma, 94, 180, 187
adenomas, 94, 97, 98, 198, 336
adenopathy, 382
adenovirus, 379
adhesion, 20, 76, 93, 214, 281, 284, 285, 318
adjudication, 114
adjunctive therapy, 138, 188, 235, 236, 247, 249, 263
administration, 205, 206, 208, 215, 217, 233, 244, 252, 259, 262, 264, 285, 287, 298, 299, 318, 325, 346
adolescence, 321
adolescent patients, 44
adrenal insufficiency, 220
adulthood, 321
adults, 7, 53, 149, 152, 155, 183, 216, 222, 267, 274, 276, 277
adventitia, 60, 61
adverse event, 225, 230, 249, 272, 273, 299, 301
Africa, 308
age, 7, 38, 97, 145, 149, 151, 192, 193, 246, 249, 335, 355, 369
age related macular degeneration, 246
agents, 85, 102, 139, 144, 198, 205, 213, 230, 233, 234, 235, 236, 255, 257, 260, 263, 264, 270, 273, 283, 284, 288, 295, 296, 300, 308, 345, 346, 353, 375, 388, 390, 396
agglutination, 150
aggregates, 22, 56, 133
aggregation, 23, 30, 105, 342
agonist, 312
agranulocytosis, 209

aid, 37
aiding, 351
AIDS, 380, 386, 387, 391, 392, 395
air, 66, 67, 72, 102, 114, 243, 317
air embolism, 243
albumin, 168, 214
alcohol, 127, 200, 359, 360
alendronate, 220
algorithm, 188
alimentary canal, 18, 29, 151
allele, 199
allergic, 145, 183, 227, 300, 321, 322
allergic reaction, 183, 227, 322
allergy, 313, 321, 323
allogeneic, 349
alternative, 76, 111, 186, 207, 220, 230, 238, 260, 261, 272
amebiasis, 77, 391
amelioration, 239
amino, 241, 242, 243, 244, 288
amino acid, 241, 242, 243, 244, 288
aminoglycosides, 368
Aminosalicylates, 182, 203, 256, 259, 264
amylase, 315
amyloidosis, 312
anabolism, 239
anaemia, 76
anaerobic, 255, 368, 395
anaesthetics, 236
anal fissures, 154, 179, 180, 187
anastomosis, 171
anatomy, 66
anemia, 31, 152, 158, 208, 239, 255, 323, 342, 359
aneuploidy, 195, 199
anger, 249
angiodysplasia, 333
angiogenesis, 90, 96
angiography, 315
animal models, 197
animal studies, 209
animals, 224, 283, 387
ankylosing spondylitis, 148, 296, 299, 301
anorectal fistula, 69, 179
anorexia, 55, 240, 321, 369, 382
antacids, 33
antagonists, 302, 303
antibacterial, 204
antibiotic, 240, 255, 272, 339, 357, 358, 367, 369, 370, 371

antibiotics, 137, 138, 183, 188, 203, 255, 264, 265, 266, 274, 317, 340, 353, 357, 367, 368, 371, 385, 387, 388, 390
antibody, 270, 291, 298, 353, 375, 380
anticancer, 294
anticoagulant, 317
antigen, 7, 195, 281, 284, 285, 289, 369
anti-inflammatory, 135, 139, 204, 205, 213, 214, 215, 233, 252, 253, 261, 287, 313, 341, 357
anti-inflammatory drugs, 233, 313, 341
antimetabolites, 183, 230, 274
antinuclear antibodies, 183, 309
antiretroviral, 385
antisense, 283, 285, 290, 295
antisense oligonucleotides, 283, 295
antithrombin, 312
Anti-tumor, 139, 352
antiviral, 380, 385
antrum, 55
anus, 3, 17, 26, 30, 53, 151, 153, 177
anxiety, 249
APC, 71, 199, 286
aphthous ulcers, 47, 48, 81, 85, 153, 171, 280, 345, 390
apoptosis, 7, 139, 206, 252, 294, 297, 341, 351
apoptotic, 342, 351, 352
appendicitis, 323
appetite, 153, 217
application, 61, 80, 102, 103, 106, 227, 231
arachidonic acid, 205
argon, 360
Army, 121, 122
arrhythmias, 312
artery, 312, 313
arthralgia, 152, 167, 168, 226, 301
arthritis, 148, 204, 308, 312, 327
AS, 140, 234, 236, 337, 372
ascending colon, 15, 205, 215, 234, 279, 322
ascites, 322, 364
aseptic, 135
Asia, 8, 25, 30, 33, 131, 132, 135, 139, 143, 163, 165, 267, 340, 371
aspergillosis, 184, 298
aspirate, 393
aspiration, 54
aspiration pneumonia, 54
aspirin, 205
assessment, 44, 56, 59, 60, 61, 69, 84, 85, 92, 93, 99, 159, 160, 162, 163, 165, 166, 169, 172, 173, 175, 180, 220, 225, 242, 262, 276

associations, 143, 156
assumptions, 86
asthma, 221
asymptomatic, 37, 85, 86, 317, 323, 365, 368, 369, 387, 388, 389, 392, 396
atrophy, 13, 30, 172, 216, 243, 244, 316, 323, 377, 384
attacks, 14, 43, 44, 174, 222
attention, 134, 242
Australia, 308
autoantibodies, 125, 128, 262
autoimmune, 125, 308
autoimmunity, 294
availability, 204, 206, 215
avoidance, 235
Azathioprine, 138, 183, 228, 260

B

B cells, 227, 280, 286
babies, 266
bacilli, 135
bacillus, 368
back pain, 287
bacteria, 245, 256, 280, 291, 312, 368, 388, 390
bacterial, 154, 203, 204, 206, 243, 256, 257, 280, 289, 308, 361, 370, 379, 381, 384, 387
bacterium, 389, 395
barium, 59, 84, 86, 132, 173, 313
barium enema, 59, 132, 173, 313
barrier, 136, 293
basal cell carcinoma, 180, 187
basement membrane, 308
basophils, 213
B-cell, 214
beef, 388
behavior, 145, 166
Beijing, 115
benchmark, 230, 273
beneficial effect, 139, 197
benefits, 98, 196, 214, 231, 259, 273
benign, 51, 155, 321, 323, 335
bias, 84
bile, 126, 127, 153, 197
bile duct, 126, 127, 153
binding, 213, 214, 280, 371
bioavailability, 204, 214, 221, 261
biochemical, 155, 157
biochemistry, 243
biologic, 269, 295, 301

biologic agents, 269, 295
biological, 137, 138, 139, 174, 283, 284, 286, 288, 296, 303
bismuth, 236
black hole, 104
bleeding, 12, 38, 39, 40, 41, 42, 76, 77, 132, 133, 147, 152, 159, 160, 161, 162, 314, 316, 317, 322, 329, 330, 335, 336, 339, 342, 350, 351, 352, 354, 364, 376, 387, 388
blocks, 271, 300
blood, 55, 90, 103, 136, 147, 150, 158, 159, 161, 224, 228, 240, 243, 252, 256, 260, 264, 311, 314, 315, 339, 355, 359, 360, 363, 368, 389, 390, 392
blood flow, 90, 311
blood transfusion, 264
blurring, 41, 148
body temperature, 168
body weight, 168, 228
Bohr, 309
bone, 216, 220, 221, 227, 228, 246, 256, 260, 261, 353, 354, 389, 396
bone marrow, 227, 228, 256, 260, 261, 353, 354, 389, 396
borderline, 197
bowel obstruction, 31, 153, 155, 279, 323, 340, 364
bowel perforation, 376
bowel sounds, 315
brain, 382
branching, 38, 40, 47, 133, 178, 346, 377
brick, 388
broad spectrum, 317
buttons, 103
bypass, 144, 312, 313

C

C reactive protein, 170, 174
Ca^{2+}, 243
cachexia, 273
calcium, 220, 240
caliber, 39, 194
Canada, 28
cancer, 37, 90, 96, 97, 101, 107, 111, 114, 115, 122, 137, 145, 154, 177, 180, 191, 192, 194, 195, 196, 199, 200, 205, 262, 294, 324, 330, 380
cancer screening, 199
cancers, 91, 115, 192, 194, 199
Candida, 395
candidates, 314
capacity, 240

capillary, 90, 92, 93, 94, 96, 316, 360
capsule, 38, 71, 76, 77, 79, 80, 81, 84, 85, 86, 87, 204
carbohydrates, 154
carcinogenesis, 197, 200
carcinoma, 27, 51, 54, 55, 67, 68, 92, 97, 121, 133, 149, 154, 155, 191, 192, 193, 94, 95, 198, 199, 315, 355
CARD15, 280
cardiovascular, 312, 314
carrier, 204, 257, 288, 368
case study, 150, 247, 337, 358, 398
Cataracts, 216
catheter, 69, 127, 242, 243
catheterization, 242, 243
cattle, 389
causation, 357
cavities, 66
C-C, 354
CCR, 281
CD3, 262, 286, 291
CD4, 203, 281, 286, 380, 384
CD40, 280, 286
CE, 71, 76, 79, 80, 84, 85, 222
cecum, 6, 28, 29, 73, 136, 322, 359, 360, 382, 389, 392
cell, 6, 8, 15, 22, 104, 105, 117, 133, 139, 172, 180, 199, 214, 228, 243, 280, 286, 288, 289, 290, 294, 312, 350, 353, 354, 377
cell adhesion, 139
cell membranes, 280
cell transplantation, 354
centigrade, 244
central nervous system, 214
certainty, 20
cesarean section, 187
CFA, 346
chemistry, 256
chemokines, 281
chemoprevention, 196, 198, 210, 205
chemotherapeutic drugs, 368, 370
chemotherapy, 352, 353, 395
childhood, 154, 220
children, 7, 31, 56, 149, 152, 153, 172, 174, 183, 189, 216, 246, 274, 303, 321, 337, 369, 388
Chinese, 8, 16, 23, 25, 26, 28, 30, 33, 34, 40, 44, 45, 52, 69, 77, 78, 121, 122, 140, 146, 150, 165, 189, 209, 211, 221, 231, 239, 246, 247, 249, 251, 252, 253, 254, 276, 314, 318, 319, 324, 337, 343, 354, 371, 397, 398

Chinese medicine, 249
Chlamydia trachomatis, 382, 383, 385
cholangiocarcinoma, 126, 127, 128
cholangiography, 128
cholangitis, 38, 98, 125, 126, 128, 148, 153, 191, 192, 200
cholesterol, 224, 312, 328
chromatin, 127
chromoendoscopy, 89, 92, 94, 95, 97, 98, 99, 102, 107, 108, 192, 195
chromosomal instability, 192
chronic disease, 256, 294
ciliate, 391
ciprofloxacin, 137, 183, 266, 274, 368, 387, 390
circulation, 252, 283, 289, 295, 318
cirrhosis, 224, 334
CL, 175, 340
classical, 112, 147
classification, 28, 33, 61, 90, 92, 94, 96, 98, 106, 107, 113, 122, 143, 145, 146, 150, 156, 158, 163, 178, 180, 181, 182, 189, 197, 330, 334
classified, 28, 61, 92, 95, 108, 113, 139, 178, 180, 204, 250, 283, 333
cleaning, 72
cleavage, 206
clinical diagnosis, 76
clinical presentation, 72, 144, 189, 309, 361
clinical symptoms, 77, 136, 158, 163, 204, 220, 251
clinical trial, 79, 157, 161, 163, 167, 174, 211, 236, 257, 269, 284, 287, 300, 301
clinically significant, 92, 206
clinicians, 143, 180, 220, 266, 296, 301, 308
clinicopathologic, 252, 307, 354
closure, 183, 184, 187, 274, 275, 301
CML, 351, 352
CMV, 350, 351, 379, 380, 381, 382, 383, 385
coagulation, 71, 283, 295, 360
coccidioidomycosis, 183
Cochrane, 210
cognitive, 90
cohort, 156, 196, 370
colectomy, 136, 137, 144, 146, 149, 193, 195, 261, 264, 265, 297, 313
collagen, 288, 307, 308
colon cancer, 97, 99, 108, 135, 154, 191, 196, 323
colon carcinogenesis, 192
colon polyps, 80
colonoscopy, 37, 38, 39, 43, 44, 60, 72, 84, 94, 95, 97, 99, 100, 101, 102, 106, 107, 108, 109, 112, 115, 121, 122, 132, 140, 149, 154, 175, 191, 193,

194, 195, 198, 313, 314, 316, 345, 346, 351, 354, 364, 381
colorectal surgeon, 178, 182
colorectum, 29, 97, 101, 103, 382
colors, 91
colostomy, 186, 346
combination therapy, 234, 263
common bile duct, 55
common symptoms, 350
competition, 256, 314
complement, 195, 298
complementary, 86, 92
complete blood count, 225, 229
complete remission, 137
complexity, 116, 131
compliance, 200, 207, 234, 263
complications, 55, 63, 66, 76, 97, 135, 136, 138, 154, 155, 167, 173, 184, 185, 216, 220, 221, 222, 241, 245, 251, 255, 260, 262, 266, 270, 272, 297, 301, 311, 339, 346, 349, 364
components, 256, 308
composite, 159, 161
composition, 90
compounds, 206, 214, 236, 284, 286, 288
computed tomography, 182
concentration, 114, 197, 206, 210, 214, 237, 243, 244, 245, 260, 261, 287, 289
concordance, 92
configuration, 40, 114
connective tissue, 102, 321, 322
consensus, 26, 33, 52, 135, 146, 150, 155, 195, 209, 237, 276
constipation, 147, 314, 322, 339, 343, 355, 357, 363, 382
consumption, 197, 388
contaminated food, 389, 390, 391
contamination, 387
contiguity, 55
continuing, 112
continuity, 132, 133, 186, 346
contraceptives, 214
contrast agent, 102
conversion, 214
correlation, 8, 15, 40, 62, 146, 163, 167, 170, 173, 233, 324, 350, 378, 397
corticosteroid therapy, 160, 216, 220, 221, 277, 298, 328
corticosteroids, 203, 214, 215, 216, 217, 218, 219, 220, 221, 223, 225, 226, 231, 235, 238, 240, 256,

259, 260, 261, 263, 266, 271, 272, 273, 289, 301, 353, 392
Cortisone, 165, 218
costimulatory molecules, 286
costs, 207, 244
coupling, 60
coverage, 94, 98, 255
covering, 207
CRC, 37, 101, 191, 192, 193, 194, 196, 197, 198
C-reactive protein, 270
creatinine, 184, 261
creep, 18
crops, 49
cross-sectional, 59, 60
CRP, 170, 171, 173
crust, 330
CS, 140, 200, 237, 238, 291
CSF, 288
CT, 66, 77, 84, 85, 86, 99, 155, 173, 315, 318, 334, 369
CT scan, 315, 318, 369
culture, 136, 364, 369, 384, 389, 395, 396
cumulative frequency, 181
curable, 101, 346
Curcumin, 252, 254
cyanotic, 179, 316
cyclooxygenase, 252, 254
cyclophosphamide, 227, 228, 231, 324
Cyclosporin, 174
cyclosporine, 136, 165, 184, 188, 224, 229, 230, 231, 261, 264, 265, 275, 324
Cyclosporine A, 261
cystitis, 228
cysts, 391, 392
cytokine, 139, 205, 214, 281, 283, 287, 290, 293, 294, 295, 300, 349
cytology, 127, 128
cytomegalovirus, 298, 312, 350, 354
cytoplasm, 103
cytosol, 280
cytotoxic, 342
cytotoxicity, 214, 369

D

DA, 56, 69, 189, 199, 318
dairy, 363
dairy products, 363
database, 196
de novo, 342

death, 126, 350
decisions, 75, 91, 157
defecation, 148, 153, 335, 355, 357
defects, 54, 55, 60, 62
defenses, 293
deficiency, 138, 198, 242, 243, 250, 312, 323, 346
deficits, 239, 240, 244
definition, 26, 111, 134, 151
deflation, 72, 73
deformities, 266
degradation, 294
degree, 3, 20, 49, 92, 108, 114, 159, 172, 193, 196, 264, 323, 345, 380
dehydration, 264, 315
delays, 207
delirium, 216
delivery, 187, 207, 209, 210, 236, 244, 256
dendritic cell, 203, 283
density, 59, 93, 118, 220
deposition, 18, 308
depressed, 96, 97, 111, 116, 121
depression, 90, 114, 216, 260
deregulation, 125, 128
dermatomyositis, 322
descending colon, 28, 49, 206, 340, 384
desensitization, 211
destruction, 7, 15, 105, 108, 163, 164, 165, 179, 316, 322, 351
detection, 22, 54, 67, 84, 91, 92, 95, 97, 98, 99, 101, 102, 106, 107, 108, 109, 121, 122, 191, 195, 369
detoxifying, 250
developing countries, 361, 391, 392
dexamethasone, 259
diabetes mellitus, 215, 216, 314
diabetic coma, 243
diagnostic, 23, 25, 37, 54, 59, 71, 76, 77, 79, 80, 84, 85, 86, 93, 94, 95, 98, 99, 106, 107, 109, 112, 122, 131, 132, 135, 140, 182, 250, 280, 323, 346, 350, 351, 352, 387
diaphragm, 180
diarrhea, 31, 37, 55, 71, 132, 133, 147, 151, 153, 158, 159, 168, 208, 214, 224, 226, 239, 240, 244, 245, 249, 250, 251, 293, 307, 308, 314, 317, 321, 322, 328, 329, 339, 341, 342, 346, 349, 350, 353, 355, 359, 363, 379, 380, 382, 384, 387, 389, 390, 391, 392, 393, 398
diet, 244, 245, 255
dietary, 239, 240, 246, 293, 336
dietary fiber, 336
dietary intake, 239, 240

diets, 138, 240, 244
differential diagnosis, 16, 37, 62, 92, 94, 98, 99, 140, 175, 315, 327
differentiation, 59, 61, 93, 94, 96, 116, 120, 203, 250, 283, 286, 322, 350, 364
diffusion, 207
digestion, 240, 244
digitalis, 313
dilation, 44, 71, 75, 76, 127, 128, 185, 264
discomfort, 153, 160, 256, 260, 314, 391
disease activity, 15, 37, 62, 80, 136, 157, 158, 160, 161, 162, 163, 166, 168, 169, 170, 173, 175, 247, 252, 261, 265, 286, 290, 298
diseases, 29, 279, 314, 324, 339, 342
Disease-specific, 161
Disinfectant, 346
disorder, 125, 126, 148, 151, 308, 321, 328, 335, 355, 357, 358
distal, 15, 17, 28, 29, 30, 31, 39, 54, 55, 73, 80, 81, 102, 103, 136, 160, 165, 174, 194, 206, 208, 210, 217, 218, 233, 234, 235, 236, 237, 244, 257, 258, 259, 260, 263, 264, 265, 329, 345, 384, 388
distress, 55
distribution, 13, 17, 19, 21, 23, 28, 29, 30, 47, 63, 80, 81, 104, 105, 119, 120, 135, 145, 169, 210, 215, 227, 234, 279, 316, 322, 369, 375, 396
diversity, 26, 34
diverticulitis, 26, 315, 339, 342
dizziness, 287, 298
DNA, 135, 183, 195, 199, 213, 298, 370, 382, 396
doctor, 168, 198
donor, 236
dosage, 207, 218, 224, 235, 244, 256
dosing, 207, 217, 230, 270, 299
DP, 108, 109, 189, 222, 267, 343, 360
drainage, 126, 138, 186, 272, 273, 297
drinking water, 388
drug history, 341
drug therapy, 33
drug toxicity, 266
drug treatment, 198, 222, 342
drug-induced, 128, 183, 298, 308
drug-induced hepatitis, 183
drug-induced lupus, 183, 298
drugs, 159, 191, 196, 204, 209, 210, 214, 227, 230, 238, 240, 245, 256, 257, 264, 266, 269, 273, 284, 297, 312, 313, 321, 322, 341, 342, 353, 387
DSS, 252, 254
duodenum, 29, 31, 33, 53, 55, 73, 81, 258, 381

duration, 97, 112, 149, 191, 192, 193, 194, 215, 216, 256, 260, 261, 262, 370
dyeing, 121
dyes, 93, 95
dyspepsia, 55, 240
dysphagia, 54
dysplasia, 37, 89, 92, 96, 98, 99, 108, 137, 149, 191, 192, 193, 194, 195, 196, 197, 198, 200
dyspnea, 298
dysregulation, 203, 308

E

E. coli, 368, 388
eating, 387, 390
economic, 233, 263
ectopic pregnancy, 313
edema, 11, 15, 20, 23, 39, 41, 42, 44, 47, 48, 49, 51, 52, 73, 80, 81, 117, 155, 242, 283, 295, 315, 329, 330, 333, 339, 350, 359, 364, 370, 376, 387, 389, 390, 393, 394
education, 112
efficacy, 107, 163, 197, 204, 206, 207, 211, 223, 224, 226, 227, 229, 230, 231, 234, 235, 236, 237, 245, 251, 252, 260, 261, 262, 263, 265, 276, 285, 295, 297, 299, 300, 301, 370, 391, 395
efflux transporters, 204, 209
effusion, 119
EGB, 252, 254
EGF, 236, 288
eicosanoid, 205
elaboration, 388
elderly, 311, 318, 340, 387
electrolyte imbalance, 224, 264
electrolytes, 240, 288, 315, 389
electron, 111, 115, 381, 384
electron microscopy, 381, 384
electronics, 90
emboli, 312
embolism, 312
embolus, 312
emission, 90
emotional, 161, 249
endogenous, 215, 368
endoscope, 40, 53, 72, 90, 95, 98, 102, 103, 111, 112, 116, 119, 122, 193, 322, 330
endoscopic retrograde cholangiopancreatography, 125
endoscopy, 38, 44, 45, 51, 53, 54, 55, 67, 71, 75, 77, 78, 79, 81, 84, 85, 86, 87, 90, 91, 93, 94, 95, 97, 98, 99, 101, 102, 107, 109, 113, 115, 116, 117, 118, 119, 120, 121, 122, 133, 163, 173, 187, 316, 352, 370, 376
endothelial cells, 213, 281, 285, 295
endothelium, 370
enemas, 40, 44, 160, 174, 182, 217, 233, 234, 235, 236, 257, 259, 260, 288, 341, 345, 346
energy, 220, 250
engagement, 286
England, 196
enlargement, 119
enteric, 139, 211, 226, 257, 341, 350
enteritis, 85, 315, 363, 367
enterocolitis, 145, 367, 371, 390
enthusiasm, 230
environmental, 151, 203, 279, 293, 321
enzymes, 204, 209, 214, 257
eosinophilia, 323, 359
eosinophils, 6, 163, 164, 213, 322, 323
epidemic, 134
epidemiologic studies, 369
epidemiological, 139
epidemiology, 131, 140, 156, 318, 324
epidermal, 236, 262, 288
epidermal growth factor, 236, 262, 288
episcleritis, 148
epithelia, 90
epithelial cells, 6, 7, 14, 103, 104, 105, 204, 205, 280, 309, 356, 370, 382, 384, 388
epithelium, 5, 6, 7, 14, 25, 30, 163, 164, 165, 172, 177, 308, 346, 356, 370, 389, 390, 391, 392
equipment, 94, 111, 391
erosion, 15, 41, 80, 82, 119, 165, 330, 350
erythema multiforme, 390
erythema nodosum, 135, 168, 327, 387, 390
erythematous, 41, 135, 323, 384
erythrocyte, 152, 168
erythrocyte sedimentation rate, 152, 168
Escherichia coli, 134
esophageal, 33, 54, 93, 328
esophagus, 29, 30, 53, 54, 57, 79, 90, 91, 153, 245, 327, 382
ESR, 158, 168, 170, 173
esters, 328
estimating, 69, 92, 237
estrogens, 313
etanercept, 296
etiologic agent, 382
etiology, 134, 143, 151, 180, 255, 279, 293, 307, 308, 321, 341, 357, 360

eukaryotes, 393
Europe, 132, 308, 390
European, 26, 52, 79, 86, 155, 222, 237, 276
European Union, 79
evacuation, 322
evidence, 14, 26, 52, 76, 80, 86, 94, 132, 145, 155, 158, 182, 185, 186, 188, 192, 195, 198, 208, 215, 219, 224, 228, 229, 230, 231, 234, 236, 237, 245, 262, 272, 276, 285, 293, 316, 321, 335, 342
evil, 250
evolutionary, 210
examinations, 193, 194, 220, 308, 351
exchange transfusion, 313
excision, 114, 184
excitation, 102
exclusion, 132, 133, 134
excretion, 206, 240
exercise, 314
exocrine, 128
exogenous, 102
expansions, 47
expert, 235, 399
explosive, 392
exposure, 210, 367
extravasation, 13
exudate, 39
eyes, 125, 279

F

factorial, 293
faecal, 151
failure, 126, 137, 138, 153, 300, 303, 312
false, 66
family, 192, 194, 196, 321
fat, 18, 19, 25, 215, 240, 242, 266, 384
fat embolism, 266
fatigue, 301
fatty acids, 236, 247, 346
FDA, 80, 225, 272, 296, 299, 301
fear, 239, 249
fecal, 66, 144, 147, 158, 188, 195, 206, 346, 347, 387
feeding, 245, 259, 273, 333
females, 167
fetal, 209, 265
fetus, 265, 266
fever, 31, 126, 134, 158, 226, 227, 240, 272, 287, 299, 317, 339, 346, 359, 363, 382, 387, 389, 390, 392, 395

fiber, 121, 255
fibrin, 18, 20, 162
fibroblasts, 281, 308
fibrosis, 13, 19, 20, 23, 51, 56, 73, 128, 155, 209, 316, 336, 342, 394
film, 13, 207, 318
filters, 89, 90, 91, 92, 95
filtration, 105
fish, 239, 262
fish oil, 262
fistulas, 23, 32, 48, 51, 66, 139, 141, 153, 154, 155, 178, 179, 180, 181, 182, 183, 184, 185, 186, 187, 188, 189, 218, 223, 274, 275, 279, 297, 301, 376, 395
flare, 226, 272, 322
flora, 203, 279, 368, 387, 388, 389
flow, 347
fluid, 264, 315, 370, 381
fluorescence, 109, 195
fluoroquinolones, 368
flushing, 298
foams, 217, 233, 235, 259
focusing, 89, 92, 252, 294
folate, 196, 197, 200, 256, 265
folic acid, 192, 197, 200
follicle, 21, 47
follicular, 346
food, 153, 239, 242, 255, 336, 363, 387, 388
Food and Drug Administration (FDA), 79, 296
food intake, 153, 239, 242
foodstuffs, 324
forceps, 72
Fox, 251
fragility, 329
fungal, 361
fusion, 119, 121

G

gamma globulin, 371
gangrene, 311, 317
gas, 315
gastric, 55, 334, 359
gastroenteritis, 321, 324, 325
gastroenterologist, 198
gastroesophageal reflux disease, 54
gastrointestinal, 26, 30, 33, 53, 57, 59, 60, 68, 71, 75, 90, 91, 95, 98, 99, 125, 134, 151, 153, 203, 205, 224, 227, 240, 242, 243, 244, 279, 308, 323, 324, 349, 350, 352, 354, 363, 380

gastrointestinal bleeding, 71, 240, 354
gastrointestinal tract, 26, 30, 57, 60, 75, 90, 91, 95, 134, 151, 153, 203, 205, 244, 279, 349, 352, 363
gastroscopy, 72
GC, 69, 199, 210, 237, 271
GCS, 136, 137, 138, 213, 214, 215, 217, 218, 219, 220
G-CSF, 288
gel, 207, 233, 242
gender, 309
gender gap, 309
gene, 199, 280, 281, 289, 300
gene expression, 300
general anesthesia, 72, 182
generation, 111, 115, 252, 318
genes, 213, 282, 356
genetic, 151, 156, 191, 203, 215, 290, 293, 321
genotype, 156, 225, 290
geography, 6
gingival, 184
globulin, 353
glucocorticoid receptor, 213, 215, 221
glucocorticoids, 136, 213, 221
glucocorticosteroids, 221, 222, 236
glucose, 214, 220, 241, 242, 243
glucose metabolism, 214
glutamine, 247
glutaraldehyde, 346
glycerin, 313
glycine, 258
glycol, 295, 296, 299
glycoprotein, 214
GM-CSF, 288
goals, 136, 272
goblet cells, 5, 7, 13, 14, 25, 103, 104, 105, 356
gold, 76, 97, 101, 155, 313, 341, 369
grades, 169, 193, 350, 353
grading, 104, 105, 107, 165, 175, 350, 351, 354
graft-versus-host disease, 353, 354
gram-negative bacteria, 353
granules, 204, 395
granulocyte, 288
granulomas, 20, 21, 22, 23, 49, 54, 56, 76, 132, 133, 134, 155, 280, 283, 295
groups, 28, 30, 107, 167, 169, 252
growth, 31, 153, 220, 241, 245, 288
growth spurt, 153
Guangdong, 122, 123
guidance, 66, 399
guidelines, 97, 112, 194, 267

Guillain-Barré syndrome, 387
gut, 24, 139, 203, 205, 280, 281, 284, 285, 288, 294, 328, 350, 352, 368, 370, 391
GVHD, 144, 349, 350, 351, 352, 353, 354
gyrus, 113

H

HA, 8, 15, 40, 146, 324, 378, 397
half-life, 206, 299
harmful, 85, 294
HDTV, 111
head, 216
headache, 184, 208, 286, 287, 298, 299, 301
healing, 13, 32, 44, 66, 77, 80, 153, 182, 185, 216, 226, 286, 297, 302, 317
health, 168, 265, 297
Heart, 158
heat, 249, 250, 389
height, 50, 168, 169
Helicobacter pylori, 357, 358
helper cells, 282
hematemesis, 55
hematochezia, 32, 152, 314, 340, 342, 359, 364, 365
hematocrit, 152
hematologic, 309, 312
hematologic disorders, 312
hematological, 314
hematopoietic stem cell, 287, 349, 354
hematoxylin-eosin, 6, 381
hemodialysis, 314
hemoglobin, 89, 90, 92, 264, 287
hemolytic uremic syndrome, 388, 389
hemorrhage, 6, 11, 12, 132, 155, 161, 315, 316, 329, 350, 376
hemorrhoidectomy, 185
hemorrhoids, 40, 177, 179, 180, 185, 187
hemostatic, 360
hemothorax, 243
Henoch-Schonlein purpura, 135
hepatic fibrosis, 224
hepatitis, 208, 227, 312
hepatosplenomegaly, 328, 387, 395
hepatotoxicity, 184, 224
herbs, 249, 250, 251
herpes simplex, 379
herring, 321
heterogeneous, 151
heterozygotes, 225
high density lipoprotein, 328

high resolution, 71, 102
high risk, 15, 226, 193
hirsutism, 184
histological, 8, 15, 40, 54, 59, 94, 101, 106, 114, 117, 132, 133, 145, 146, 155, 163, 165, 175, 235, 323, 324, 335, 336, 355, 357, 370, 378, 397
histology, 92, 101, 132, 133, 140, 163, 173, 199
histopathology, 308
histoplasmosis, 183, 298, 395, 396, 398
HIV, 85, 379, 380, 382, 383, 385, 393
HLA, 287, 309, 390
HLA-B, 390
homogeneous, 41, 103, 104, 105
homosexuals, 391
hookworm, 321
hormone, 215
hospital, 112, 115, 140, 197, 228, 255, 370, 393
hospitalization, 160, 218, 264, 302
hospitalizations, 236, 276, 297
hospitalized, 136, 217, 218, 273
host, 144, 349, 353
household, 387
HSCT, 349, 350, 351, 352, 353
hue, 93, 179
human, 90, 92, 183, 203, 210, 261, 266, 279, 286, 287, 288, 290, 295, 296, 298, 299, 301, 303
hydro, 207
hydrocortisone, 215, 217, 218, 219, 220, 221, 235, 236, 259, 263
hydrogen, 346
hydrogen peroxide, 346
hydrophilic, 207
hydroxylation, 206
hygiene, 179
hyperalimentation, 273
hyperbilirubinemia, 209
hypercoagulable, 317
hyperemia, 17, 40, 44, 330, 333, 387, 388, 389, 393, 394, 395
hyperglycemia, 215, 245
hyperlipidemia, 215
hyperphosphatemia, 287
hyperplasia, 13, 15, 23, 96, 184, 346, 360
hyperplastic polyps, 94
hypersensitivity, 183, 227, 262
hypertension, 184, 224, 261, 314, 334
hypertensive, 333, 334
hypertrophy, 336, 395
hyperuricemia, 287
hypoglycemia, 243, 245, 287

hypokalemia, 245
hypoperfusion, 144, 311, 314, 317
hypothesis, 197
hypovolemia, 218

I

iatrogenic, 313
ICAM, 252, 281, 284, 285
identification, 62, 101, 120, 242, 364, 369, 375, 384, 391, 392, 393
idiopathic, 15, 25, 128, 143, 144, 145, 157, 179, 321, 322, 327, 342, 345, 376, 377, 378, 397
idiosyncratic, 208
IFN, 281, 286, 288, 289, 293, 324
IgE, 323
IL-1, 205, 252, 282, 286, 287, 289, 293, 353
IL-2, 205, 252, 262, 281, 282, 286, 289, 290
ileostomy, 186, 346
ileum, 17, 25, 28, 29, 30, 31, 42, 48, 53, 55, 73, 106, 169, 172, 174, 205, 206, 207, 215, 258, 279, 342, 382, 388, 389, 390
illumination, 90, 92, 98
images, 60, 79, 89, 90, 91, 92, 96, 102, 103, 104, 106, 111, 336
imaging, 38, 59, 62, 66, 68, 86, 89, 92, 94, 96, 97, 98, 99, 100, 101, 106, 125, 126, 144, 174, 182, 264
imaging modalities, 86, 182
imaging systems, 99
imaging techniques, 100
immigration, 284
immune cells, 139, 280, 281
immune function, 227, 239, 379
immune reaction, 213, 293
immune response, 203, 280, 287, 294
immune system, 279
immunity, 290, 353
immunocompromised, 395, 396
immunodeficiency, 380, 382, 383, 385
immunoglobulin, 214, 236
immunohistochemical, 308, 384
immunology, 283
immunomodulation, 200
immunomodulatory, 223, 252, 261
immunopathology, 281
immunosuppressive, 223, 224, 230, 313, 340, 352, 383
immunotherapy, 371
in situ, 286

in vitro, 281
in vivo, 92, 101, 106, 108, 109
inactivation, 371
inactive, 15, 51, 155, 160, 163, 169, 187, 205, 229, 322
incidence, 30, 49, 97, 131, 132, 138, 139, 140, 149, 184, 193, 200, 230, 260, 297, 307, 309, 321, 350, 353, 354
inclusion, 196
incubation period, 387
incurable, 193
indication, 220, 224, 342, 346
indicators, 170, 173
indices, 136, 163, 173, 180
induction, 80, 137, 138, 141, 183, 188, 218, 219, 220, 229, 231, 249, 259, 264, 269, 270, 274, 275, 280, 282, 286, 288, 295, 297, 299, 301, 303
industrialized countries, 388
inefficiency, 259
inert, 288
infarction, 312, 315, 317, 318
infectious disease, 131, 134
inflammatory cell migration, 283
inflammatory cells, 7, 14, 21, 22, 23, 103, 133, 221, 283, 297, 300, 322, 351, 352, 356, 377
iinflammatory mediators, 293
inflammatory response, 246, 282, 358
inflation, 72, 73
infliximab, 137, 138, 139, 141, 189, 220, 226, 295, 296, 297, 298, 300, 301, 303, 353, 357, 358
influenza, 301
infusions, 219, 262, 274, 297
ingestion, 86, 205, 214, 256, 272, 341, 363, 367, 391
inguinal, 382
inhibition, 198, 214, 318, 342
inhibitor, 214, 290, 385
initiation, 89, 92, 225, 226, 280
injection, 251, 253, 271, 276, 287, 298, 299
injuries, 240
injury, 21, 30, 47, 155, 186, 240, 314, 318, 353, 367, 388, 390
insects, 250
insertion, 72, 112, 243, 245
insight, 303
insomnia, 184
inspection, 182, 250
instability, 192, 198, 199
institutions, 112
instruments, 53, 60, 73, 76, 157, 159, 161
insulin, 242, 288

integration, 102
integrins, 281, 283, 285
integrity, 117, 244
intensity, 89, 92, 96, 147, 163, 216, 279, 286
interaction, 151, 284, 285, 321
intercellular adhesion molecule, 252, 290
interference, 90, 91, 265
interferon, 262, 313
interleukin, 236, 252, 253, 291
international, 132, 297
interpretation, 59, 96
interval, 194
intervention, 66, 85, 144, 185, 301
intestinal flora, 293
intestinal obstruction, 71, 154, 241, 244, 272
intestinal perforation, 244, 384
intestinal tract, 204
intestine, 3, 5, 22, 26, 73, 143, 144, 182, 204, 244, 281, 288
intracranial, 150
intramuscularly, 229, 271
intraocular, 221
intraocular pressure, 221
intravenous, 102, 184, 215, 217, 218, 219, 221, 222, 227, 228, 229, 231, 261, 264, 275, 297, 298, 299, 318, 370
intussusception, 360
invasive, 68, 193, 298, 391, 392
iridocyclitis, 327
iritis, 148, 154
iron, 152, 247, 323, 342, 359
irradiation, 353
irrigation, 391
irritable bowel syndrome, 8, 163, 308
irritation, 298, 317
ischemia, 133, 311, 312, 314, 315, 316, 317, 318, 319, 368, 370, 372
ischemic, 132, 134, 135, 312, 314, 315, 316, 318, 319, 369, 370, 372, 384, 388
island, 50

J

JAMA, 56
Japanese, 111, 113, 132, 133, 246
jaundice, 126, 349, 395
jejunum, 31, 81, 244, 256, 258
joints, 148, 204, 279
JT, 99, 303
judge, 163

judgment, 163
Jun, 122, 151, 276
Jung, 26

K

K^+, 243
keratinocyte, 288
kidney, 243
kinases, 303
KL, 33, 40, 165, 343, 347, 371, 378, 397
Korea, 140

L

laboratory studies, 308
lactation, 266
lactose, 86
lamina, 6, 7, 13, 14, 21, 61, 91, 103, 117, 133, 134, 163, 172, 203, 252, 281, 282, 284, 286, 287, 293, 308, 336, 340, 370, 377
laparoscopy, 315, 328
laparotomy, 22, 133, 317
large intestine, 3, 5, 8, 29, 30, 113, 114, 115, 121, 122, 154, 358
laser, 101, 102, 109, 195
latex, 72
laxatives, 8, 313, 341
LDH, 315
lead, 12, 13, 21, 31, 108, 133, 179, 182, 198, 239, 240, 243, 245, 266, 279, 287, 289, 298, 324, 329, 341, 349, 388
leakage, 105
leukemia, 321, 353
leukocytes, 134, 163, 281, 284, 285
leukocytosis, 152, 317, 339
leukopenia, 208, 224
levator, 177, 178, 180
LFA, 281
life expectancy, 43
life quality, 266
life-threatening, 149, 311
lifetime, 97
ligand, 294
likelihood, 273
limitations, 85, 98, 163
linear, 17, 25, 48, 60, 73, 81, 155, 167, 316, 364, 376
lipid, 154, 240
lipoid, 241, 242
lipophilic, 207
lipoxygenase, 205
literature, 169, 193, 237, 238, 297, 322, 337
liver, 8, 22, 33, 125, 126, 197, 205, 225, 229, 243, 256, 279, 300, 328, 334, 347, 349, 392
liver abscess, 392
liver disease, 33, 347
liver enzymes, 243, 300
liver function tests, 197
localization, 53, 76
location, 60, 145, 153, 169, 178, 180, 187, 192, 250, 272, 322, 342
London, 16, 231, 238, 378, 397
long distance, 114
long period, 138
long-term, 107, 137, 196, 208, 219, 220, 224, 230, 233, 235, 242, 256, 261, 264, 270, 273, 274, 297, 298, 302, 303, 311, 314, 385
losses, 42, 198
Louisiana, 146, 378, 397
LPS, 353
lumbar, 313
lumen, 13, 18, 39, 42, 43, 50, 103, 112, 133, 154, 205, 208, 257, 280, 329, 330, 364, 389
luminal, 47, 103, 104, 105, 205, 229, 233, 279, 280, 289, 296, 316, 346, 370
lungs, 395
lupus, 228
lymph, 18, 22, 60, 62, 63, 66, 68, 134, 328, 364, 395
lymph node, 18, 22, 60, 62, 63, 66, 68, 134, 328, 364, 395
lymphadenopathy, 395
lymphocytes, 13, 21, 23, 155, 213, 271, 285, 289, 295, 307, 308, 309, 394
lymphogranuloma venereum, 134, 382
lymphoid, 13, 14, 15, 21, 23, 25, 47, 56, 85, 133, 345, 377
lymphoid hyperplasia, 25, 85
lymphoma, 77, 85, 116, 133, 135, 227, 260, 262, 298
lysis, 298

M

mAb, 285, 286, 288, 295, 296, 298, 299
macrocytosis, 227
macrolide antibiotics, 261
macromolecules, 280
macrophages, 13, 21, 23, 203, 213, 280, 281, 289, 294, 300, 328, 360
magnetic, 69, 128, 173, 174, 182

magnetic resonance imaging, 69, 173, 174, 182
maintenance, 137, 138, 141, 183, 188, 205, 208, 211, 219, 224, 227, 229, 230, 231, 234, 236, 249, 256, 259, 260, 261, 262, 264, 265, 273, 274, 275, 276, 277, 282, 288, 295, 297, 301, 302, 303
malabsorption, 31, 154, 240, 384
malaise, 31, 55, 226, 387
males, 167
malignancy, 38, 68, 114, 125, 127, 154, 395
malignant, 13, 40, 68, 90, 96, 97, 99, 127, 135, 180, 191, 194, 198, 323, 324, 336
malnutrition, 240, 241
management, 26, 52, 59, 62, 66, 80, 108, 121, 131, 135, 155, 165, 169, 182, 195, 199, 203, 208, 209, 210, 222, 229, 237, 239, 243, 245, 255, 262, 264, 267, 271, 272, 275, 276, 287, 295, 302, 324, 331, 336, 351, 354, 357, 364, 380
mania, 216
manipulation, 112
manure, 388
MAPK, 300
market, 244
marketing, 79
marrow, 328
mast cell, 13, 213, 253
maternal, 265
meals, 153
measurement, 225
measures, 157, 194, 314
media, 390
median, 62, 309
mediators, 214
medications, 86, 183, 196, 223, 225, 234, 240, 247, 261, 269, 274, 313, 314, 317
medicine, 228, 275
MEK, 300
membranes, 297, 369
mesenchymal, 213
mesentery, 18, 22, 31
meta-analysis, 84, 86, 183, 206, 237, 238, 274
metabolic, 204, 209, 215, 220, 241, 242, 245, 315
metabolic acidosis, 315
metabolic changes, 245
metabolic rate, 241
metabolism, 196, 205, 214, 246, 260
metabolite, 205, 226, 260
metalloproteinase, 294
metals, 241
metastases, 68
methamphetamine, 313

methionine, 200
Methotrexate, 138, 224, 228, 229
methylene, 95
methylprednisolone, 215, 217, 218, 219, 220, 222
Mg^{2+}, 243
mice, 251, 253, 282, 285, 287, 289
Microbial, 280, 290, 302
microscopy, 102, 109, 113, 393
microvascular, 89, 92, 93, 94, 96, 103, 104, 214, 221
middle-aged, 308, 309
migration, 18, 295
military, 22
milk, 239, 321, 323, 363, 388
mimicking, 246, 324, 336, 342, 388, 390
mimicry, 337
mineralocorticoid, 215
minerals, 240
minority, 311, 322
mitogen, 300
mitogen-activated protein kinase, 300
mitral, 359
mitral valve, 359
ML, 33, 40, 140, 343, 347, 371, 378, 397
MMW, 246
modalities, 38, 59, 84, 86, 127
modality, 59, 66, 68, 71, 76, 80, 85, 86
models, 252, 283
modulation, 246
Mofetil, 230
molecular biology, 221
molecular changes, 195
molecular markers, 192, 195
molecules, 139, 281, 283, 284, 285, 287, 289
monoclonal antibody, 141, 261, 270, 271, 291, 295, 296, 303, 353
monocytes, 213, 271, 285, 289, 297
mononuclear cell, 163, 252, 287, 293
morbidity, 192, 193
morphological, 54, 91, 95, 116, 120, 121
morphology, 19, 90, 91, 114, 174
mortality, 38, 101, 193, 197, 241, 317, 352, 387, 395
mothers, 266
mouse, 266, 270, 271, 296
mouth, 30, 53, 148, 151, 153, 154, 255, 256, 275, 327, 395
movement, 67, 159, 336
MPS, 60, 69, 357
MRI, 66, 85, 155, 173, 182, 187, 188, 189
mRNA, 252
MS, 33, 99, 146, 150, 199

MSI, 192, 195
MUC4, 356
mucin, 13, 15, 25, 103, 105, 195, 341, 377
mucoid, 382
mucosal barrier, 279
mucous membranes, 93
mucus, 5, 13, 93, 133, 147, 162, 249, 355, 356, 358, 375, 390, 392
multiple regression analysis, 166
multiplicity, 116
Municipal Hospital, 3, 5, 11, 17, 27, 37, 143, 223, 249, 341, 345, 367, 375, 379, 399
muscle, 3, 178, 186, 242
musculoskeletal, 216
mutation, 281, 289, 312
Mycobacterium, 363, 379
Mycophenolate, 224, 230
myopathy, 216

N

NA, 226, 227, 386
Na⁺, 243
N-acety, 205, 206
nasogastric tube, 317
national, 69, 112
nationality, 45
natural, 14, 91, 139, 189, 192, 296, 302, 387
nausea, 55, 153, 208, 245, 286, 298, 299, 322, 350, 369, 382, 387, 389
necrosis, 139, 148, 216, 280, 302, 303, 317, 329, 330, 346, 350, 370, 384
needle aspiration, 68
neglect, 341
neonatal, 265
neoplasia, 91, 92, 95, 97, 98, 99, 102, 104, 105, 106, 107, 108, 109, 193, 194, 197, 199, 200
neoplasms, 199, 228, 266
neoplastic, 90, 91, 93, 94, 95, 97, 98, 99, 101, 103, 106, 114, 199
Neoplastic, 96, 113, 199
neoplastic tissue, 101
neovascularization, 91
nephrotoxicity, 184, 209, 261
nerve, 25, 341, 343
nerve growth factor, 341, 343
nervous system, 25, 341
network, 38, 40, 43, 47, 89, 90, 91, 93, 94, 95, 103, 104, 105
neuropathy, 298

neurotoxicity, 209, 224
neutralization, 301
neutropenia, 352
neutrophils, 13, 15, 21, 163, 164, 213, 342, 370, 377
New Orleans, 146
New York, 16, 231, 238, 371, 378, 397
Ni, 309
nicotine, 236, 262
nitric oxide, 236
nitrogen, 240, 242, 244
NK cells, 280, 285
nocardiosis, 298
nodes, 22
nodules, 22, 40, 50, 135, 154, 316, 364
non-Hodgkin's lymphoma, 183
North America, 132, 218, 308, 390
NSAIDs, 85, 341, 342
nuclear, 127, 214, 252
nuclei, 102
nutrient, 240, 241, 244
nutrition, 138, 174, 239, 240, 241, 242, 244, 245, 246, 266, 275, 277
nutritional deficiencies, 31

O

obligate, 393
observations, 160
obstruction, 55, 73, 93, 133, 138, 144, 154, 273, 334, 339, 350, 364
occlusion, 311, 314
odds ratio, 196
odynophagia, 54
ofloxacin, 389
old age, 314
oligomerization, 280
Oman, 139
Omega-3, 247
operator, 93
opioid, 264
optic neuritis, 298
optical, 89, 90, 92, 95, 98, 102, 111
OR, 196
oral, 72, 73, 76, 135, 136, 137, 165, 182, 184, 204, 205, 208, 210, 214, 217, 218, 219, 220, 221, 222, 224, 230, 234, 235, 237, 238, 241, 244, 245, 255, 257, 259, 260, 261, 263, 264, 265, 266, 271, 272, 275, 287, 313, 327, 345, 370, 371, 387, 388
organ, 215, 298, 349

organism, 363, 364, 375, 387, 389, 390, 391, 392, 396
orientation, 105
oropharynx, 382
osteoporosis, 216, 220, 222, 324, 325
oxygen, 205
oxygenation, 317

P

PA, 200
Pacific Region, 131, 139
pain, 31, 54, 55, 71, 76, 112, 126, 147, 148, 151, 152, 153, 158, 159, 162, 167, 168, 179, 181, 185, 239, 240, 249, 251, 293, 298, 299, 307, 308, 309, 314, 318, 321, 322, 335, 339, 342, 350, 355, 359, 363, 369, 382, 387, 390, 392
palpation, 182, 250
pancreatic, 125, 128
pancreatitis, 55, 125, 127, 128, 183, 208, 227, 260, 312
paper, 39, 117
parasites, 312, 321, 323, 380, 381, 391, 393
Parasites, 144
parasitic infection, 379
parenteral, 138, 218, 219, 220, 230, 235, 241, 246, 259, 264, 266, 273
paresthesias, 184
Paris, 90
partnership, 198
pathogenesis, 125, 128, 141, 156, 175, 203, 209, 255, 279, 280, 290, 293, 302, 335, 353, 357, 358, 363
pathogenic, 388
pathogens, 280, 381
pathologist, 198
pathologists, 144
pathology, 173, 327, 331
Pathophysiological, 146
pathophysiology, 91, 351
pathways, 192, 285, 290, 302
pattern recognition, 280
PCR, 364, 380, 384
PD, 175, 277, 318
PE, 84, 189, 210
pediatric, 44, 152, 194, 221, 296
pediatric patients, 221, 296
pelvic, 182, 187, 188, 358
penicillin, 313, 368
peptic ulcer, 55, 323

peptic ulcer disease, 323
peptides, 288, 295
perception, 90, 180
perforation, 12, 20, 44, 76, 149, 154, 155, 316, 317, 322, 327, 329, 330, 342, 364, 369
performance, 160
perfusion, 252, 317
perianal abscess, 177, 179, 180, 185, 186, 187, 188
periodic, 195
Peripheral, 323
peripheral blood, 281
peripheral neuropathy, 328
peripheral vascular disease, 317
peritoneal, 317, 365, 369
peritoneum, 22
peritonitis, 316, 317
permeability, 85, 214, 221, 288, 342
permit, 93, 155
peroxide, 346
personal, 314
pets, 387
PG, 252
pH, 207, 215, 257, 258, 347
pharmaceutical, 80
pharmacodynamics, 257
pharmacokinetic, 206, 210
pharmacological, 196, 252
pharmacology, 209, 238
phenotype, 140, 156, 177, 225
phenotypic, 145
pheochromocytoma, 312
Philadelphia, 15, 16, 25, 26, 34, 40, 44, 146, 222, 231, 238, 342, 343, 347, 371, 377, 378, 397
phlebitis, 300
phosphate, 345
photophobia, 148
physicians, 217
physiology, 221
pigs, 391
pilot study, 95, 99, 303
placebo, 160, 197, 219, 231, 237, 238, 262, 269, 273, 274, 276, 285, 287, 290, 297, 298, 299, 300, 301, 303, 330
placenta, 221, 266
planning, 265, 266
plaques, 368, 369
plasma, 6, 7, 13, 14, 15, 22, 23, 71, 155, 206, 214, 261, 299, 328, 360, 377, 394
plasma levels, 206
plasmapheresis, 262

platelet, 134, 253, 352
play, 76, 79, 86, 96, 192, 205, 280, 282, 350, 353, 357, 376
plexus, 39, 341
pneumocystis carinii, 184
pneumonia, 183, 184, 245
pneumonitis, 224
poison, 246
polarization, 283
polycythemia vera, 312
polyethylene, 242, 295, 296, 299
polygons, 119
polymer, 380
polymorphonuclear, 21, 134, 163, 370
polypectomy, 71, 94, 106, 193, 357
polyps, 13, 20, 21, 40, 94, 96, 99, 323, 355, 356, 357, 358
poor, 162, 167, 168, 184, 185, 242, 350
population, 140, 149, 156, 181, 194, 196, 197, 307, 308, 309, 361, 391
pork, 390
portal hypertension, 39, 334
portal vein, 334
postoperative, 174, 184, 185, 216, 221, 223, 226, 237, 241, 274, 327
potassium, 244
pouches, 3
poultry, 389
powder, 244, 250, 251, 253
power, 102, 111
precancerous lesions, 97
preconditioning, 350, 351, 352
prediction, 62, 96, 104, 105, 108
predictors, 189
predisposing factors, 279
Prednisolone, 235, 236
prednisone, 138, 214, 217, 218, 219, 220, 221, 222, 228, 259, 266, 269, 272, 273
pre-existing, 327, 342
preference, 233
pregnancy, 221, 229, 265, 266
pregnant, 187, 265, 266
preoperative, 330
preparation, 40, 44, 60, 72, 244, 262, 317, 345
prevention, 191, 194, 196, 198, 199, 205, 353
priming, 286
probability, 13, 193
probe, 69, 396
probiotics, 137, 203, 262, 265, 266
Probiotics, 137, 266, 267

procedures, 112, 186, 188, 236, 243, 276
proctitis, 28, 29, 31, 42, 145, 147, 165, 208, 223, 234, 237, 238, 321, 341, 375, 379, 382, 388, 396
proctosigmoidoscopy, 160
prodrugs, 210, 257
production, 205, 214, 215, 252, 253, 286, 287, 289, 293, 300, 368
progestins, 313
prognosis, 127, 230, 317, 323, 349, 350
program, 193, 270, 274
progressive, 115, 148, 149, 314, 380, 384
proinflammatory, 203, 205, 281, 283, 287, 290, 294, 295
prolapse, 337, 357, 358, 360
proliferation, 25, 206, 230, 281, 288, 294
promote, 91, 239, 245, 286, 317
prophylactic, 353
prophylaxis, 352, 393
propofol, 72, 122
prostaglandin, 252, 342
prostate cancer, 330
protection, 198, 294, 356
protein, 184, 199, 214, 240, 252, 294, 299, 301, 312, 315, 321, 323, 355, 359, 389
protocol, 96, 194
proton pump inhibitors, 138, 276
protozoa, 381
proximal, 11, 27, 28, 29, 30, 55, 75, 81, 182, 193, 194, 206, 244, 257, 259, 263, 315, 329
pruritus, 126, 298
pseudo, 76
pseudomembranous colitis, 369, 371
psoriasis, 296
psoriatic, 296, 299, 301
psoriatic arthritis, 296, 299, 301
psychosis, 216
psychotropic drugs, 313
puberty, 153
pulse, 158, 228, 231, 250, 371
purpura, 216
pus, 12, 39, 147, 240
pylorus, 359, 360
pyoderma gangrenosum, 167, 168
pyrosis, 54

Q

quality of life, 136, 161, 297
questionnaire, 161

R

RA, 57, 237, 238
radiation, 85, 132, 133, 135, 144, 315, 329, 330, 331
radio, 86
radiography, 54, 84, 85
radiological, 53, 55, 71, 132, 155, 315, 316, 317
radiotherapy, 329, 330
random, 192
range, 89, 91, 92, 102, 152, 154, 158, 161, 163, 186, 187, 206, 219, 220, 223, 224, 261, 309, 368, 370
ras, 199
rash, 226, 349
rats, 252, 253, 254, 266, 318, 319
RB, 156, 209, 211, 290, 302, 319
RC, 146, 199, 221, 378, 397
RDP, 288
reactive oxygen species, 206, 252
real-time, 101, 109
rebound tenderness, 273
receptors, 260, 280, 294
recognition, 111, 204, 266, 280, 286
reconstruction, 62, 90, 313
recovery, 234, 353
rectal examination, 355
rectal prolapse, 360
rectosigmoid, 29, 186, 187, 311, 391
rectum, 6, 11, 27, 28, 29, 31, 39, 41, 42, 47, 48, 61, 73, 115, 122, 133, 147, 177, 179, 180, 181, 182, 185, 186, 193, 194, 200, 208, 233, 234, 236, 257, 259, 260, 263, 311, 328, 333, 335, 336, 345, 347, 355, 360, 369, 384, 387, 389, 390, 393, 398
recurrence, 172, 223, 226, 237, 247, 262, 273, 327, 357
reduction, 108, 137, 160, 184, 198, 206, 208, 214, 297, 311
reflectance spectra, 96
refractory, 66, 136, 225, 228, 230, 231, 232, 260, 261, 263, 265, 285, 287, 291, 297, 300, 302
regeneration, 7, 15, 105
regional, 19, 364
regression, 169, 196, 357
regular, 77, 103, 104, 105, 138, 193, 196, 198, 230, 245, 273
regulation, 294, 336
rejection, 353
relapse, 15, 62, 136, 137, 173, 174, 219, 230, 231, 245, 259, 262, 264, 265, 273, 274, 353, 370, 371, 387
relationship, 178, 319, 358, 380

relevance, 45, 180, 334
reliability, 323
renal, 184, 224, 266
repair, 21, 283
reporters, 352
research, 33, 98, 146, 195, 265, 266, 290, 302
resection, 72, 92, 114, 115, 121, 122, 168, 195, 240, 317, 357
resin, 257
resistance, 312, 324
resolution, 60, 101, 102, 172, 272, 316, 317, 358, 370
respiratory, 299
responsiveness, 233
restoration, 240
retardation, 31, 153, 216, 220
retention, 30, 76, 85, 174, 259, 260
Reynolds, 246
RF, 173, 198, 199, 347
rheumatoid arthritis, 203, 296, 299, 301, 321
rheumatoid factor, 308
rigidity, 112, 323
risk, 13, 27, 38, 44, 66, 67, 76, 85, 96, 97, 101, 149, 154, 184, 186, 191, 192, 193, 194, 195, 196, 197, 198, 200, 205, 216, 217, 220, 221, 224, 228, 230, 234, 256, 262, 264, 266, 297, 301, 314, 352, 369, 380, 388
RNA, 382
rods, 389
Rome, 145

S

SA, 109, 174, 189
safety, 206, 230, 231, 265, 270, 277, 297, 303
saline, 102, 259, 313, 380
saliva, 383
salmon, 38, 40
Salmonella, 134, 375, 379, 381, 389
salts, 243
sample, 53, 243, 352, 393
sampling, 49, 92, 195
Sao Paulo, 246
scattering, 91, 162
schistosomiasis, 334, 398
scholarship, 399
scintigraphy, 173, 175
scleroderma, 322
sclerosis, 114
scores, 158, 160, 161, 163, 169, 172, 173, 301

SD, 16, 25, 26, 33, 52, 251, 378, 397
SD rats, 251
search, 175
Seattle, 166
second generation, 115
secondary syphilis, 396
secretion, 203, 207, 240, 282, 287, 290, 295
sedation, 72
sedimentation, 339
seizures, 184, 224, 261
selecting, 59
Self, 373, 375, 376
sensitivity, 84, 94, 95, 106, 127, 193
sepsis, 181, 183, 185, 317
septum, 48
sequelae, 311, 314
series, 8, 84, 128, 139, 183, 184, 187, 196, 274, 275, 297, 315
serologic test, 384, 392
serology, 396
serum, 76, 152, 171, 184, 239, 242, 243, 252, 261, 262, 289, 290, 299, 315, 323, 375
serum albumin, 76, 239, 243
SES, 171, 174
severe asthma, 324
severity, 44, 47, 59, 61, 63, 71, 75, 76, 135, 138, 147, 148, 157, 159, 163, 166, 169, 171, 173, 192, 233, 237, 245, 259, 262, 272, 323, 345, 351
sex, 168
sexually transmitted disease, 388
SH, 108, 199
Shanghai, 79, 115
shape, 81, 86, 92, 105, 114, 117, 119, 120, 126, 330
Shigella, 134, 379, 381, 388, 389
shock, 312, 315
short period, 399
shortage, 158
short-term, 141, 219, 270, 288, 330
side effects, 197, 207, 208, 218, 235, 236, 256, 259, 260, 261, 264, 287, 299
sigmoid, 28, 50, 147, 194, 206, 233, 260, 263, 280, 340, 345, 355, 369, 393
sigmoid colon, 50, 147, 233, 260, 355, 393
sigmoidoscopy, 37, 132, 160, 314
sign, 316, 319, 346, 357
signaling, 286, 289, 294, 300
signals, 21, 294
signs, 40, 41, 148, 250, 264, 296, 299, 315, 369
silica, 242
silver, 381

similarity, 134
Singapore, 140, 336
sinus, 23, 180, 187
sites, 21, 28, 31, 180, 206, 283, 293, 295, 322, 355, 359, 360
skeletal muscle, 177
skills, 112
skin, 31, 32, 125, 135, 148, 153, 154, 177, 179, 180, 181, 184, 251, 256, 279, 349
skin tags, 153, 177, 179, 180, 181, 184
small intestine, 3, 5, 29, 30, 71, 76, 77, 152, 154, 206, 209, 210, 382, 391
smoking, 137, 196
smooth muscle, 177
smoothness, 40
social, 161
sodium, 102, 150, 214, 252, 253, 259, 318, 319, 324, 345, 347
solutions, 242, 346
sores, 153
soy, 321
SP, 52, 155, 189, 334
species, 390, 391
specificity, 84, 94, 95, 106, 127, 350, 369
spectroscopy, 100, 195
spectrum, 89, 90, 91, 96, 102, 199, 255, 264, 342, 358, 368
speed, 98, 234, 243, 245
sperm, 256
spheres, 258
sphincter, 177, 178, 186
spider angiomas, 333
spine, 148
splenectomy, 334
sporadic, 101, 192, 196, 197, 199, 205, 322
sputum, 363
squamous cell carcinoma, 187
SR, 141, 290, 324
St. Louis, 16, 231, 238, 371, 378, 397
stages, 47, 54, 163, 193, 250, 314, 316, 370, 387
stasis, 6, 154, 252
steady state, 234
steatorrhea, 31, 328
stem cells, 7
stenosis, 43, 49, 80, 81, 128, 153, 169, 170, 171, 172, 173, 181, 185, 329, 330, 382
stent, 38, 127
sterile, 135, 242
stiffness, 20
stimulant, 341

stomach, 26, 29, 30, 53, 55, 56, 90, 153, 252, 357, 359, 360
stomatitis, 167
stool culture, 350, 387, 388, 390
strains, 368, 370, 388
strangulated hernia, 312
strategies, 191, 198, 199, 203, 371
strength, 207
stress, 214, 220, 242, 303
stretching, 149
striae, 216
strictures, 13, 49, 51, 60, 76, 85, 126, 127, 133, 138, 154, 155, 179, 180, 185, 187, 193, 194, 276, 317, 323
stroma, 103, 104, 105, 346
stromal cells, 281
structuring, 194
subcutaneous injection, 270, 287, 288, 299
subcutaneous tissue, 216
subjective, 168, 169
submucosa, 5, 11, 12, 14, 15, 17, 21, 22, 23, 25, 38, 48, 60, 61, 133, 186, 360, 395
substances, 280
subtraction, 251
success rate, 187
sulfate, 251, 253
sulfonamides, 385
sulfur, 395
sumatriptan, 313
Sun, 253
superiority, 208
supplements, 265
supply, 139, 242, 243, 244
suppository, 204, 205, 208, 215, 235, 236
suppression, 138, 215, 216, 227, 228, 235, 256, 261
suppressor, 214, 227
supraventricular tachycardia, 359
surface area, 106
surface layer, 103
surface structure, 119
surgeries, 153, 236, 276, 297, 346
surgery, 27, 32, 59, 62, 69, 86, 136, 138, 153, 195, 203, 219, 220, 224, 227, 240, 259, 264, 266, 276, 302, 312, 315, 317, 336, 340, 357, 358, 376, 380
surgical, 22, 32, 61, 69, 96, 132, 148, 182, 186, 188, 189, 193, 220, 222, 244, 272, 273, 313, 315, 317, 334, 337, 346, 357
surgical intervention, 32, 220, 315, 317
surgical resection, 132, 148, 193, 244, 318, 357

surveillance, 37, 43, 45, 94, 96, 97, 98, 99, 106, 108, 125, 154, 191, 192, 193, 194, 195, 196, 198, 199
survival, 127, 128, 353, 354
susceptibility, 290
suture, 186
swallowing, 153, 363
Sweden, 309
swelling, 18, 117, 118
switching, 98, 208
Switzerland, 296
syndrome, 140, 144, 153, 240, 301, 307, 315, 321, 324, 335, 336, 337, 355, 357, 358, 360
synthesis, 230, 288
synthetic, 215, 312
syphilis, 134
systematic, 146, 192, 235, 297
systemic lupus erythematosus, 312
systemic sclerosis, 359
systems, 91, 163, 169, 207, 256, 349

T

T cell, 203, 230, 280, 281, 282, 283, 284, 285, 286, 287, 290, 294, 297, 352, 353
tachycardia, 149, 158
tacrolimus, 184, 261, 274, 275, 353
target organs, 352
targets, 233
TCR, 286
teaching, 140
technological, 90
technology, 80, 90, 91, 92, 207
telangiectasia, 329, 330, 333
tenascin, 308
teratogenic, 224, 266
tetracycline, 102, 385, 390, 392
TGF, 282
Th cells, 286
Thalidomide, 284, 300
therapeutic, 38, 66, 71, 72, 75, 76, 85, 112, 135, 141, 144, 156, 157, 163, 165, 166, 167, 203, 207, 209, 218, 221, 236, 237, 250, 251, 252, 255, 256, 260, 262, 266, 270, 284, 286, 289, 322, 370, 371
therapeutic agents, 209, 262
therapeutic approaches, 371
therapeutic benefits, 38, 260
therapeutic goal, 255
therapeutic interventions, 71
Thomson, 109
threshold, 351

throat, 53, 245
thrombocytopenia, 352
thrombocytopenic purpura, 388
thromboembolic, 148
thromboembolism, 264
thrombophlebitis, 327
thrombosis, 150, 243, 312, 316, 317, 360
thrombotic, 314, 350
thromboxane, 205
thymus, 328, 353
time, 20, 62, 93, 94, 97, 101, 106, 112, 127, 132, 153, 159, 175, 183, 187, 193, 194, 206, 216, 229, 230, 243, 257, 258, 261, 266, 272, 273, 275, 329, 367, 370, 399
timing, 266
tissue, 22, 30, 53, 59, 73, 80, 85, 89, 90, 92, 98, 100, 102, 103, 105, 106, 151, 165, 186, 195, 203, 207, 213, 214, 281, 307, 315, 316, 330, 336, 346, 364, 391
titration, 347
TJ, 221, 291
TLR, 280, 289
TLR4, 289
TNF, 139, 252, 261, 270, 281, 283, 286, 287, 289, 290, 293, 294, 295, 296, 297, 298, 299, 300, 301, 302, 353, 357
TNF-α, 261, 270, 353
Tokyo, 102, 121
tolerance, 207, 282
Toll-like, 280
tonsils, 328
top-down, 276
total body irradiation, 352
total parenteral nutrition, 239, 255, 273
toxic, 12, 136, 149, 208, 228, 249, 256, 264, 317, 345, 368, 376
toxic megacolon, 149, 256, 264, 368, 376
toxicities, 224, 260
toxicity, 138, 184, 204, 207, 223, 224, 226, 228, 230, 250, 260, 264, 273
toxin, 313, 368, 369, 371, 381, 388, 390
trace elements, 241
trachea, 245
tracking, 178
training, 94
transducer, 60
transduction, 295
transfer, 294
transformation, 198
transfusion, 242, 243, 314

transgenic, 291
transition, 245, 316
translational, 290, 302
translocation, 243
transmembrane, 294
transparent, 38, 93
transplantation, 349, 350, 353, 354
transverse colon, 39, 43, 117, 208, 234
trauma, 313, 356, 360
tremor, 184
trend, 185, 198
trial, 80, 107, 135, 141, 157, 160, 165, 174, 184, 188, 197, 211, 217, 228, 231, 237, 269, 274, 275, 276, 285, 288, 290, 291, 298, 300, 301, 302, 303, 330
triggers, 295
Tsuga, 61, 68
TT, 290, 302
tuberculosis, 52, 77, 85, 116, 119, 131, 133, 140, 183, 298, 363, 364, 365
Tuberculosis, 363
tubular, 3, 113, 180
tumor, 90, 92, 96, 104, 114, 115, 121, 122, 139, 141, 252, 261, 294, 303, 318, 357
tumor invasion, 93
tumor necrosis factor, 139, 141, 252, 261, 318, 357
tumors, 77, 80, 92, 99, 114, 115, 121, 122, 329
tumour, 302, 303
turnover, 13
typhoid fever, 389, 398

U

ulcer, 20, 24, 25, 48, 49, 50, 54, 55, 56, 73, 74, 80, 81, 83, 120, 132, 133, 144, 162, 171, 177, 179, 315, 316, 327, 328, 330, 335, 336, 337, 350, 355, 360, 384, 392, 398
ulceration, 12, 13, 21, 30, 42, 73, 76, 119, 132, 135, 148, 160, 163, 165, 170, 172, 179, 180, 181, 185, 317, 330, 335, 346, 364, 391
ultrasonography, 38, 59, 60, 66, 69, 182, 187
ultrasound, 68, 69, 273
ultrastructure, 356
unclassified, 79, 145
undifferentiated cells, 7
uniform, 7, 47, 85, 242, 369, 376
United States, 80, 166, 217, 257, 296, 299, 392
unmasking, 97, 215
upper respiratory tract, 298
urea, 243

Index

urinary, 31, 154, 206, 234, 298, 299, 382
urinary bladder, 31, 154
urinary tract, 298, 299
urine, 206, 228
urticaria, 323
users, 198
uveitis, 135, 148, 167, 168

V

vaccines, 385
vagina, 154, 180
vaginal, 139, 187
validation, 174
values, 25, 127, 170, 171
vancomycin, 370, 371, 372
variability, 167, 175
variable, 11, 27, 42, 160, 163, 172, 173, 279, 296, 345, 346
variables, 158, 160, 166, 167, 169, 196
variation, 44, 90
vascular, 6, 11, 13, 14, 15, 38, 39, 41, 42, 43, 47, 48, 49, 90, 91, 94, 95, 103, 117, 133, 144, 160, 315, 333, 345, 359, 360
vasculature, 39, 98, 102, 103, 104, 271, 311
vasculitis, 135, 227, 312, 321, 327
vasopressin, 313
vasospasm, 311
VCAM, 284, 285
vein, 150, 243, 312, 317, 334
velocity, 242
venous pressure, 242
vessels, 38, 39, 40, 60, 62, 63, 91, 103, 105, 329, 333
Victoria, 102
video, 38, 79, 86, 90, 91, 95
vincristine, 324
viral, 361, 379, 381, 382, 384
virus, 379, 382, 383, 384, 385
viruses, 312
viscera, 250
visible, 38, 40, 91, 96, 102, 103, 104, 107, 108, 117, 158, 173, 308
vision, 114, 148
visual, 85, 114, 182
visualization, 39, 59, 60, 71, 79, 91, 92, 94, 95, 364

vitamin B1, 154
vitamin D, 220
vitamin E, 246
vitamin K, 240
vitamins, 240, 241, 242, 243
VLA, 285
voiding, 382
volvulus, 312, 323
vomiting, 55, 153, 208, 224, 272, 321, 322, 350, 369, 382, 389

W

Wales, 196
warfarin, 317
Washington, 166
water, 60, 102, 207, 214, 240, 242, 244, 255, 388, 389, 391
water absorption, 214
water supplies, 391
watershed, 311
weight gain, 217, 272
weight loss, 31, 54, 55, 151, 153, 154, 239, 242, 307, 321, 322, 382, 391, 393, 395
well-being, 158, 159, 160, 167, 214
Western countries, 28, 30, 131, 135, 139
Western societies, 143
wet, 11, 48, 376
wild type, 225
withdrawal, 73, 229, 230, 273
women, 187, 227, 308
worm, 321
wound healing, 179, 184, 185, 217

X

xenon, 90
x-ray, 13, 220, 315

Y

yield, 49, 75, 84, 85, 86, 95, 98, 107, 109, 173, 347
young adults, 303